Introduction to
Visual Optics

Introduction to Visual Optics

A Light Approach

Samantha Strong, PhD, BSc (Hons)

Lecturer, Optometry
Vision Sciences
Aston University
Birmingham, UK

ELSEVIER

Senior Content Development Manager: Somodatta Roy Choudhury
Senior Content Strategist: Kayla Wolfe
Senior Content Development Specialist: Priyadarshini Pandey
Publishing Services Manager: Shereen Jameel
Project Manager: Vishnu T. Jiji
Design Direction: Bridget Hoette

Printed in United Kingdom

Last digit is the print number: 9 8 7 6 5 4 3 2 1

Working together to grow libraries in developing countries

www.elsevier.com • www.bookaid.org

To Howard, for everything;
To Decaf and Alex, for believing in me;
To my students, for supporting me with enthusiasm and a willingness to learn;
To my cats Muffin and Cookie, for their love and company every step of the way;
And to tea, because this book would not exist without tea.

Acknowledgements

Writing a textbook involves the support of several people, so I'd like to take a moment to thank everyone who helped me with this endeavour.

Firstly I'd like to thank Professor Leon Davies (Aston University) for handing me the optics module that's fulfilled my love of teaching ever since I joined Aston, and I'd like to thank Dr. Rob Cubbidge (ABDO College) and Dr. Rebekka Heitmar (University of Huddersfield) for helping me get to grips with the practical side of optics when I was learning.

I'd also like to thank Dr. Howard Collins (Aston University) and Dr. Elaine Hallam (Aston University) for their suggestions on the content of the book and for their essential help with my understanding of the clinical side of optics.

I should also thank Kayla Wolfe at Elsevier for helping me put forward this proposal and for advising and supporting me along the way.

I'd also like to thank my family and friends for putting up with me talking about this for such a long time, but special thanks go to my sister Catherine (Decaf) Strong for her motivating messages, endless stream of love-heart emojis, and such a passionate investment in me finishing the book that I felt it would have let her down not to do it!

Finally, I'd like to express an extra set of humongous thanks to Dr. Howard Collins for being my kind and patient proofreader, for believing in me even when I struggled to believe in myself and, importantly, for helping me to recognise when I went a bit 'too Yorkshire for a textbook'.

Preface

This book has been an idea I've been nurturing since I first started trying to learn about optics myself. I remember sitting at my desk, surrounded by black-and-white textbooks that I considered too difficult to even *attempt* to read and deciding in that moment that probably I just really hated science, or possibly that I just didn't have the right type of brain or capacity or intelligence for understanding physics (*this probably sounds quite dramatic but if you're a student you may empathise a little with me here*). However, through necessity, I had to persevere, and once I managed to break through the initial off-putting nature of the content, I began to find the content fascinating, inspiring and all-together very appealing. This obviously required a re-think of my capacity for science, and I realised that actually, quite contrary to hating science, I absolutely loved it! It turns out that I just was very easily de-motivated as a student, and with not much of a science background (I studied art, graphic design, philosophy and psychology at A-level), I found it difficult to understand content that was written with the assumption that I had prior knowledge that I really didn't possess – which, when you think about it, is fair enough really.

When I first started teaching optics, it seemed sad to think that some students (like myself) might be put off by a subject because it feels too difficult or because it feels too boring, and so the first thing I did was scour the web for resources that made optics sound fun or used lots of colourful diagrams to help explain the concepts. It didn't take me long to realise that nothing available quite seemed to live up to what I wanted, and so I started to design A4-sized handouts for my students (I dubbed them 'mini-guides'), and the feedback was far better than I could ever have hoped for! Students told me they stuck them up in their accommodation to help them revise, and said they made it look 'less frightening', which eventually inspired me to write this little book.

The beginning of the book covers fundamental principles of light and geometrical optics (chapters 1–9), before moving on to discuss physical optics (chapter 10), clinical applications (chapters 11–17) and then attempting to inspire a love of science by providing you with an opportunity to do some experiments at home (chapters 18–23).

I hope that this book will serve as a way of showing all students that optics doesn't have to be extremely complicated and can instead be interesting (possibly even fun). To that end, I've attempted to make this book a light-hearted, simplified introduction to the topic in the hopes that it will inspire you to do some further reading of the more advanced content once you realise how lovely optics can be.

So, without further ado, I wish you a lovely time reading my book, and if you have any feedback for me, please do be encouraged to reach out and share your thoughts.

Samantha Strong, PhD, BSc (Hons)

Contents

CONTENTS

Video Table of Contents

Video 1.1: Light is comprised of different wavelengths, and these wavelengths can combine to produce different colours of light. This video shows an example of additive colours, demonstrating that red, green and blue light make white light, whereas different combinations of two of the lights (e.g. red and blue or red and green) produce different colours (e.g. magenta or yellow). This same principle also explains how shadows can be colourful, which is demonstrated towards the end of the video.

Video 2.1: This video teaches you about refraction and images, as seen through curved refractive surfaces (in this case, a round glass of water). Real and virtual images are considered (with reference to the object's distance relative to the surface), and we also consider how the refractive index and curvature of the glass can make objects appear to look different when placed in water.

Video 10.1: Diffraction is a process by which light 'bends' round the corners of apertures or obstacles, given the right circumstances, and the amount of bending is determined by what's called the diffraction angle. Crucially, if diffracting through an aperture (or slit), the diffraction angle will depend on how large the wavelength is relative to the size of the slit. In general, large wavelengths (e.g. red) will have a larger diffraction angle than shorter (e.g. blue) wavelengths when passing through the same slit. This video utilises a diffraction grating (comprising many tiny slits) to demonstrate this effect.

Video 19.1: This video shows you an example of a completed 'blue sky' experiment, as described in chapter 19. Initially the torchlight appears white when shone through the water, but when a small amount of milk is added to the water, the particles in the milk 'scatter' the short (blue) wavelengths out of the torchlight, making it appear yellowy-orange. If you complete this experiment at home and obtain different results, please see the troubleshooting table in chapter 19 for help.

Video 20.1: This video shows successful completion of the 'create a prism' experiment, using water, a mirror and a torch to demonstrate dispersion at home. If you complete this experiment at home and obtain different results, please see the troubleshooting table in chapter 20 for help.

Video 21.1: This video shows clearly how to complete the 'speed of light' experiment by melting chocolate in a microwave and measuring the distance between the melting 'hot-spots' that form. The video contains several advice to help you complete it at home if you'd like to. If you complete this experiment at home and obtain different results, please see the troubleshooting table in chapter 21 for help.

Video 22.1: This video shows how to prepare materials and complete the 'create a cornea' experiment from the textbook. This experiment should demonstrate how refractive index changes and curvature can impact the appearance of the final image. Screenshots from this video can be seen in the textbook. If you complete this experiment at home and obtain different results, please see the troubleshooting table in chapter 22 for help.

Introduction to
Visual Optics

SECTION 1

Geometric and Basic Optics

1

Basics of Light and Colour

CHAPTER OUTLINE

OBJECTIVES

After working through this chapter, you should be able to:

Explain what light is in relation to the wave-particle duality

Explain what the wavelength of light means in terms of appearance and energy

Explain how light interacts with objects

Explain how we perceive colours

Introduction

If you're anything like me, then at some point in your life you will have had one of those moments when you have a deep, philosophical thought about what light is, or what a shadow is, or how colours are produced, or why things look distorted in water. Alternatively, if you've never thought in too much detail about this – have a think about it now.

What even *is* 'light' anyway?

This chapter will seek to answer these questions by reviewing some key physical principles and defining some very important terms. To this end, this chapter will lay the foundation for the rest of the book, so please make sure to obtain a solid understanding of this content before moving on.

What Is Light?

When we talk about 'light' as something that allows us to see objects that exist in the real world, we are actually talking specifically about something referred to as 'visible light'. The special feature of visible light is that it's detectable by the sensory receptors in the human eye, which is how we use light to help us to see. It can originate from natural (e.g. from the sun), or artificial (e.g. from a lamp) sources, but in all cases, visible light will illuminate (light up) objects, allowing us to perceive their existence.

However, when we start to think more deeply about what light is, or what it's composed of, things start to become a little more complicated. For example, research into whether light could be classed as 'particles' or as 'waves' went on for centuries before scientists finally agreed that light must possess something called **wave-particle duality,** meaning it exhibits properties of both particles *and* waves (Box 1.1), and this is particularly relevant when we start to think about the energy associated with the **electromagnetic spectrum**.

It can be slightly bizarre to think of 'light' as a type of energy, so let's discuss that in more detail. The energy packets (quanta) associated with the electromagnetic spectrum are called **photons**, and these are considered the basic unit of all light. The amount of energy emitted per photon is dictated by its wavelength.

Wavelength is a term to describe the *distance* between two equal points on a wave. In Fig. 1.1, you can see that on the shorter wavelength, if I take the distance between two peaks (the very top of a wave), then it should be identical to taking the distance between two troughs (the very bottom of a wave). Typically we measure distances from peak to peak because it is easier to identify the peak of a wave in a diagram than somewhere halfway up. Also, because it is a measure of distance, we need to use distance-related units, for example, nanometres, millimetres, centimetres, or metres.

Importantly, the wavelength of a light source is also related to its **frequency**. Frequency is defined as the number of complete cycles of the wave that pass any given point in 1 second. So, for example, if we shine a laser light at a wall and measure how many full cycles pass a point halfway along the beam within 1 second, we can calculate the wavelength

• BOX 1.1 **What Is the Difference Between a Particle and a Wave?**

Let's start by using a football as an example particle. If you have a football sitting stationary on the ground in front of you, then the particle is 'at rest', but if you approach the football at speed and kick it like Harry Kane, then it will (hopefully) go flying off into the distance. This happens because you have transferred energy to the football – in this case, kinetic (movement-related) energy. This energy allows the football to travel the distance required to land safely between two goalposts (or a neighbour's garden).

However, waves are different. For this example, let's think of dropping a stone into a still pond. We would expect the kinetic energy from the stone to move the water and produce a ripple, emanating outwards and taking the energy with it. However, even in a single ripple, the energy is contained within the full 'wave', meaning that with waves the energy is much more spread out (Fig. B1.1).

The key difference, then, is that particles will collide with each other and change direction, whereas waves will pass through one another (imagine two footballs colliding relative to two ripples in a pond). This idea will be covered in more detail in later chapters of the book.

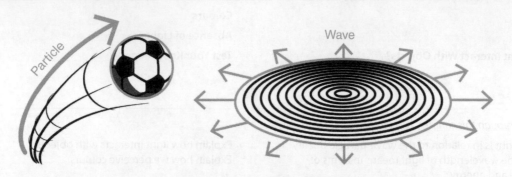

• **Fig. B1.1** Diagram showing the difference in how energy transfers in a particle relative to a wave. Blue arrows indicate the direction of the energy.

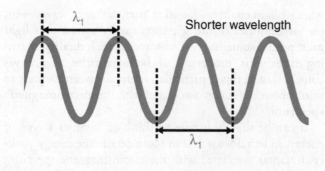

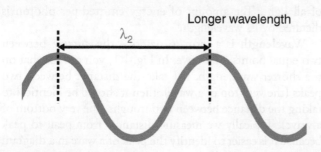

• **Fig. 1.1** Two example waves, showing identification of wavelength.

(λ; lambda) by using Equation 1.1 to divide speed of light (c) by frequency (v; nu) (Box 1.2). This equation also highlights that as wavelength *decreases*, frequency should *increase*, which makes sense because if the distance between two corresponding points of the wave is small, more

complete cycles should pass through a particular point within a second, specifying a higher frequency.

Equation 1.1
$$\lambda = \frac{c}{v}$$

Equation 1.1 (explained)
$$wavelength = \frac{speed\ of\ light}{frequency\ of\ light}$$

Let's consider the relationship between wavelength and energy in more detail. If you look at Fig. 1.2, you can examine the entirety of the electromagnetic spectrum, with visible light sitting roughly in the middle.

Importantly, in the electromagnetic spectrum, as wavelength increases (to the right of Fig. 1.2), energy will decrease. This is because wavelength and energy are inversely proportional. In Equation 1.2 below, energy (E) is equal to Planck's constant (h) multiplied by the speed of light (c), all divided by the wavelength of the light source (λ). This shows that as the value for wavelength increases, the value for energy gets smaller, and vice versa.

Equation 1.2
$$E = \frac{hc}{\lambda}$$

Equation 1.2 (explained)
$$energy = \frac{planck's\ constant \times speed\ of\ light}{wavelength\ of\ light}$$

If we apply this principle to Fig. 1.2, we can see that cosmic rays have more energy than radio waves. As a top tip,

The speed of light, denoted in equations by the letter c (which stands for 'constant'), is a known speed, recorded to be: 299,792,458 m/s. However, it is important to note that this is the speed that light is recorded to travel in a vacuum, such as that found in outer space. When light is on Earth (in the atmosphere), it travels almost as fast as it would in a vacuum, but if the light comes into contact with any object/material, then it can be slowed down if it is made to change direction slightly. One easy way to think about this is that when light is in a vacuum, there are no electrons or particles to get in the way – it's just smooth sailing. However, in the Earth's atmosphere, or in water, the light will need to take very minuscule detours every time it comes into contact with an atom – which inevitably slows it down (Fig. B1.2).

For example, if light passes through a diamond (a high-density object), it will be slowed down to 124,000,000 m/s, which is still a great deal faster than you or I could ever hope to run, but it's been reduced to less than half of the speed of light in a vacuum!

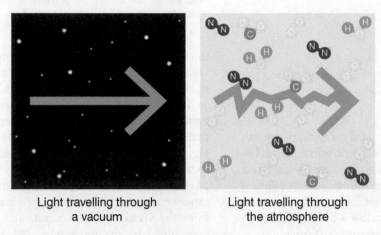

Light travelling through a vacuum

Light travelling through the atmosphere

• **Fig. B1.2** Diagram showing difference in how light (blue arrow) travels unimpeded in a vacuum (left), relative to small detours in the Earth's atmosphere (right).

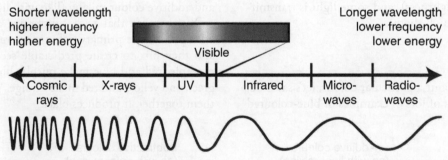

Shorter wavelength higher frequency higher energy

Longer wavelength lower frequency lower energy

Visible

Cosmic rays | X-rays | UV | Infrared | Micro-waves | Radio-waves

• **Fig. 1.2** Schematic of electromagnetic spectrum. As wavelength increases, energy decreases.

one way to remember this is to apply it to existing knowledge. For example, we know that x-rays can damage tissue and that UV (ultraviolet) light can burn the skin over reasonably short exposure times. This suggests that they possess higher energy levels than visible light or radio waves (for example) because they do not cause damage to tissue in the same way.

How Does Light Interact With Objects?

We have already discussed that light allows us to see objects, but in order to understand how that happens, we need to first think about the way that light can interact with objects. In simple terms, when light falls on an object, one of three things can happen: (1) the light is **transmitted** and passed through the material, (2) the light is **absorbed** and stopped by the material, or (3) the light is **reflected** backwards by the material (Fig. 1.3).

Let's consider an example object, like window glass. Window glass is transparent, meaning it's see-through, so what do you think happens to the light in this instance? Is it transmitted, absorbed, or reflected?

I'll bet that you've gone for 'transmitted', suggesting that light travels through the glass in order for you to see through it, and in a way this is correct. However, in most circumstances and with most objects, light experiences a combination of all three possible interactions.

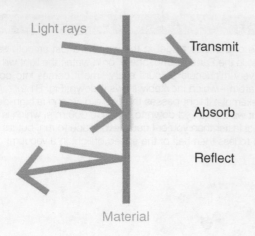

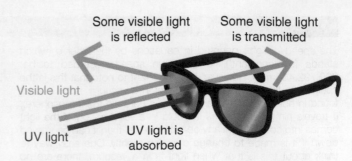

• **Fig. 1.4** Simple diagram showing how light (blue arrow) interacts with materials.

• **Fig. 1.3** Simple diagram showing how light (blue arrow) interacts with materials.

For example, when we look out of a car window, we can see through it, clearly indicating that some of the light is being transmitted through; however, we can usually also see a reflection of the inside of the car, meaning that some light is being reflected back towards us as well. Similarly, the reason we can't get sunburnt through a window is because the harmful UV rays are absorbed by the glass and can't reach us!

This means the correct answer to what happens to light when it reaches window glass would be that some light is transmitted, some is reflected and some is absorbed.

A nice, easy-to-remember example of this is a sunglasses lens (Fig. 1.4), as UV rays are absorbed (to prevent them from reaching our eyes), some light is reflected (to contribute to reducing the brightness), and some light is transmitted (so we can see through them).

Colours

If I ask you to think about a particular colour, let's say blue, you can probably think of lots of examples of blue-coloured things, for example, the sky, forget-me-not flowers, sapphires. . . . However, if I ask you to tell me what 'blue' is, that's where things start to get a little tricky.

To start with, we need to understand that natural, white light (e.g. from the sun) contains every wavelength within the visible light spectrum, from ~380 to ~700 nm (see Fig. 1.2). These wavelengths mix together (as waves can), so when they reach the receptor cells in our eyes, they are processed at the same time. This means that colours, as we experience them, are simply combinations of light waves from the visible light spectrum, and the *perceived* hue is determined by the wavelength. So, for example, a short (~400 nm) wavelength will appear blue, whereas a long (~650 nm) wavelength of light will appear red.

When light waves combine together, '**additive' colours** are created, which can be quite counterintuitive if you have any art experience. In Fig. 1.5, I have sketched out the differences between subtractive colour mixing (like with paint) and additive colour mixing (like with light).

You can see that with subtractive colour mixing (e.g. with paint), the primary colours are red, yellow and blue, and they mix to create predictable secondary colours; for example, red and blue make purple, blue and yellow make green and yellow and red make orange. When you mix all of them together, it produces black.

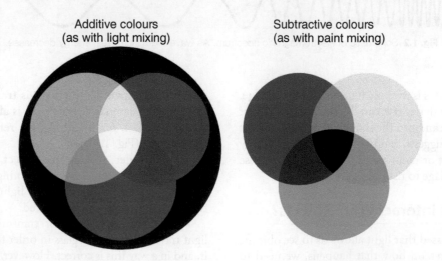

• **Fig. 1.5** Examples of colour mixing, showing the difference between additive mixing (left) and subtractive mixing (right).

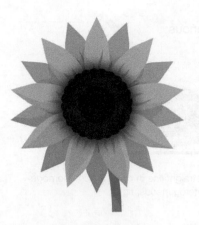

• **Fig. 1.6** Illustration depicting a yellow sunflower.

However, with additive colour mixing, the primary colours are red, green and blue, which correspond to the long (red), middle (green) and short (blue) wavelengths of light that make up the visible light spectrum. When these colours mix together, they produce different colours from what might be expected; for example, red and blue make magenta (pink), blue and green make cyan (light blue) and green and red make yellow. Importantly, when all of these colours mix together, they produce white. The reason this type of mixing is called 'additive' colour is that when the wavelengths of light combine together to produce the new colour, all wavelengths are still detectable by our eyes – therefore suggesting that the perceived colour is the result of the combination of the individual wavelengths.

When we view an object, such as that shown in Fig. 1.6, providing we have typical colour vision, we are able to easily detect the colour, and we can describe the object in the figure as a yellow sunflower. But how do we perceive it as being yellow if the light is white?

When we look at any object, the colour we perceive is a result of the reflecting wavelengths. As depicted in Fig. 1.7, the white light (containing all possible wavelengths) reaches the object, and depending on the object's physical structure, some of the wavelengths are absorbed and some are reflected. The reflected wavelengths 'add' together to produce the resultant wavelength that the receptor cells in our eyes detect. This is what gives rise to colour perception!

Absence of Light

Before we end the chapter on the basics of light, we need to talk a little bit about what happens when light is stopped in its path. Generally speaking, light travels in straight lines in a homogeneous medium – this means that if light stays in one (constant) medium, it won't deviate (this is called the **rectilinear propagation of light**). However, we should note that if there are density changes within that medium, then it is possible for light to change direction within a single medium (see chapter 2, 'The Weird and Wonderful World of Refraction Through a Single Material', for more information), but for now let's assume the simple explanation that if light stays within a single medium, it won't deviate. For example, if light travels from a lamp in your house to the physical (or digital) pages of this book, it will travel in a straight line from the lamp to the book. However, if you place the book in a bucket of water, the light will deviate slightly as it enters the water, as illustrated in Fig. 1.8.

This is important because it means that if light is not transmitted through a material, then it will be either absorbed or reflected, meaning that the light will be stopped in some way by that material. This is how **shadows** are produced.

The type of shadow produced depends on the light source and the distance of the object from the source. If, for example, we have a point light source, where light originates from a small point, then the straight light rays will be stopped by the object and produce a well-defined shadow called an umbra (from the Latin for *shade*), as shown in Fig. 1.9A. In clear conditions, the sun acts as a point light source because it's so far away from us, which is why we get such crisp shadows of ourselves on sunny days. However, in most artificially lit environments (e.g. a home or workplace), there are extended light sources (Fig. 1.9B), which produce two types of shadow – an umbra and a penumbra (from the Latin for *almost shade*).

With an extended light source, the light is emanating from a source that covers a wider area than the point light source. This means that light from one side of the source will fall on the object from one direction and light from the other side of the source will fall on the object from a slightly different direction. This means that there will be an

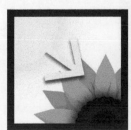 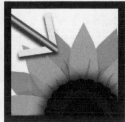 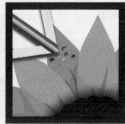 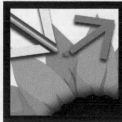 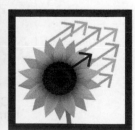

| White light from the sun reaches the object | White light is made up of lots of different wavelengths (colours) | Some of the wavelengths get absorbed by the object | And some wavelengths are reflected by the object | The reflected wavelengths are what we perceive as colour |

• **Fig. 1.7** Illustration explaining how objects appear to have a 'colour'.

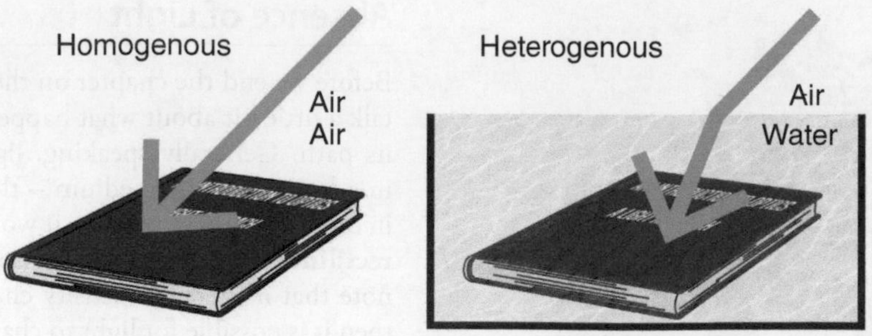

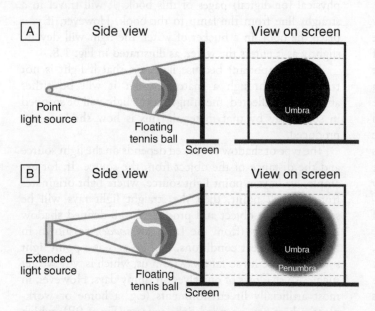

Homogenous
Air
Air

Heterogenous
Air
Water

• **Fig. 1.8** Illustration showing that light (blue arrow) will travel in a straight line in one medium (homogeneous, left) but will bend if moving from one medium to another (heterogeneous, right).

[A] **Side view** | **View on screen**

Point light source

Floating tennis ball

Screen

Umbra

[B] **Side view** | **View on screen**

Extended light source

Floating tennis ball

Screen

Umbra
Penumbra

• **Fig. 1.9** Illustration showing how point light sources (A) produce crisp, tidy shadows, whilst extended light sources (B) produce two types of shadows – an umbra and a penumbra.

area where none of the light can reach, because the object obstructs the light from all parts of the source, and there will be an area where only *some* of the available light is stopped by the object. This produces a dark area where no light from the source can reach (**umbra**) and an area with a lighter, less defined shadow (**penumbra**). Typically, the more extended the light source is, the less defined the shadow will be, because more light will have the opportunity to travel past the object.

Another thing to think about is that shadows are almost always black or grey, because they represent the blockage of white (or white-ish) light, meaning that the shadow represents an absence of white light.

However, it is also absolutely possible to have coloured shadows in the right lighting conditions. For example, we can replace our single point light source with three light sources, and instead of using white light, we can make sure each one is a different colour representing each wavelength – red, green and blue (Fig. 1.10). In typical conditions, these three light sources 'add' together to produce white light (see Fig. 1.5 for

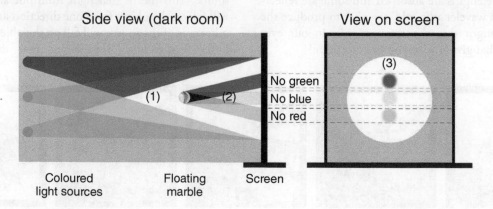

Side view (dark room)

(1)   (2)

Coloured light sources

Floating marble

Screen

View on screen

(3)

No green
No blue
No red

• **Fig. 1.10** Illustration showing how coloured light sources can produce coloured shadows if one or more is blocked by an object. When light from all three sources combines, it produces white light (1), whereas when light from all three sources is blocked, it produces a black shadow (2). On the screen, there are sections where light from all three sources is reaching the screen (white) and areas where one of the sources is blocked, leaving a shadow that exhibits the additive colour of the other two sources (3).

a reminder of this), but in our scenario, there is a small marble in the way! This means that there will be parts of the screen where one of the lights is blocked, which in turn means that the resultant light falling in the shadow of that blocked light will be the sum of the two remaining lights. So, for example, if the green light is blocked (see Fig. 1.10, *no green*), then the red and the blue will combine to produce a magenta shadow. You can see an example of this in the video content related to this book through the Elsevier website.

Test Your Knowledge

Try the following questions to determine whether you need to review any sections again. All answers are available in the back of the book.

TYK.1.1 How do we measure 'wavelength'?

TYK.1.2 Does ultraviolet light have higher or lower energy than visible light?

TYK.1.3 Does ultraviolet light have a larger or smaller wavelength than visible light?

TYK.1.4 Think about a regular table. Do you think light approaching the table is absorbed, reflected, transmitted or a combination of a few of these?

TYK.1.5 What colour would be produced if we combined green and red wavelengths?

TYK.1.6 What is a shadow?

2

Vergence and Refraction

OBJECTIVES

After working through this chapter, you should be able to:

Explain what vergence and refraction are

Explain how sign convention works, and be able to determine whether a distance should be positive or negative

Understand how refractive index and curvature of a surface can affect the emergent vergence

Be able to calculate use vergence equations to determine where an image will form after refraction

Introduction

In chapter 1 we began to learn about light – what it is, how it interacts with materials and how light allows us to see colour and objects.

The current chapter will seek to explore these elements a little further by going over some key terms and introducing the principles of how light changes direction when it meets certain materials (vergence and refraction).

Key Terms Relating to Light

Let's start with some discussion of 'light'. As discussed in chapter 1, light possesses **wave-particle duality**, meaning it exhibits characteristics of both waves *and* particles. If we take a point light source, we can imagine that light will be emitted in all directions, and we can liken this to ripples on a pond after throwing a pebble into the water. However, with light, these 'ripples' are referred to as **wavefronts**. Much like our water ripples, these wavefronts remain consistently spaced (unless interfered with – see chapter 10), and as the

distance from the light source increases, the wavefronts will start to get relatively 'flatter'. In terms of describing the path of the light, this can be depicted as a **wave** (a wiggly line) or a **ray** (an arrow), as shown in Fig. 2.1.

This book uses wavefronts, waves and rays interchangeably in diagrams to illustrate key points, but please remember that they are all connected.

Vergence

As discussed in chapter 1, when light travels unimpeded in a homogenous medium, it will travel in a straight line (rectilinear propagation of light); however, this is a slight over-simplification. As you can see from Fig. 2.1, any individual light ray will be travelling in a straight line, but if we draw a number of light rays to show how the light is truly leaving the light source, we can see that the light would be travelling in straight lines in *all* directions (Fig. 2.2A). So, if we select a few rays close together, known as a **pencil**, the individual rays travel in their respective straight lines, but this means that they are actually travelling further away from each other (Fig. 2.2B).

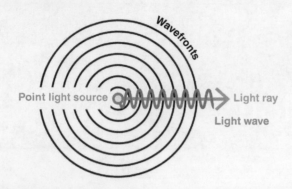

• **Fig. 2.1** Diagram showing a light source producing wavefronts in all directions. The direction of the light can be represented as waves or rays. Wavefronts are typically considered to correspond to the peaks of the waves.

The difference in direction of each ray within a pencil represents the **vergence**, which can be classified as one of three types (Fig. 2.3):

- **Divergence** (diverging rays) – individual light rays travel *away* from one another
- **Parallel** (parallel rays) – individual rays remain *in line* with one another (this requires a light source at infinity)
- **Convergence** (converging rays) – individual light rays travel *towards* one another

It is important to note that the vergence of the rays is associated with the wavefronts and how they are sampled (Fig. 2.4) – all wavefronts are curved (like ripples from throwing a stone in a pond), but the closer they're sampled to the source, the more curved they will appear to be. In Fig. 2.4 you can see that the closer the observer is to the light source, the more curved the wavefronts will be when they reach the observer's pupil. Ultimately, then, if the sampled wavefronts appear to be curved, then divergence or convergence is indicated, whereas wavefronts that appear to be flat indicate parallel vergence. This also shows that the further away the wavefronts are from the source, the flatter they *appear* to become, so parallel vergence is most often associated with sources that are a reasonable distance away, referred to in optics as **infinity**. Therefore, for example, light from the sun, which is pretty far away, would be considered to have parallel vergence when it finally reaches the Earth. However, if the object is closer to the observer than optical infinity (<6 metres), then wavefronts will appear to be diverging, as shown in Figs 2.3 and 2.4 (and this also nicely highlights how distance is related to vergence, which we will discuss in the next section).

Now, just to make things slightly more complicated, in optics, as well as thinking of light as being emitted from a light source (e.g. a lamp), we can also consider the light to be coming *from* an **object**, as we know that in order for us to be able to see an object, we need light to be reflecting off

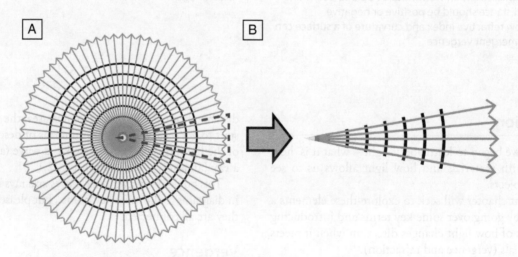

• **Fig. 2.2** Diagram showing a point light source producing light rays (blue) that travel in straight lines in all directions (A) and showing that individual rays are travelling away from each other (B).

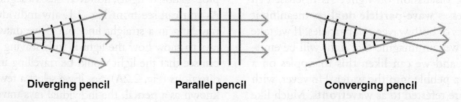

Diverging pencil **Parallel pencil** **Converging pencil**

• **Fig. 2.3** The three types of pencil: diverging (rays are travelling away from each other), parallel (rays are staying in line with each other), and converging (rays are travelling towards each other).

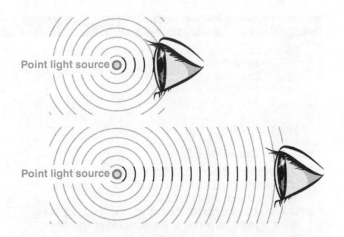

• **Fig. 2.4** Diagram showing position of observer (eye) relative to light source will alter the relative vergence sampled by the pupil of the eye. In the top image, the observer is very close and so the wavefronts reaching the eye are very curved (diverging), whereas in the bottom image, the observer is further away and so the wavefronts from the same light source are relatively much flatter.

it. Helpfully though, just like with a light source, the light reflected from objects has parallel vergence when the object is at infinity and diverging rays when it's in proximity, so the principle remains the same.

Vergence Calculations

Up to this point, we have only considered vergence in descriptive terms, but it's also important to be able to calculate values of vergence. Now, we already know that vergence is associated with the distance of wavefront from the light source/object, as a greater distance will lead to flatter wavefronts. So you'll be pleased to know that the calculation for object vergence (the vergence of light reflected from an object) mostly revolves around the distance of the object from the point of measurement.

Mathematically, vergence is given the symbol L, is measured in **dioptres (D)**, and is calculated using Equation 2.1. However, in order to calculate vergence we need to know two things: the **refractive index of the primary medium** (in which the object exists), indicated by n and, as mentioned above, the **distance of the object** from the point of measurement (usually a surface of some kind, e.g. a lens), represented by l.

Equation 2.1

$$L = \frac{n}{l}$$

Equation 2.1 (explained)

$$\frac{object}{vergence} = \frac{refractive\ index\ of\ medium}{object\ distance\ from\ surface}$$

Refractive index is a term that relates to the density of the material that the light is moving through, so the value of the refractive index indicates how fast (or slow) light will travel through that particular material, relative to how fast it would travel in a vacuum. The refractive index of air is 1.00, meaning that light will travel (approximately) as fast in air

TABLE 2.1	Common Refractive Materials and Their Respective Refractive Indices (n)[1]	
Material	**Refractive Index (n)**
Air	1.00
Water	1.333
Plastic (CR39)	1.498
Crown glass	1.523

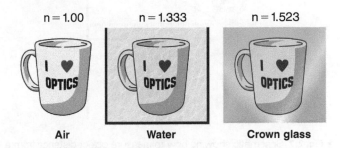

• **Fig. 2.5** Illustration highlighting that the primary refractive index (refractive index that the object exists in – here the object shown is a mug) will change depending on what material it starts in, for example, air, water and glass.

as it would in a vacuum, whereas the refractive index of crown glass is 1.523, meaning light would travel 1.523 times slower in crown glass compared to a vacuum. Importantly, this means that refractive index of a material will *never* be below 1.00. Some of the most common examples of materials and their respective refractive indices are listed for your information in Table 2.1.[1]

Now, when we say that the letter n in Equation 2.1 indicates the refractive index of the primary medium, we mean the refractive index of the medium in which the *object* exists. So, for example, in Fig. 2.5 the refractive index changes when the mug is placed in water or encased in glass.

Finally, as a top tip, if an optics question doesn't state otherwise, it is safe to assume that the object exists in air (so, if you are not provided with a material or a refractive index, assume a value of n = 1.00).

When considering object distance (l) we need to remember that, in optics, distances are always measured from the surface/lens to the object and are *always* measured in **metres**. This is because dioptres are SI (International System) Units and so the distance also needs to be the correct SI unit in order for the numbers to come out correctly. Distance measures will also need to be assigned either a positive or negative value depending on the location of the object from the surface. In typical optics convention, we assume that light will always travel from left to right across the page, as shown in Fig. 2.6, and this is called **linear sign convention**. The reason we do this is because it helps to make diagrams easy to read, and it helps to make the mathematical equations work.

Now, assuming a direction of light where light begins on the left and travels to the right, and understanding that distances are always measured from the surface/lens *to* the

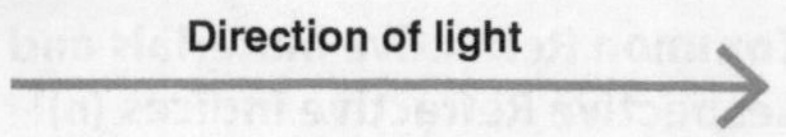

Direction of light →

• **Fig. 2.6** In optics, light is always assumed to travel from left to right.

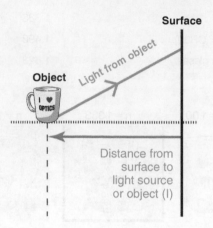

• **Fig. 2.7** Schematic showing how to measure object distance from a surface in this example the distance would be assigned a negative value as the distance is measured against the direction of light according to our linear sign convention. Note that the light is diverging as it leaves the object.

object, if a distance is measured *with* the direction of light (e.g. from left to right) then the distance is assigned a positive value or 'sign' (e.g. +0.16 m). However, if the distance is measured in the opposite direction of that of light, then the distance is assigned a negative value or 'sign' (e.g. −0.08 m). Be very careful not to forget the minus sign when recording these measurements in your calculations, as it's one of the most likely areas for errors to occur! In the example image (Fig. 2.7) the object is left of the surface, which means that we measure from the surface on the right to the object on the left, a direction that is opposite to the direction of light (Fig 2.6). Thus the distance (l) would be recorded as negative.

Assuming a refractive index of 1.00 then, Equation 2.1 tells us that any object distance which is negative should produce a negative vergence value, and any positive distance should produce a positive vergence value. Importantly, negative values for vergence (e.g. −2.00 D) describe diverging rays, and positive values (e.g. +3.00 D) describe converging rays.

DEMO QUESTION 2.1

If an object is placed 10 cm in front of a surface, what is the object's vergence at the point where light from the object meets the surface?
   Step 1: Determine what we need to calculate
   object vergence, L
   Step 2: Define variables
$l = -0.10$ m *(the question stated the object was 10 cm 'in front of', meaning it's to the left of, the surface. Therefore, it will have a negative distance and we need to convert to metres)*
$n = 1.00$ *(nothing is specifically mentioned so we assume the object is in air)*

DEMO QUESTION 2.1—cont'd

   Step 3: Determine necessary equation
$L = n/l$ *(Equation 2.1)*
   Step 4: Calculate
$L = n/l$
$L = 1.00/-0.10$
$L = -10.00D$
   (don't forget the ± sign and the units!)

Practice Questions 2.1:

2.1.1 If an object is placed 12 cm in front of a surface, what is the object's vergence at the point where light from the object meets the surface?
2.1.2 If an object is placed 7 cm in front of a surface, what is the object's vergence at the point where light from the object meets the surface?

However, it is important to note that as we always assume light is travelling from left to right, and that light will always originate from a light source or an object, this means that our sources and objects will always be pictured on the left in any diagrams (which will be important to remember in future chapters). This means that the source or object should always have a negative (or infinite) distance and will therefore always have diverging or parallel light rays – so how do we produce convergence? The answer is that when a light ray travels through a surface (e.g. a lens or a glass block or water), it's path may be altered by either a change in refractive index or a change in power (see 'Spherical Curved Surfaces') The view of the object after the rays change direction is called the **image**, and an image can have converging, diverging or parallel rays. The **distance of the image** from the surface is denoted as **l'** (pronounced little el prime or little el dash).

In Fig. 2.8, the image is on the right of the surface, which gives it a positive distance and indicates the light rays are converging to produce it.

Now, although light usually travels in straight lines, it can change direction if it travels into a different medium. This change in direction is called **refraction** and is one of the core underlying principles of visual optics.

Refraction

If a light ray changes direction, this is called **refraction**. This can occur if there is a change in velocity of the light as it travels from one material (primary medium, e.g. air) to another (secondary medium, e.g. glass) where the refractive indices of the materials are different. A real-life example of this is when you try to look at your arms or legs under water when you're in a swimming pool – water has a different refractive index to the air and so the image of your limbs looks distorted. This is refraction in action! You can try it at home by placing a pencil in a glass of water (or by watching the demo video on the associated Elsevier web content) – does it look distorted in any way? Please also see chapter 22

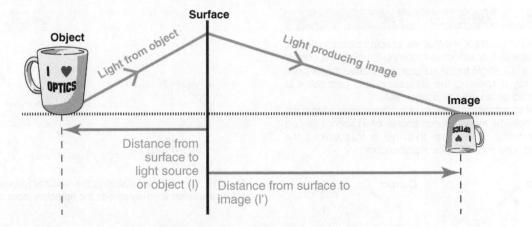

• **Fig. 2.8** Schematic showing a surface can change the direction of light to alter the vergence. In this example it has produced converging rays and a minified, upside-down image (magnification will be discussed in more detail in chapter 3).

• BOX 2.1   **Why Can We See Ice in Water?**

As a general rule, when light travels within a single medium it travels in a straight line, providing the refractive index doesn't change (see section on 'The Weird and Wonderful World of Refraction Through a Single Material' for more discussion on this). Similarly, if light travelled from one medium to another of an identical refractive index, no refraction (bending of the light) would occur.

Now, in the case of ice cubes in a glass of water, ice is literally made of water, and yet it refracts light differently – this suggests it probably has a different refractive index somehow (which indeed it does). This is because refractive index is determined by both density and temperature. Ice is less dense than water (we know this because ice floats in water – a clear indication of lower density) and usually a lot colder, which means its refractive index is lower, sitting at approximately 1.309 (relative to water's 1.333). This means light can technically travel slightly faster through ice than it can through water – which will affect the refraction that we see. Next time you have an ice cube in a drink, see if you can link it back to what you've learned here!

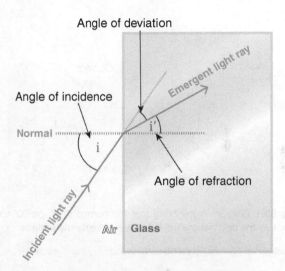

• **Fig. 2.9** Diagram showing how light rays can refract (bend) when entering a material with a different refractive index.

---

to complete your own demonstration of how refractive index can influence an image, and see Box 2.1 to investigate why we can see ice in water.

In Fig. 2.9, light rays are seen approaching a glass block. Another way of phrasing this is to say the light rays are **incident** upon the surface of the glass block, and so these are called the **incident light rays**. You will hopefully notice that the incident light rays are approaching the glass block at a particular angle relative to the **normal**, which is a hypothetical line drawn perpendicularly to the surface itself (Box 2.2). This particular angle between the incident ray and the normal is known as the **angle of incidence** (i). Now, because the glass block (n′ 1.523) has a different refractive index to air (n 1.00), the light rays will change direction (refract) as they enter it and thus alter the angle of the light ray relative to the normal. This new angle is called the **angle of refraction (i′)**, but please be careful here, as students often confuse the angle of refraction with the angle of deviation, so it is important to remember that both the angle of incidence and the angle of

refraction are always measured relative to the normal. In this example, the light rays have refracted (or bent) *towards* the normal, meaning that the **angle of refraction** (i′) (Box 2.3) is smaller than the angle of incidence. In contrast to this, the angle of deviation describes the angular difference between the emergent (refracted) light ray and the original path of the incident light ray, but don't worry too much about that right now.

Calculating Angles

In order to mathematically calculate the angles of incidence or refraction, we can use something called **Snell's law** (Equation 2.2) to work out one from the other if we know the refractive indices of the materials (see Table 2.1). Also, just as a word of caution, in this text I have defined the angles of incidence and refraction as i and i′ respectively, but you may encounter other resources that refer to them as θ and θ′ instead – they represent the same thing and simply depend upon whichever convention the author prefers to use!

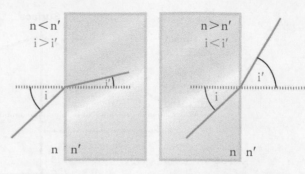

• **Fig. 2.10** Diagram demonstrating the relationship between angles of incidence and refraction relative to the refractive index of the medium.

Snell's law helpfully shows us that the refractive indices of the primary (without the primes) and secondary (with the primes) mediums will affect the size of the angles. Essentially, without getting into too much detail, if the light ray moves from a low refractive index to a high one, the light ray will bend towards the normal (producing a smaller angle of refraction), whereas if the light ray moves from a high refractive index to a low one, the light ray will bend away from the normal (producing a larger angle of refraction). This is shown in Fig. 2.10.

BOX 2.2 What Is the 'Normal'?

The 'normal' is a hypothetical line that we imagine exists relative to the surface of refractive or reflective material. Crucially the normal *always* exists at a 90° angle to the surface and intersects the point where the light ray is meeting the surface. In this textbook it is always represented as an orange dashed line.

It is important to remember how to draw the normal so that we can remember how to measure our angles of incidence (i) and refraction (i') correctly. Remember that this is true even if the surface is curved. See Fig. B2.1 for a demonstration.

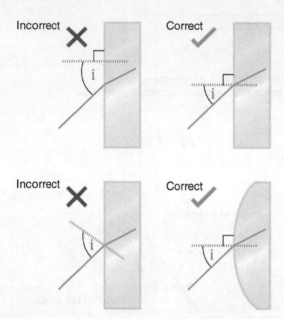

• **Fig. B2.1** Diagram highlighting that the normal must be 90° to the surface at the point where the light ray intersects the surface.

BOX 2.3 Why the Little Apostrophe?

In optics, the apostrophe is a prime (or dash), meaning that if we were talking about the angle of refraction, for example, represented as (i'), we would pronounce this as 'i prime' (though I like to call it '*little* i prime' to save myself the confusion when we sometimes use capital letters). As a handy tip for you, try to remember that the apostrophe usually means that the variable is representing something *after* a refractive or reflective process has taken place, and so it is related to the secondary (after refraction) variables.

As an example of this, the refractive index of air might be written as n = 1.00, but if the light moves from air (the primary medium) to a glass block (the secondary medium) we would write the refractive index of the glass block as n' = 1.523.

Equation 2.2 $n(\sin i) = n'(\sin i')$

Equation 2.2 (explained)
$$\frac{primary\ refractive\ index}{(\sin \times angle\ of\ incidence)} = \frac{secondary\ refractive\ index}{(\sin \times angle\ of\ refraction)}$$

DEMO QUESTION 2.2

If a light ray is incident on a glass block (refractive index 1.523) at an angle of 28°, what is the angle of refraction?

Step 1: Determine what we need to calculate angle of refraction, i'

Step 2: Define variables

i = 28° *(angle of incidence)*

n = 1.00 *(nothing is specifically mentioned so we assume the primary medium is air)*

n' = 1.523 *(refractive index of secondary medium – glass block)*

Step 3: Determine necessary equation

n (sin i) = n' (sin i') *(Equation 2.2)*

Step 4: Calculate

n (sin i) = n' (sin i')

1.00 (sin 28) = 1.523 (sin i')

0.4695.. = 1.523 (sin i') *(solve the left side)*

0.4695../ 1.523 = (sin i') *(rearrange n')*

0.3083.. = (sin i') *(solve the left side)*

sin-1 (0.3083..) = i' *(rearrange sin – this makes it an inverse sin)*

i' = 17.95°

(don't forget the units!)

Also remember to double check your answer. If n' is larger than n (as in this case) then i' should be smaller than i.

Practice Questions:

2.2.1 If a light ray is incident on a glass block (refractive index 1.523) at an angle of 35°, what is the angle of refraction?

2.2.2 If a light ray is incident on a piece of plastic (refractive index 1.498) at an angle of 25°, what is the angle of refraction?

2.2.3 If a light ray refracts out of a glass block (refractive index 1.523) at an angle of 20°, what was the angle of incidence?

Lateral Displacement

If a light ray enters a glass block, chances are it will leave the glass block on the other side. The term *lateral displacement* describes a phenomenon when a ray of light enters a material and, upon leaving the material, has exhibited a parallel shift to the side. If you've ever played a video game involving the use of portals, it can be likened to entering a portal at the first surface of a glass block and then leaving a portal shifted slightly to the side on the second surface of a glass block, as shown in Fig. 2.11. It also means that the angle of incidence at the first face will be identical to the angle of emergence at the second face.

Importantly, when an emergent ray is parallel to the incident ray, the emergent ray forms two hypothetical right-angled triangles within the material that we can use to calculate how much displacement (s) has taken place (Fig. 2.12).

In Fig. 2.12, we can see that the displacement (s) is actually the same distance as the side BD of our triangle ABD, so in order to calculate the displacement, we're going to need to investigate our triangles, and as we'll see below, the key component is the path of the light through the block (side AB). Firstly, though, we need to do a little bit of revision of vertically opposite angles (Box 2.4), because we can use this principle to determine the angle 'BAD' ($\angle$BAD). This principle tells us that $i_{1'}$ and the mystery angle (?) should add up to equal i_1 on the opposite side of the surface (Fig. 2.13). This means that *subtracting* $i_{1'}$ from i_1 should reveal the size of the mystery angle.

$$\angle BAD = i_1 - i_1'$$

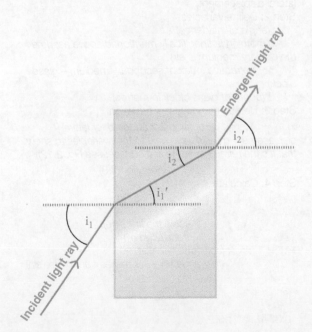

• **Fig. 2.11** Diagram showing that even though refraction occurs here at two surfaces (the front and back surface of the glass block), the incident and emergent light rays are parallel, just displaced slightly to the side from the original path of the light ray.

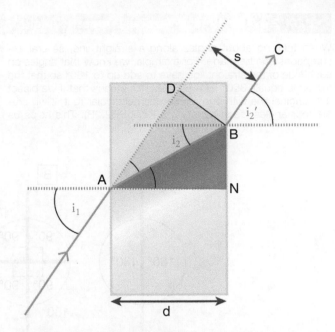

• **Fig. 2.12** Diagram showing that when the emergent light ray exiting a material is parallel to the incident light ray, it forms two hypothetical right-angled triangles (highlighted in colour) within the glass block.

Once we know the angle $\angle$BAD, we can then use trigonometry to solve for triangle ABD – all we have to do is substitute in our calculation for finding the mystery angle:

$\sin (\text{angle}) = \text{opposite/hypotenuse}$
$\sin (\angle\text{BAD}) = \text{BD/AB}$ *(remember, we can substitute*
BAD for $i_1 - i_1'$)
$\sin (i_1 - i_1') = \text{BD/AB}$

which can be rearranged to show that

$$AB = BD/ \sin (i_1 - i_1')$$

Magic! We've managed to find one way of expressing side AB. Let's now use the same principles of trigonometry to solve for triangle ANB, but for this triangle we know the angle:

$\cos (\text{angle}) = \text{adjacent / hypotenuse}$
$\cos (i_1') = \text{AN / AB}$

which can be rearranged to show that

$$AB = AN / \cos (i_1')$$

Perfect! What we've managed to achieve here is two different ways of calculating the length of the side AB, which represents the path the light ray takes within the glass block. This means that these equations are equivalent and can be written without needing to know AB at all.

$$(AN / \cos (i_1')) = BD/ \sin (i_1 - i_1')$$

This rearranges to:

$$BD = (AN (\sin (i_1 - i_1'))) / (\cos (i_1'))$$

•BOX 2.4 Revision of Vertically Opposite Angles

When thinking about angles along a straight line, several assumptions can be made. For example, we know that angles on each side of the straight line have to add up to 180° so that the full circle equals 360° (Fig. B2.2A). This means that if we bisect that original line with one running perpendicular to it, it will create four angles, each equalling 90° (Fig. B2.2B). This helps us see that if we rotate that second line by 25°, two of the angles will increase to equal 90° + 25°, whilst two of the angles will decrease to equal 90° − 25°, but crucially the total angles all still add up to 360° (Fig. B2.2C). This means that vertically opposite angles (angles opposite each other at a vertex) will be identical (Fig. B2.2D).

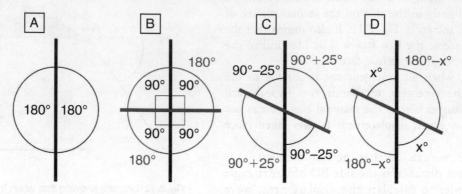

• **Fig. B2.2** Illustration showing angles along a straight line equal 180° (A), so if a second line is placed on top at a perpendicular angle, all angles will now equal 90° (B). If we then rotate the bisecting line by 25°, two angles will increase by 25° and two will shrink by 25° (C), showing that vertically opposite angles will be identical (D).

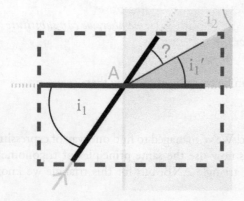

• **Fig. 2.13** Illustration applying the principle of vertically opposite angles to angle BAD from Fig. 2.11.

As a final step, we just need to substitute in the variables from Fig. 2.13 to obtain our calculation for determining lateral displacement (Equation 2.3):

Equation 2.3
$$s = \frac{d \sin\left(i_1 - i_1{}'\right)}{\cos i_1{}'}$$

Equation 2.3 (explained)
$$lat.\ disp. = \frac{width\ of\ block \sin\left(i_1 - i_1{}'\right)}{\cos i_1{}'}$$

DEMO QUESTION 2.3

Calculate the lateral displacement of a light ray that enters a 3 cm wide glass block (refractive index 1.523) at an angle of 25°.

Step 1: Determine what we need to calculate lateral displacement, s

Step 2: Define variables

i_1 = 25° *(angle of incidence)*

n = 1.00 *(nothing is specifically mentioned so we assume the primary medium is air)*

n' = 1.523 *(refractive index of secondary medium – glass block)*

d = 0.03 *(depth of glass block in metres)*

Step 3: Determine necessary equation

n (sin i_1) = n' (sin i_1') *(Equation 2.2 adapted for lateral displacement q (I put 1s in next to the i variables to show that it's the refraction at the first surface; see Fig. 2.12))*

s = (d (sin ($i_1 - i_1'$)) / (cos (i_1')) *(Equation 2.3)*

Step 4: Calculate

n (sin i) = n' (sin i')

1.00 (sin 25) = 1.523 (sin i')

0.4226.. = 1.523 (sin i') *(solve the left side)*

0.4226../ 1.523 = (sin i') *(rearrange n')*

0.2775.. = (sin i') *(solve the left side)*

$\sin^{-1}$ (0.2775..) = i' *(rearrange sin – this makes it an inverse sin)*

i' = 16.11°

s = (d (sin ($i_1 - i_1'$))) / (cos (i_1'))

s = (0.03 (sin(25−16.11))) / (cos (16.11))

s = 0.0046.. / 0.9607

s = 0.004825 m

s = 0.4825 cm

(don't forget the units!)

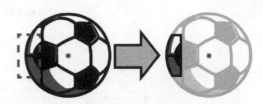

• **Fig. 2.15** Example showing the centre of curvature (pink star) remains the same distance away for the whole football (left) and for a small section of the football (right).

Spherical Curved Surfaces

Up to this point we have only considered flat, 'plane' surfaces, but we also need to understand how light interacts with curved surfaces. In optics, a ***spherical curved surface*** is any surface or boundary between two refractive materials that forms part of a sphere in its shape (Fig. 2.14). This section will go through some important elements of vergence and refraction at spherical curved surfaces.

Power

Spherical curved surfaces can alter the vergence of incoming light through refraction, and the degree of change they are capable of introducing is indicated through their **power**, measured in dioptres (D). For example, if a spherical surface increases convergence, this suggests it is making the vergence more positive (see 'Vergence' section), thereby indicating they have a positive power (e.g. +6.00 D). Whereas if a spherical surface increases divergence, this suggests it is making the vergence more negative (see 'Vergence' section), thereby indicating they have a negative power (e.g. −6.00 D). The power of a surface determines the degree to which the light will converge or diverge. For example, a surface with a power of +10.00 D will converge light to a greater extent than a surface of power +1.00 D.

Importantly, spherical curved surfaces will also have a **centre of curvature**, which we can liken to the very central point of a sphere. Let's consider an example of a football which is spherical and therefore easy to identify the

central-most point, termed the centre of curvature (Fig. 2.15). It is reasonable then to assume that any distance measured from the outer edge of the football to the centre of curvature would equate to the football's radius. If we then cut out a small section of the football, as shown in Fig. 2.15, although it no longer makes the completely spherical, football shape, you can see that the curvature of the outer surface still falls along the 'sphere' of the original shape. This means that it will maintain the same centre of curvature as the original football.

With spherical refractive surfaces the idea is the same – although we only see part of the sphere in the surface, it will still possess a centre of curvature (C) whose distance from the surface equates to the **radius of curvature** (Fig. 2.16). You will also notice that Fig. 2.16 has a line called the **optical axis** – this is a straight line drawn in optical diagrams that passes through the centre of curvature of the system.

As discussed previously, because the radius of curvature will be a measure of distance, the radius will need to be assigned a positive or negative value depending on which side of the surface it is on and how it is measured relative to the direction of light (see Fig. 2.6), and it will also need to be reported in metres. Remember, because we always assume that light travels from left to right across the page and all distances are measured from the surface, if radius of curvature is measured from left to right with the direction of light, then the distance is positive (e.g. +0.16 m). However, if the radius of curvature is measured from right to left against the direction of light, then the distance will be negative (e.g. −0.16 m). Typically this means that if a surface is **convex** and the centre of curvature is on the right, then the radius will be positive, whereas if the surface is **concave** with a centre of curvature on the left, then the radius will be negative. This assignment of a positive or negative sign is crucial for calculations determining the power of the surface, so make sure you have a good understanding of this before proceeding (Box 2.5).

Logically, a small radius of curvature would predict a higher degree of curvature in the surface than a larger radius of curvature, meaning that the radius of curvature must predict the curve of the surface which is intrinsically linked to the power of the surface. It is therefore no surprise to see that the radius of curvature (r) can be used to calculate the

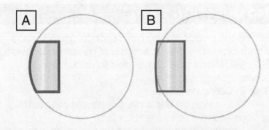

• **Fig. 2.14** Diagram highlighting that spherically curved surfaces will fit along a circle (A), whereas aspherical (not spherical) curved surfaces will not (B).

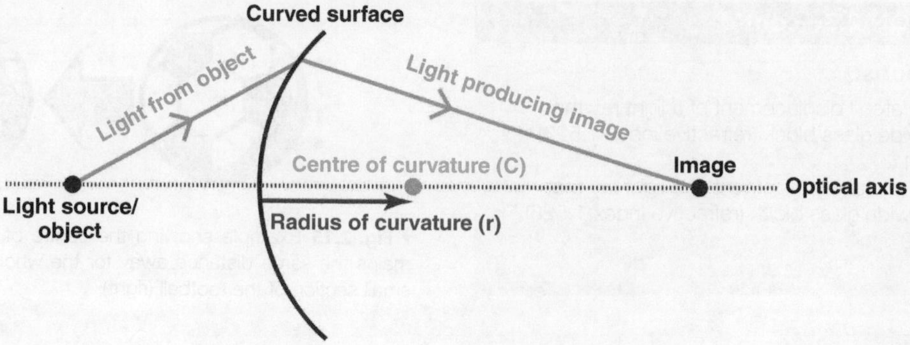

Curved surface

Light from object

Light producing image

Centre of curvature (C)

Image

Optical axis

Light source/
object

Radius of curvature (r)

• **Fig. 2.16** Diagram showing vergence of light from an object and its constituent image following refraction through a spherically curved surface. The radius of curvature (distance from surface to centre of curvature 'C') is on the right because this surface is convex.

• BOX 2.5   Is the Centre of Curvature on the Right or the Left?

In terms of how to determine on which side to put the centre of curvature, we can pretend the spherical surface is part of a full sphere and then just draw a dot in the centre like in Fig. B2.3.

In the example on the left in Fig. B2.3, the surface is convex (it bows out towards the direction we assume light to be originating from – the left), which means the centre of curvature is on the

right and will therefore have a positive value. The opposite would be true if the surface was concave, as that would produce a centre of curvature on the left-hand side with a negative distance. Logically then, using Equation 2.4, we can assume that:

• Convex spherical surfaces are positively powered
• Concave spherical surfaces are negatively powered

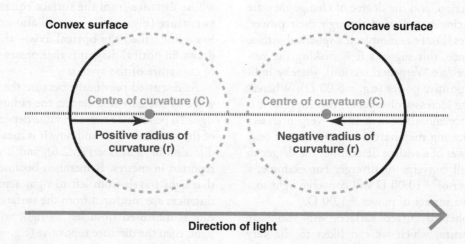

Convex surface

Centre of curvature (C)

**Positive radius of
curvature (r)**

Concave surface

Centre of curvature (C)

**Negative radius of
curvature (r)**

Direction of light

• **Fig. B2.3** Diagram showing relationship between convex and concave surfaces and their centre of curvature.

---

power using Equation 2.4. Remember that distances always need to be measured in metres so that the power is calculated correctly.

Equation 2.4
$$F = \frac{n' - n}{r}$$

**Equation 2.4
(explained)**
$$power = \frac{secondary\ refr.index - primary\ refr.index}{radius\ of\ curvature}$$

DEMO QUESTION 2.4

Determine the power of a convex spherical glass surface (refractive index 1.523) with a radius of curvature of 12 cm.
   Step 1: Determine what we need to calculate power, F
   Step 2: Define variables
r = +0.12 m *(because the surface is convex the radius is positive and in metres (see Box 2.5))*
n = 1.00 *(nothing is specifically mentioned so we assume the primary medium is air)*

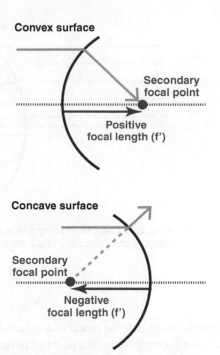

• **Fig. 2.17** Diagram showing how parallel light can help decide whether the secondary focal point is on the right of the surface (convex, top) or the left (concave, bottom).

Focal Length and Focal Points

As discussed previously, the power of a surface indicates the degree of vergence it will add to or remove from incoming light rays, but the value assigned for power is based on what happens to incoming parallel light (from infinity). Parallel light possesses zero vergence as the rays are neither diverging away nor converging towards one another. When these rays refract through a spherical surface, they will form an image at a point referred to as the **secondary focal point** (F′) whose distance away from the apex (tip) of the surface is referred to as the **secondary focal length** (f′). We will cover how to calculate focal length in chapter 3, so for now just make sure you understand what it is (Fig. 2.17).

Importantly, as focal length is measured as a distance, it needs to be recorded in metres, and it needs to be measured from the refracting surface. Therefore it will have a positive value if the secondary focal point is on the right of the surface, and it will have a negative value if the secondary focal point is on the left of the surface. To decide which side the secondary focal point will be on, you can think about what happens to light when it meets a convex (positively powered) or concave (negatively powered) surface.

When parallel light enters a positively powered (convex) surface, the surface converges the light towards the optical axis. This means that light will bend towards the optical axis on the right-hand side of the surface, indicating the secondary focal point will be on the right (see Fig. 2.17, *top*). However when parallel light enters a negatively powered (concave) surface, the surface will diverge the light away from the optical axis, meaning that the light rays need to be projected backwards (left) to ever meet the optical axis. This is referred to as the point where the light rays *appear* to originate from,

and it means the secondary focal point will always be on the left of a concave surface (see Fig. 2.17, *bottom*).

Limiting Spherical Aberration

With a curved surface, the normal needs to remain at 90° to the surface at every position on the surface. Typically, we'd expect that parallel light (from infinity) should form a lovely, focused image at the secondary focal point of the system. However, light rays within a *wide* beam of light from infinity will all refract *slightly* differently depending on where they intersect the surface (as shown in Fig. 2.18) as their angles of incidence (i), relative to the normal, will all be slightly different. In this case, light will be focused along the optical axis instead of producing at a single focus, and the light rays will follow what's called a ***caustic curve***. Importantly, the tip of the caustic curve will coincide with the focal point of the surface. This is called **spherical aberration,** which means the quality of the image will be poor because it will be blurred along this section of the optical axis (we will discuss aberrations in more detail in chapter 16).

The good news, however, is that **paraxial rays** (rays very close to the optical axis) are negligibly affected by these increasingly large differences in vergence, and so we will always use paraxial rays in our equations to make the maths easier, hooray!

Object and Image Vergence

Thinking back to 'Vergence', we know that object vergence (L) defines the path of the light rays leaving the object, and

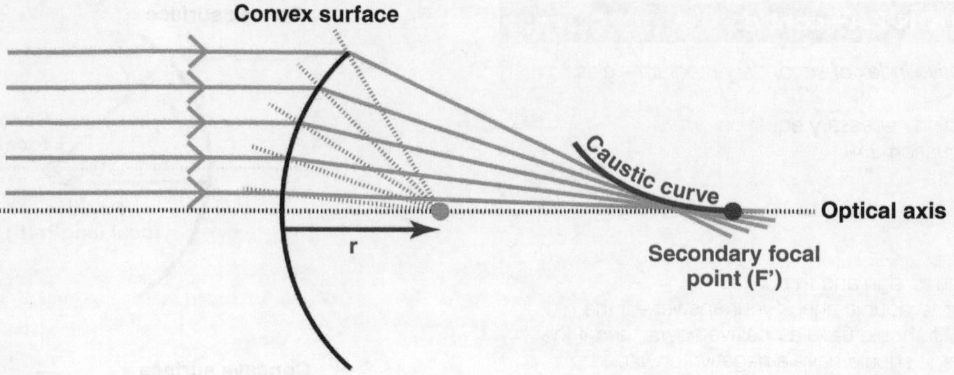

Convex surface

Caustic curve

Optical axis

r

Secondary focal point (F')

• **Fig. 2.18** Diagram showing a wide pencil of parallel rays will fail to focus at a single point, instead producing a caustic curve and spherical aberration (blurring).

we have recently learnt that the power of a spherically curved surface can alter the vergence at the point of refraction. This means that we also need to be able to calculate the vergence of the image rays (image vergence; L′), which represents the path of the light rays (following refraction) that form the image (this is also true for reflection at curved surfaces, which will be discussed in chapter 6). Previously we learnt only how to calculate object vergence (see Equation 2.1), because we hadn't yet learnt about power, but luckily for us we can now learn the full set of equations! Image vergence (L′) is calculated from the sum of the object vergence (L) and the power (F) of the surface (Equation 2.5), which then allows us to determine where the image will form (the image distance, l′; Equation 2.6).

Equation 2.5 $$L' = L + F$$

Equation 2.5 (explained) $$image\ vergence = object\ vergence + power$$

Equation 2.6 $$L' = \frac{n'}{l'} \quad l' = \frac{n'}{l'}$$

Equation 2.6 (explained) $$image\ distance = \frac{secondary\ refr.index}{image\ vergence}$$

If you are thinking that Equation 2.6 looks very similar to Equation 2.1 then you're right, because it relies on the same principles – that vergence depends on distance and the refractive index of the material. However, notice all the prime symbols (which look like little apostrophes) indicating that these are all **secondary variables** this time, so for example, n′ would be the refractive index of the material into which the light travels.

Importantly, the surface is curved so we need to ensure we always measure distances (e.g. for object, image, radius) from the apex (the peak) of the surface because we are using paraxial rays which lie close to the optical axis.

DEMO QUESTION 2.5

An object is placed 15 cm in front of a convex spherical glass surface (refractive index 1.523) with a radius of curvature of 6 cm. Where does the image form?

Step 1: Determine what we need to calculate image distance, l′

Step 2: Define variables

l = −0.15 m *(the question stated the object was 15 cm 'in front of', meaning it's to the left of the surface. This means it will have a negative distance (see Fig. 2.7), and we need to convert to metres)*

r = +0.06 m *(because the surface is convex the radius is positive and in metres (see Box 2.5))*

n = 1.00 *(nothing is specifically mentioned so we assume the primary medium is air)*

n′ = 1.523 *(refractive index of secondary medium – glass block)*

Step 3: Determine necessary equation(s)

L = n / l *(Equation 2.1)*

F = (n′ − n) / r *(Equation 2.4)*

L′ = L + F *(Equation 2.5)*

L′ = n′ / l′ *(Equation 2.6)*

Step 4: Calculate

F = (n′ − n) / r

F = (1.523 − 1.00) / 0.06

F = +8.72 D

L = n / l

L = 1.00 / −0.15

L = −6.67

L′ = L + F

L′ = −6.67 + 8.72

L′ = +2.05

L′ = n′ / l′

l′ = n′ / L′ *(rearrange to get l′)*

l′ = 1.523 / 2.05

l′ = +0.7429 m

The image forms 74.29 cm right of the surface.

(don't forget the ± sign and the units!)

We know the image forms to the right of the surface because the distance is positive.

DEMO QUESTION 2.5—cont'd

Practice Questions:

2.5.1 An object is placed 10 cm in front of a convex spherical glass surface (refractive index 1.523) with a radius of curvature of 8 cm. Where does the image form?

2.5.2 An object is placed 30 cm in front of a concave spherical glass surface (refractive index 1.523) with a radius of curvature of 15 cm. Where does the image form?

In Fig. 2.19 we can see that the surface is convex, meaning it is positively powered, which also means that the surface will add convergence to the rays after they pass through it. You can see that there is an object drawn on the left, illustrated as an arrow pointing upwards. In optics, we usually draw objects to look like this to help make diagrams easier to understand (see chapter 7 for more information on optical diagrams). Similarly the image is drawn on the right-hand side and is also depicted as an arrow. One crucial thing to note is that in this example illustration, the image formed is upside down, or 'inverted' (Box 2.6). When describing image characteristics in optics, we need to take special care to determine which way up the image is, it's position relative to the surface, and whether it is bigger (magnified) or smaller (minified) than the object.

The Weird and Wonderful World of Refraction Through a Single Material

In this final section of the chapter, we will discuss specific requirements that cause light to change direction and refract even when within a homogenous medium (i.e. staying within one material).

A Load of Hot Air

Have you ever noticed that on a really hot day, there seems to be 'invisible' wiggly lines emanating off warm surfaces (e.g. the road or cars, or above a fire in a fireplace)? (If not then it might be worth looking for this effect next time it's really warm out). This distortion occurs because the light travelling through the 'heat' to get to your eyes is travelling through different temperatures of air, which have different **densities**. For those of you who aren't natural experts in thermal physics, it's important to know that warm air is less dense than cold air, and the difference between the densities of warm and cold air results in small refractive index differences. As we learned in sections on 'Vergence' and 'Refraction', if light passes through materials with different refractive indices, then it may refract (change direction). In a way, then, we can assume that if there is a pocket of hot air within a larger pocket of cold air, then the hot pocket of air will kind of behave as if it's a very weak lens. Thus if an object is on the opposite side of the hot air pocket to you, even though it is only travelling through one material (air), it will produce a refracted image as it passes through the hot pocket. Another key factor here is that the heat coming off the warm surface in these examples varies rapidly over time, hence the density also varies over time, which ultimately varies the refractive index difference over time. This results in the moving 'wiggly' image that you can see on a hot day or above a hot item, for example, a candle flame heating the air around it.

The cool thing about this is that, because the differences in air density affect the light that travels through it, we can photograph the density changes associated with heat using specialised **Schlieren imaging**[2] (also see Box 2.7). Schlieren imaging is the name ascribed to imaging systems that can detect density changes within a material (and thereby can detect patterns of heat). The setup required to get a Schlieren image is quite complex because we need to somehow get rid of the light that isn't passing through the density changes – as otherwise the density changes will be obscured by the rest of the light. One way to do this is outlined in Fig. 2.20, which shows a laser light source in front of a positively powered lens, a candle, another positively powered lens, a pin and a screen (to view the image). Importantly, the laser light source (producing divergent light) is placed at the focal point of the first positively powered lens (for content on lenses, please see

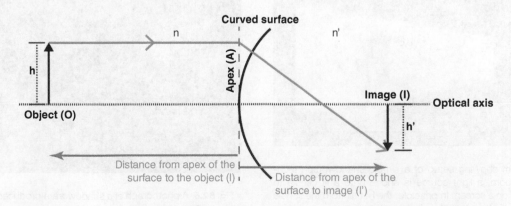

• **Fig. 2.19** Simplified diagram showing formation of image on the right of a positively powered spherical surface.

• BOX 2.6   Image Characteristics

Images produced following refraction (or reflection) will either be real or virtual (Fig. B2.4).
The following is always true about **real** images:
- inverted (upside down)
- can be projected onto a screen
- drawn with solid line

The following is always true about **virtual** images:
- erect (upright)
- cannot be projected onto a screen
- drawn with dashed line

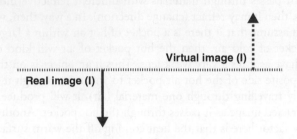

Virtual image (I)

Real image (I)

• **Fig. B2.4** Diagram showing real vs virtual images.

---

chapters 3, 4, 5 and 7). At this point in the book, we know that parallel light entering a surface (or lens) will focus at the focal point (see section on 'Focal Length and Focal Points'), but for lenses, the opposite is also true. If an object (or light source) is placed at the focal point of a lens, it will produce parallel vergence leaving the lens. Therefore, as the laser light travels through the positively powered lens, it leaves the first lens with zero vergence (parallel rays). The light then travels past the candle, and still has zero vergence as it approaches the second positively powered lens, meaning the light will focus at the focal point of that lens. However, in our setup we've sneakily placed a pin at the focal point of the second lens in order to block the light that travels unimpeded through the system. However, we know the heat near the candle will lower the density of the air around it, which will alter the path of any laser light that travels through the pocket of hot air. This light will have altered vergence as it approaches the second lens (see Fig. 2.20), which means it doesn't focus at the pin and instead carries on to produce an image on the screen. This image will be a wiggly image, showing that the density profile of the air changes with time, but a rough approximation of the image is shown in Fig. 2.20.

• BOX 2.7   Shadowgraph

So far this chapter has taught us that density differences in air can cause light to refract differently, and that this can be viewed as 'wiggly' images above a hot surface, or through a Schlieren image (in a lab setting). However, there is another way to view these changes in air density, and that's through a method called **shadowgraph.**[2] Now, if we examine the etymology of the word 'shadowgraph', we can see it breaks down as 'shadow' and 'graph' (which means a way of producing images), so we can safely assume that this method will produce an image of a shadow – which is called a **shadowgram**. More specifically, though, this technique can be used to identify the density changes within a single material, for example, density changes in air associated with differences in temperature.

For this to work, light must be shone onto a heat source and onto a screen (see Fig. B2.5). As the light travels through the

different densities of air, it will change direction and leave areas where less (or no) light is able to reach the screen, which produces shadows associated with the density changes. Fig. B2.6 shows an example shadowgram that I produced at home with a candle. From this you can see that the hot air from the candle is rising relatively straight for a while, before then becoming very wiggly and interesting. This shows us that there are density changes in

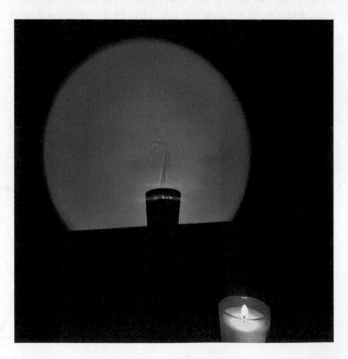

• **Fig. B2.6** A photograph of a shadowgram produced by the air above a lit candle.

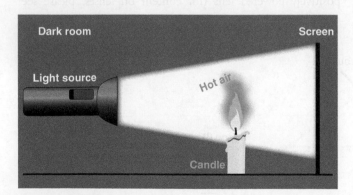

• **Fig. B2.5** Diagram showing setup of a simple shadowgraph technique. In a dark room, a light source is shone onto a lit candle to produce a shadow on a screen. In principle, the hot air from the candle should produce a shadowgram showing the density changes.

• BOX 2.7 Shadowgraph—cont'd

the air above the candle (and all I used was a torch – how fun is that!).

For another (slightly less dangerous) example, see Fig. B2.7 – this time I produced a shadowgram of a wine glass (can you see the different patterns of concentric lines appearing in the shadow on the desk?). This shows that the density of the glass is variable from the bottom to the top – you can try this one at home and see if you can find your 'best' optical glass!

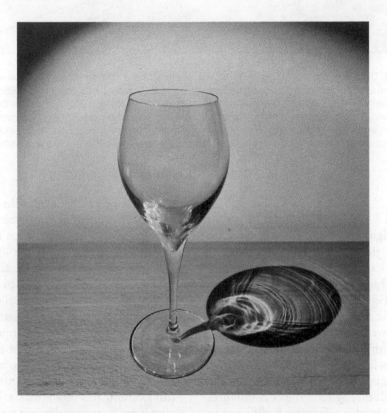

• Fig. B2.7 A photograph of a shadowgram produced by glass.

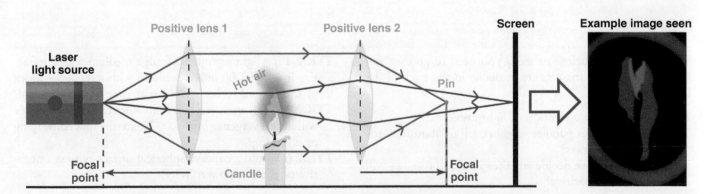

• Fig. 2.20 A diagram showing one possible setup required to produce a Schlieren image. Here you can see that laser light source is placed at the focal point of the first positive lens, which (if no heat was present) would produce parallel light that would focus at the focal point of the second positive lens (lighter red light). However, in this case a pin is placed in exactly the same point that the light focuses, meaning only light that has been refracted (changed direction) through air temperature changes (caused by the candle) will be visible (darker red light). A rough approximation of the type of image you might see is shown on the right.

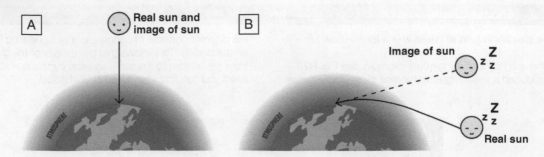

• **Fig. 2.21** Diagram showing exaggerated effects of atmospheric refraction using the sun as the light source. The atmosphere is made up of gradually increasing density as it gets closer to the Earth, producing a gradient of refractive index changes (shown in purple). When the sun is directly above the observer (A) it will travel in a straight line through the atmosphere, but when it is in any other location, the light will bend as it travels through the refractive indices within the atmosphere. This is particularly evident at sunset and sunrise, as the sun will be visible above the horizon even when it is below the horizon (B).

The Atmosphere

Another example of how light can change direction within a single medium is when light from the sun (or moon or a star) travels through the Earth's atmosphere. For this to make sense, we need to picture the Earth, surrounded by an atmosphere, as shown in Fig. 2.21 where we are using the sun as our example, but the same principle applies to light from the moon or stars as well. Fig. 2.21 demonstrates that there is a density change within the atmosphere – the atmosphere closer to the Earth is denser than the atmosphere further away, and this change in density can change the direction of light that travels through it if the circumstances are appropriate. Interestingly, this refraction is different to that which occurs when light travels directly from one material into another (e.g. light moving from air into water), because the refractive index change within the atmosphere is gradual, like a gradient. This can produce a similarly gradual change in the direction of light, which is called **atmospheric refraction**.

For example, if light from the sun travels in a straight line (along the normal) through the atmosphere, like it does at noon on a summer's day (when in a zenith position directly above the observer), then the light will travel in a straight line through the different densities within the atmosphere (see Fig. 2.21A). However, when the sun is in any other position relative to the observer, the light will gradually bend (and curve gradually towards the Earth) as it travels through the refractive indices within the atmosphere. This is particularly evident when the sun is below the horizon, at which point the light from the sun will curve so much that it will produce an image of the sun which appears much higher up than its actual location. This means that, at sunset, the sun is still visible after it has disappeared below the horizon (see Fig. 2.21B).

As a little bonus thought to end the chapter – we also know that temperature of the air can affect the way light travels through air (and the atmosphere), which means that on a warm day (with lower overall air density) the sun may appear to set faster than on an equivalent day that is slightly cooler in temperature.

Test Your Knowledge

Try the questions below to see if you need to go over any sections again. All answers are available in the back of the book.

TYK.2.1 What is a collection of light rays called?

TYK.2.2 What does parallel vergence tell us about the origin of the light rays?

TYK.2.3 How do we decide whether an object distance will be negative or positive?

TYK.2.4 If a light ray moved from a medium with a refractive index of 1.00 into a medium with a refractive index of 1.523, would it bend towards or away from the normal?

TYK.2.5 If you work out that following refraction an image will have a vergence of $+4.00$ D, are the rays converging or diverging?

TYK.2.6 Would a concave spherical surface possess a negative or positive power? Why?

References

1. Tunnacliffe AH, Hirst JG. *Optics*. 2nd ed. London, UK: Association of British Dispensing Opticians; 1996.

2. Davidhazy A. Introduction to Shadowgraph and Schlieren Imaging. RIT Scholar Works; 2006. Available at: http://scholarworks.rit.edu/article/478. Accessed 20th January 2022.

3

Thin Lenses

CHAPTER OUTLINE

OBJECTIVES

After working through this chapter, you should be able to:

Define 'thin lens' and apply the vergence equations from chapter 2 to thin lenses

Determine linear magnification of an image

Understand the difference between back vertex power, front vertex power, and equivalent power

Confidently apply step-along vergence equations and Newton's Formulae to determine image formation with multiple lens systems

Introduction

In chapter 2 we covered the basics of vergence and refraction at plane and spherical curved surfaces, but within clinical optics we also need to be able to understand how light interacts with lenses.

This chapter will seek to cover the fundamentals of thin lenses for calculating image location, power, vergence and focal lengths of the system.

What Is a 'Thin Lens'?

Lenses, by definition, are refractive devices that possess two surfaces (one on the front and one at the back) (Fig. 3.1A) and are available in several **forms** (Fig. 3.1B). In the last chapter we discussed at length that the curvature of a surface and the refractive index of a material can have an impact on the refractive power of a material. However, if the thickness is slight enough (relative to the radius of curvature of each surface), then it's assumed that the refractive index of the lens material has a negligible effect on the power, so

it can be completely ignored. These types of lenses, in which we ignore the refractive index, are called **thin lenses**.

In optical diagrams, thin lenses are drawn as vertical lines with arrowheads, where positive (converging/ convex) lenses are simplified to be outward pointing arrows, and negative (diverging/ concave) lenses are simplified to be inward pointing arrows (Fig. 3.2). We will cover this in more detail in chapter 7, but it is good to be aware of this now as lenses will commonly be depicted as arrows throughout this chapter.

Power of a Thin Lens

The refractive **power** (F) of a thin lens can be determined by either knowing the power or curvature of each surface, or by knowing the focal length (f′) of the lens. Remember, power is measured in **dioptres**.

Power of a Single Thin Lens

With a single thin lens, the approximate overall power can be calculated by adding the front (F_1) and back surface

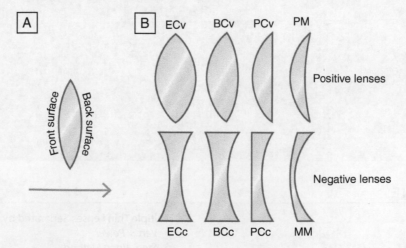

• **Fig. 3.1** Lenses possess both a front and back surface (A) relative to the conventional direction of light (blue arrow) and come in a variety of forms (B). Positive lenses can be equiconvex (ECv), biconvex (BCv), plano-convex (PCv) or plus meniscus (PM), whereas negative lenses can be equiconcave (ECc), biconcave (BCc), plano-concave (PCc) or minus meniscus (MM).

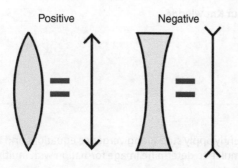

• **Fig. 3.2** Positive and negative lenses are commonly depicted as straight lines with outward- (positive) or inward- (negative) facing arrows on either end.

powers (F_2) together (Equation 3.1), for example, in Fig. 3.3, the front and back surface powers add together to suggest the lens depicted has an approximate power of $-3.50D$.

Equation 3.1
$$F = F_1 + F_2$$

Equation 3.1 (explained)
$$power = front\ surface + back\ surface$$

DEMO QUESTION 3.1

A biconvex thin lens has a front surface power of $+5.00D$ and a back surface power of $+4.25D$. What is the overall power of this lens?

    Step 1: Determine what we need to calculate power, F

    Step 2: Define variables
$F_1 = +5.00$
$F_2 = +4.25$

    Step 3: Determine necessary equation
$F = F_1 + F_2$ *(Equation 3.1)*

DEMO QUESTION 3.1—cont'd

    Step 4: Calculate
$F = F_1 + F_2$
$F = +5.00 + +4.25$
$F = +9.25D$
(don't forget the $\pm$ sign and the units!)

Practice Questions:

3.1.1 A biconcave thin lens has a front surface power of $-4.00D$ and a back surface power of $-8.00D$. What is the overall power of this lens?

3.1.2 A plus meniscus thin lens has a front surface power of $+6.50D$ and a back surface power of $-2.00D$. What is the overall power of this lens?

Focal Length

In chapter 2 we learned the basics of a surface's **focal length** by discussing that the **secondary focal length (f')** describes the distance between the surface and the **secondary focal point (F')**. We also learned that convex spherical surfaces will have a positive focal length whilst concave surfaces will have a negative focal length. For thin lenses, this principle is the same, with positively powered (convex) lenses converging light towards the optical axis, resulting in a secondary focal point on the right-hand side of the lens, and therefore a positive secondary focal length. In contrast, negatively

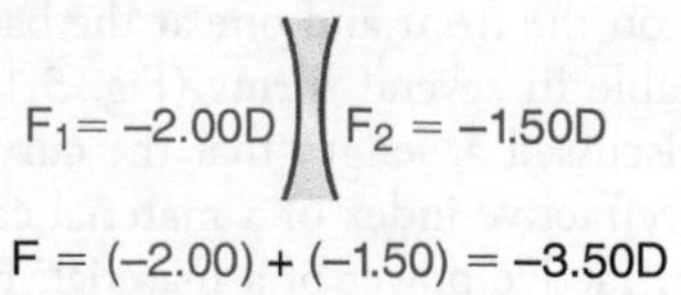

$$F_1 = -2.00D \qquad F_2 = -1.50D$$

$$F = (-2.00) + (-1.50) = -3.50D$$

• **Fig. 3.3** Diagram showing how to calculate approximate power (F) of a single thin lens by adding the front surface power (F_1) and the back surface power (F_2) together.

powered (concave) lenses diverge light away from the optical axis and therefore possess a secondary focal point on the left of the lens, leading to a negative secondary focal length. However, we now also need to start to consider what happens if light travels backwards through the system, from right to left.

With a thin lens, we assume that the lens will do the same to light travelling from either direction, so the focal length will be identical on either side. The only difference lies in the nomenclature, as when light travels backwards through the system it produces a **primary focal point (F)** at a distance corresponding to the **primary focal length (f)**. This distinction will be very important for chapter 7, but for now, please see Fig. 3.4 for an illustration of this in action.

We can use the secondary focal length (f′) and the **secondary refractive index** (of the surrounding material) (n′) to calculate the power of the lens using Equation 3.2. Assuming that refractive indices of materials will always be ≥1, then if you're a fan of maths, this equation should demonstrate that positively powered lenses will have a positive focal length (and vice versa), and negatively powered lenses will have a negative focal length (and vice versa).

Equation 3.2

$$F = \frac{n'}{f'}$$

Equation 3.2 (explained)

$$power = \frac{surrounding\ refr.index}{secondary\ focal\ length}$$

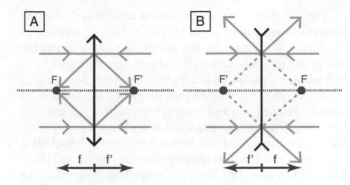

• **Fig. 3.4** Diagram showing light from the left (blue) and light from the right (green) interacting with lenses. The positive lens (A) converges light towards the optical axis and so the secondary focal point (F′) is on the right of the lens and the primary focal point (F) is on the left. The negative lens (B) diverges light away from the optical axis and so the secondary focal point (F′) is on the left of the lens and the primary focal point (F) is on the right.

Vergence Relating to a Thin Lens

For thin lenses in a homogenous material – e.g. the entire lens is in air – you can use the same vergence equations we learned in chapter 2 to calculate where the image will form (for revision, see Equations 2.1, 2.5, and 2.6), but we can also use equations to determine how big (or small) the image will be relative to the object. This is called **linear magnification** (m).

Linear Magnification

The term 'linear magnification' is a measure of how big (or small) the image is relative to the *original* object. It's important to note here that because we are using **paraxial rays** (which are, by definition, extremely close to the optical axis), the angle of incidence (i) and the angle of refraction (i′) are extremely small and hardly different from one another. Ultimately this helps us to use substitute tan into Snell's Law[1] and use trigonometry to determine the linear magnification of the image, but we don't need to worry about how that works providing we can remember how to apply the equation to calculate linear magnification (m) (Equation 3.3). It is also important here to understand that although magnification is related to power, it is not the same. For example, an object 10cm in front of a +5.00D lens will produce an image with different magnification to an object 12cm in front of the same lens. In that way, magnification is related to both the power of the lens and the distance of the object. A top tip here is to make a note to yourself to ensure you understand the difference between power of a lens and magnification of an image.

Equation 3.3

$$m = \frac{h'}{h} = \frac{l'}{l} = \frac{L}{L'}$$

Equation 3.3 (explained)

$$mag. = \frac{image\ height}{object\ height} = \frac{image\ dist.}{object\ dist.} = \frac{object\ verg.}{image\ verg.}$$

The best feature of a magnification calculation is that the answer can tell you an awful lot about the characteristics of the image. To be specific, the numerical value indicates the size of the image relative to the object, and the sign $(+/-)$ will tell you if the image is upright or inverted. For example, if the magnification is below zero (negative), the image is inverted (classified as a **real** image), whereas if it is above zero (positive), it is upright (classified as a **virtual** image). Similarly, if the magnification is between -1 and $+1$ (excluding zero), then it is **minified** (smaller than the object), and if it is below -1 or above $+1$, then it is **magnified** (bigger than the object). For example, a magnification of -0.45 would be inverted and minified, whilst a magnification of $+2.30$ would be upright and magnified. Importantly, if the magnification equates to a value of $+1$ or -1, then it is the same size as the object, and the sign will tell you if it is inverted or upright. See Fig. 3.5 for a handy way to remember this. For a real world example of magnification in action, if you know someone who wears glasses then you may have noticed that their eyes appear to be larger (magnified) or smaller (minified) when seen through their lenses. This is an example of the light from the object (in this example, the person's eyes) being refracted to produce an image a different size (the image is the view of the person's eyes that you see when you look at them). Hopefully though their eyes will always still be upright, indicating a magnification value above 0...

Image Distance

Utilising equations from chapter 2 and from the previous linear magnification section, we can calculate where an image forms after the light from the object refracts through a thin lens. Remember, with thin lenses we don't consider the refractive index of the lens at all, and so the refractive index

will usually be identical on each side $(n \equiv n')$, for example if the lens is "in air" then the refractive index would be 1.00 on both sides (Fig. 3.6).

DEMO QUESTION 3.3

An object is placed 20 cm in front of a biconvex thin lens of power +4.50D.
(a) Where does the image form?
(b) What is the magnification of the image?
    Step 1: Determine what we need to calculate
image distance, l'
magnification, m
    Step 2: Define variables
l = −0.20m *(negative distance and we need to convert to metres)*
F = +4.50D
n = 1.00 *(nothing is specifically mentioned, so we assume the primary medium is air)*
n' = 1.00 *(nothing is specifically mentioned, so we assume the secondary medium is air)*
    Step 3: Determine necessary equation
L = n / l *(Equation 2.1)*
L' = L + F *(Equation 2.5)*
L' = n' / l' *(Equation 2.6)*
m = (h' / h) = (l' / l) = (L / L') *(Equation 3.3)*
    Step 4: Calculate
L = n / l
L = 1.00 / −0.20
L = −5.00
L' = L + F
L' = −5.00 + +4.50
L' = −0.50
l' = n' / L' *(rearranged)*
l' = 1.00 / −0.50
l' = −2.00m
(a) The image forms 200.00 cm left of the lens.
m = (h' / h) = (l' / l) = (L / L')

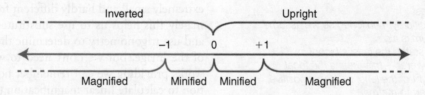

• **Fig. 3.5** Schematic for helping you remember what the magnification value tells you about the image.

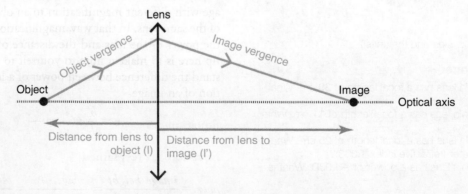

• **Fig. 3.6** Diagram showing relationship between vergence and object/image distance with a thin lens.

DEMO QUESTION 3.3—cont'd

m = L / L′ *(choose which part we want to use)*
m = −5 / −0.50
(b) m = +10.00X
   (don't forget the ± sign!)

Practice Questions:

3.3.1 An object is placed 50 cm in front of a biconvex thin lens with a power of +10.00D. Where does the image form?
3.3.2 An object is placed 35 cm in front of a biconcave thin lens with a power of −12.00D. What is the magnification of the image?
3.3.3 An object is placed 15 cm in front of a biconcave thin lens with a focal length of 20 cm. Where does the image form?

Multiple Thin Lenses

Up to this point we have considered thin lenses in isolation, but sometimes optical systems have more than one lens present, for example, in telescopes. This means we also need to think about systems with more than one thin lens, and how to calculate power, vergence and magnification for these systems.

Multiple Thin Lenses in Contact

The simplest form of system containing more than one thin lens is when all the lenses are **in contact with one another**. When positioned like this to have negligible distance between each lens, just like how we can ignore the refractive index, we can pretend the distance doesn't exist! To that end, we can simply add up the powers of each of the lenses in contact in order to work out the overall power of the system (Fig. 3.7), and then we can calculate vergence using the same equations as in the section titled "Vergence Relating to a Thin Lens". This time, however, we will refer to the calculated power as the **equivalent power** (F_e) as we are working out the equivalent *single* power of the multiple lenses, as shown in Equation 3.4.

Equation 3.4 $F_e = F_1 + F_2$

Equation 3.4 (explained)

$$equivalent\ power = lens1\ power + lens2\ power$$

DEMO QUESTION 3.4

Two thin lenses of powers +3.00D and +2.00D are in contact with each other. If an object is placed 40 cm in front of the first lens, where does the image form?
   Step 1: Determine what we need to calculate image distance, l′
   Step 2: Define variables
l = −0.40m *(negative distance and we need to convert to metres)*
F_1 = +3.00D
F_2 = +2.00D
n = 1.00 *(nothing is specifically mentioned, so we assume the primary medium is air)*
n′ = 1.00 *(nothing is specifically mentioned, so we assume the secondary medium is air)*
   Step 3: Determine necessary equation
$F_e = F_1 + F_2$ *(Equation 3.4)*
L = n / l *(Equation 2.1)*
L′ = L + F *(Equation 2.5)*
L′ = n′ / l′ *(Equation 2.6)*
   Step 4: Calculate
$F_e = F_1 + F_2$
F_e = +3.00 + +2.00
F_e = +5.00D
L = n / l
L = 1.00 / −0.40
L = −2.50
L′ = L + F
L′ = −2.50 + +5.00
L′ = +2.50
l′ = n′ / L′ *(rearranged)*
l′ = 1.00 / +2.50
l′ = +0.40m
The image forms 40.00 cm right of the second lens.
   (don't forget the ± sign (or the direction) and the units!)

Practice Questions:

3.4.1 Two thin lenses of powers +1.00D and +5.50D are in contact with each other. If an object is placed 10 cm in front of the first lens, where does the image form?
3.4.2 Two thin lenses of powers +6.50D and −4.25D are in contact with each other. If an object is placed 40 cm in front of the first lens, what is the linear magnification?
3.4.3 Three thin lenses of powers +1.00D, −3.50D and +6.75D are in contact with each other. If an object is placed 25 cm in front of the first lens, where does the image form?

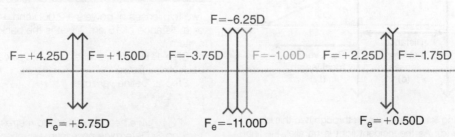

• **Fig. 3.7** Diagram showing that the equivalent power of thin lenses in contact with each other can be calculated through adding up the individual powers.

Multiple Thin Lenses Separated by a Distance

If the thin lenses are separated by a distance, then we need to take that distance into consideration when performing our calculations. This is because vergence depends on the distance from the surface, so increasing the distance (d) of the second lens will have an impact on the sampled vergence of the light as it reaches the second lens (Fig. 3.8).

Lens systems of this nature still have secondary and primary focal points, but they will no longer be equidistant on either side, as the powers of the individual lenses will likely be different, so light will travel differently in each direction. Instead, we need to consider what's called the back and front vertex power.

Vertex Power

Vertex power refers to the vergence of light as it leaves the system, assuming that the incident light is parallel (zero vergence), leading to light focusing at one of the focal points. If the light travels forwards through the system from left to right, the vergence of light leaving the second lens will be called the **back vertex power** (F_v'), sometimes referred to as emergent vergence at F_2. However, if the light travels backwards, from right to left, then the vergence of light leaving the first lens will be called the **front vertex power** (F_v), or sometimes referred to as emergent vergence at F_1. Now, because the incident (approaching) light is parallel, the light will form a focus at the secondary (F') or primary focal point (F), depending on the direction. The distance between the second lens (F_2) and the secondary focal point (F') is called the **back vertex focal length** (f_v'), and the distance between the first lens (F_1) and the primary focal point (F) is called the **front vertex focal length** (f_v). Fig. 3.9 depicts these distances in a multiple lens system.

To calculate vertex power, we need to take the distance between the lenses (d) into consideration. See Equations 3.5 and 3.6 for back and front vertex calculations, but be careful because these equations are extremely similar and easy to confuse for one another. My top tip for successful application of

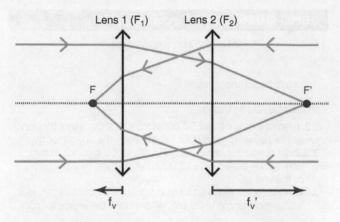

• **Fig. 3.9** Diagram showing light from the left (blue) and light from the right (green) interacting with a multiple lens system. The distance between lens 2 and the secondary focal point (F') equates to the back vertex focal length (f_v'), whereas the distance between lens 1 and the primary focal point (F) equates to the front vertex focal length (f_v). Notice that these distances are **not** identical.

these equations is to try to understand what the calculations are doing. For example, if we're determining the emergent vergence at F_2 after light has entered the system through F_1 (back vertex power; F_v'), then we need to know how the vergence from F_1 will have changed across the distance (d) between the lenses. As the incident light is assumed to be parallel, the power of the lens at F_1 will be identical to the vergence leaving it, and so the equation for back vertex power takes into account the power of F_1 in the denominator (and the opposite is true for front vertex power; F_v).

Equation 3.5 $F_v' = \dfrac{F_1 + F_2 - dF_1F_2}{1 - dF_1}$

Equation 3.5 (explained)

$$\frac{back\ vertex}{power} = \frac{lens1 + lens2 - (distance \times lens1 \times lens2)}{1 - (distance \times lens1)}$$

Equation 3.6 $F_v = \dfrac{F_1 + F_2 - dF_1F_2}{1 - dF_2}$

Equation 3.6 (explained)

$$\frac{front\ vertex}{power} = \frac{lens1 + lens2 - (distance \times lens1 \times lens2)}{1 - (distance \times lens2)}$$

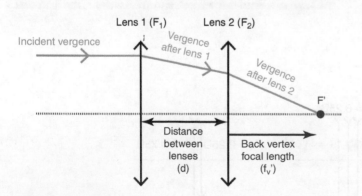

• **Fig. 3.8** Diagram showing light (blue) passing through two thin lenses separated by a distance (d). As the incident light is parallel, the final image will form at the secondary focal point (F'), but the distance between the back lens and the secondary focal point is called the back vertex focal length (f_v').

DEMO QUESTION 3.5

Two thin lenses of powers +2.00D and +8.00D are separated by a distance of 15 cm. What is the back vertex power of the system?

Step 1: Determine what we need to calculate back vertex power, F_v'

Step 2: Define variables
F_1 = +2.00D
F_2 = +8.00D
d = 0.15m *(we need to convert to metres)*

Step 3: Determine necessary equation
F_v' = (F_1 + F_2 − d$F_1$$F_2$) / (1 − d$F_1$) *(Equation 3.5)*

If we know the back or front vertex power of a lens system, then we can use that information to help us calculate the **back vertex focal length** (f_v') and the **front vertex focal length** (f_v). Equations 3.7 and 3.8 explain the difference for each. The equations refer to the surrounding refractive index (n), but usually this will be air, so you can substitute n for the number 1 in this equation. It is also important to notice the minus sign in Equation 3.8 (front vertex focal length), students often miss this, but it is crucial as we're assuming light is travelling backwards when we solve for front vertex focal length.

Equation 3.7 $\quad f_v' = \dfrac{n}{F_v'}$

Equation 3.7 (explained)

$$\frac{back\ vertex}{focal\ length} = \frac{surrounding\ refractive\ index}{back\ vertex\ power}$$

Equation 3.8 $\quad f_v = -\dfrac{n}{F_v}$

Equation 3.8 (explained)

$$\frac{front\ vertex}{focal\ length} = -\frac{surrounding\ refractive\ index}{front\ vertex\ power}$$

These equations help us a lot when there's zero vergence in the incident light, but if the incident rays don't originate from infinity, then we need to utilise something called the step-along method.

Step-Along Method

The step-along method allows us to calculate the image vergence (emergent vergence, L') of light leaving a multi-lens system if the incident vergence (L) is not equal to zero. For this method, we need to utilise (but slightly modify) the vergence equations we learned in chapter 2 (Equations 2.1, 2.5 and 2.6), and we need to learn a brand-new equation (Equation 3.9) to help us take into account that the lenses are separated by a distance (d). The idea is that we work out the incident and emergent vergence at each lens individually, as if we're 'stepping along' the lens system (Fig. 3.10).

You'll notice that, this time, we've used subscript numbers to indicate whether the vergence is related to lens 1 ($_1$) or lens 2 ($_2$), but remember, if there's a prime (') then the

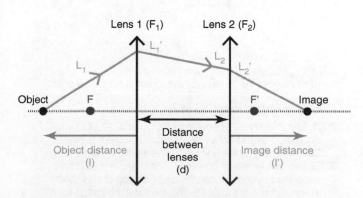

• **Fig. 3.10** Diagram highlighting the incident and emergent vergence steps at each lens when the object is closer than infinity. This example uses two positively powered lenses.

variable represents emergent vergence, otherwise it represents incident vergence.

Equation 3.9 $L_2 = \dfrac{L_1'}{1 - dL_1'}$

Equation 3.9 (explained)

$$verg.\,at\,lens2 = \frac{verg.\,leaving\,lens1}{1-(distance \times verg.\,leaving\,lens1)}$$

DEMO QUESTION 3.7

Two thin lenses of powers +2.50D and +4.00D are separated by a distance of 5 cm. If an object is placed 20 cm in front of the first lens, where will the image form?

Step 1: Determine what we need to calculate
image distance after second lens, l_2'

Step 2: Define variables
F_1 = +2.50D
F_2 = +4.00D
d = 0.05m *(we need to convert to metres)*
l_1 = −0.20m *(the question stated the object was 20 cm 'in front of' the first lens, meaning it's to the left of the surface; this means it will have a negative distance and we need to convert to metres)*
n = 1.00 *(nothing is specifically mentioned, so we assume the primary medium is air)*
n' = 1.00 *(nothing is specifically mentioned, so we assume the secondary medium is air)*

Step 3: Determine necessary equation(s)
L_1 = n / l_1 *(Modified Equation 2.1)*
L_1' = L_1 + F_1 *(Modified Equation 2.5)*
L_2 = L_1' / (1 − dL_1') *(Equation 3.9)*
L_2' = L_2 + F_2 *(Modified Equation 2.5)*
L_2' = n' / l_2' *(Modified Equation 2.6)*

Step 4: Calculate
L_1 = n / l_1
L_1 = 1.00 / −0.20
L_1 = −5.00
L_1' = L_1 + F_1
L_1' = −5.00 + +2.50
L_1' = −2.50
L_2 = L_1' / (1 − dL_1')
L_2 = −2.50 / (1 − (0.05 × −2.50))
L_2 = −2.2222...
L_2' = L_2 + F_2
L_2' = −2.2222... + +4.00
L_2' = +1.7778...
l_2' = n' / L_2'
l_2' = 1.00 / +1.7778...
l_2' = +0.5625m
The image will form 56.25 cm right of the second lens.
(don't forget the ± sign (or the direction) and the units!)

Practice Questions:

3.7.1 Two thin lenses of powers +5.00D and +1.00D are separated by a distance of 15 cm. If an object is placed 25 cm in front of the first lens, where will the image form?
3.7.2 Two thin lenses of powers −2.50D and +8.25D are separated by a distance of 8 cm. If an object is placed 10 cm in front of the first lens, where will the image form?

Equivalent Lenses

In this section we are still considering an optical system where two thin lenses are separated by a distance, but now we are going to see if we can determine a way of hypothetically replacing the two-lens system with a **single lens of equivalent power** (F_e). This single lens would be referred to as an **equivalent lens** and, importantly, although it will have a different power to the first and second lens, it will need to focus the light at the focal points (F and F′) in order to truly be 'equivalent' to the two-lens system. The appropriate equivalent power of the system can be calculated using Equation 3.10.

Equation 3.10 $F_e = F_1 + F_2 - dF_1F_2$

Equation 3.10 (explained)

$$equiv.\,power = lens1 + lens2 - (distance \times lens1 \times lens2)$$

DEMO QUESTION 3.8

Two thin lenses of powers +5.00D and +4.00D are separated by a distance of 20 cm. What is the equivalent power of the system?

Step 1: Determine what we need to calculate
equivalent power, F_e

Step 2: Define variables
F_1 = +5.00D
F_2 = +4.00D
d = 0.2m *(we need to convert to metres)*

Step 3: Determine necessary equation(s)
F_e = F_1 + F_2 − (dF_1F_2) *(Equation 3.10)*

Step 4: Calculate
F_e = F_1 + F_2 − (dF_1F_2)
F_e = (+5) + (+4) − (0.2 × (+5) × (+4))
F_e = +5.00D
The equivalent power of the system is +5.00D
(don't forget the ± sign and the units!)

Practice Questions:

3.8.1 Two thin lenses of powers +6.00D and +1.75D are separated by a distance of 10 cm. What is the equivalent power?
3.8.2 Two thin lenses of powers −2.25D and +8.00D are separated by a distance of 11.5 cm. What is the equivalent power?

However, we know from the section titled "Vertex Power" that the back vertex power (F_v') describes the vergence of light leaving the system from left to right, and we know this light would form a focus at the secondary focal point (F′). We also know that if the back vertex power of the system differed to the power of the equivalent lens (F_e), then they must also have different focal lengths. This means that, in most cases, the equivalent lens will need to be placed somewhere different to that of one of the existing lenses. So how do we determine where it should go?

Principal Planes

The answer to the question in the previous section is that the equivalent lens will need to have two unique positions along the optical axis: one position for when light is travelling left to right in order to focus light at the secondary focal point (F′), and a separate position for when light travels backwards through the system right to left to focus light at the primary focal point (F). These unique positions are called **principal planes**. The plane at which the equivalent lens would need to be located to focus light at the secondary focal point is called the **secondary principal plane** (H′P′), and the location of the equivalent lens to focus light at the primary equivalent focal point is called the **primary principal plane** (HP) (Fig. 3.11).

Once you know the equivalent power, the distance between the principal planes and the focal points can be calculated. The distance between the secondary principal plane and the secondary focal point is called the **secondary equivalent focal length** ($f_e′$), and the distance between the primary principal plane and the primary focal point is called the **primary equivalent focal length** (f_e). These can be calculated using Equations 3.11, 3.12 and 3.13.

Equation 3.11 $\quad f_e′ = \dfrac{n}{F_e}$

Equation 3.11 (explained)

$$secondary\ equiv.\ focal\ length = \frac{surround\ refr.\ index}{equivalent\ power}$$

Equation 3.12 $\quad f_e = -\dfrac{n}{F_e}$

Equation 3.12 (explained)

$$primary\ equiv.\ focal\ length = -\frac{surround\ refr.\ index}{equivalent\ power}$$

Equation 3.13 $\quad f_e = -f_e′$

Equation 3.13 (explained)

primary equiv. focal length = −secondary equiv. focal length

DEMO QUESTION 3.9

Two thin lenses of powers +2.00D and +1.75D are separated by a distance of 11 cm. What is the secondary equivalent focal length of the system?

Step 1: Determine what we need to calculate
secondary equivalent focal length, $f_e′$

Step 2: Define variables
F_1 = +2.00D
F_2 = +1.75D
d = 0.11m *(we need to convert to metres)*
n = 1.00 *(nothing is specifically mentioned, so we assume the primary medium is air)*
n′ = 1.00 *(nothing is specifically mentioned, so we assume the secondary medium is air)*

Step 3: Determine necessary equation(s)
$F_e = F_1 + F_2 - (dF_1F_2)$ *(Equation 3.10)*
$f_e′ = n / F_e$ *(Equation 3.11)*

Step 4: Calculate
$F_e = F_1 + F_2 - (dF_1F_2)$
$F_e = (+2) + (+1.75) - (0.11 \times (+2) \times (+1.75))$
$F_e = +3.365$
$f_e′ = n / F_e$
$f_e′ = 1 / +3.365$
$f_e′ = +0.2972m$
The secondary equivalent focal length is +29.72 cm. *(don't forget the ± sign and the units!)*

Practice Questions:

3.9.1 Two thin lenses of powers −3.50D and +6.75D are separated by a distance of 10 cm. What is the secondary equivalent focal length of the system?

3.9.2 Two thin lenses of powers −2.25D and +10.00D are separated by a distance of 50 cm. What is the primary equivalent focal length of the system?

3.9.3 A multiple lens system has a secondary equivalent focal length of +25 cm. What is the primary equivalent focal length of the system?

Newton's Formulae

If you can determine the equivalent focal lengths of a multiple lens system, then you can utilise a method called **Newton's formulae** in order to calculate object and image distances. However, for Newton's formulae to be useful, we need to be given the **object distance from the primary focal point** (x), which is very different to the object distance relative to the first lens (l), and we will also need to utilise the equivalent focal lengths (f_e and $f_e′$). This will allow us to calculate the image distance relative to the secondary focal point (x′). Fig. 3.12 utilises the same lens system as demonstrated in Fig. 3.10, but this time it shows the relationship between object distance (x) and image distance (x′) relative to the focal points.

Newton's formulae can be used to calculate image distance using Equation 3.14 or 3.15 (see Box 3.1 for advice

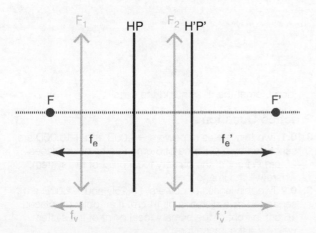

• **Fig. 3.11** Diagram highlighting the secondary (H′P′) and primary (HP) principal planes for an optical system with two positively powered lenses (grey). The primary (f_e) and secondary equivalent focal lengths ($f_e′$) are identical albeit inverted to one another, which is always true for equivalent focal lengths (see Equation 3.13).

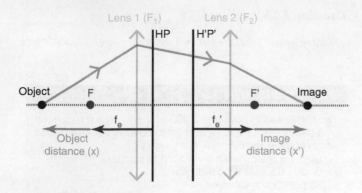

• **Fig. 3.12** Diagram highlighting the important points required for Newton's formulae. This example uses two positively powered lenses.

• **BOX 3.1** **Step-Along or Newton's Formulae?**

If presented with an optical question that provides you with an object distance in front of a multiple lens system, then you might be wondering how to decide whether it's more appropriate to use a step-along method or Newton's formulae. The answer to this riddle lies in the description of the object distance:

1. If the object distance is measured relative to the first lens, then you have been given the variable l (little l) and you need to use step-along methods. In this instance there is no need to calculate equivalent power as you will consider each lens individually.

2. If the object distance is given relative to the primary focal point, then you have been given the variable x and you need to use Newton's formulae. In this instance it is essential to calculate equivalent power to help you determine the equivalent focal lengths.

Fig. B3.1 shows the difference between the two distances.

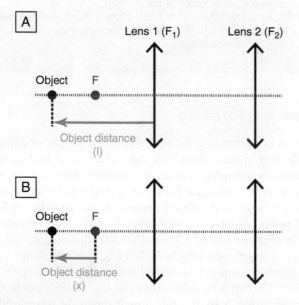

• **Fig. B3.1** Illustration showing the difference between l (A) and x (B). It might help to do a little diagram like this when solving equations to decide which method to use.

---

on how to know when to use step-along vergence or Newton's formulae).

Equation 3.14 $(f_e')^2 = -xx'$

Equation 3.14 (explained)

$(secondary\ equiv.\ focal\ length)^2 = -object\ dist. \times image\ dist.$

Equation 3.15 $f_e f_e' = xx'$

Equation 3.15 (explained)

$\begin{array}{c}primary\ equiv.\\focal\ length\end{array} \times \begin{array}{c}secondary\ equiv.\\focal\ length\end{array} = object\ dist. \times image\ dist.$

DEMO QUESTION 3.10

Two thin lenses of powers +6.00D and +1.00D are separated by a distance of 10 cm. If an object is placed 25 cm in front of the primary focal point of the system, where will the image form?

Step 1: Determine what we need to calculate
image distance (relative to secondary focal point), x'

Step 2: Define variables
F_1 = +6.00D
F_2 = +1.00D
d = 0.10m *(we need to convert to metres)*
x = −0.25m *(negative distance and we need to convert to metres)*
n = 1.00 *(nothing is specifically mentioned, so we assume the primary medium is air)*
n' = 1.00 *(nothing is specifically mentioned, so we assume the secondary medium is air)*

Step 3: Determine necessary equation(s)
$F_e = F_1 + F_2 - (dF_1F_2)$ *(Equation 3.10)*
$f_e' = n / F_e$ *(Equation 3.11)*
$(f_e')2 = -xx'$ *(Equation 3.14)*

Step 4: Calculate
$F_e = F_1 + F_2 - (dF_1F_2)$
$F_e = (+6) + (+1) - (0.10 \times (+6) \times (+1))$
$F_e = +6.4$
$f_e' = n / F_e$
$f_e' = 1 / +6.4$
$f_e' = +0.15625m$
$(f_e')^2 = -xx'$
$(0.15625)^2 = -(-0.25) x'$
$0.0244.. = -(-0.25) x'$
$0.0244.. / -0.25 = -x'$
$-0.09765625 = -x'$
$x' = +0.0977m$

The image will form 9.77 cm right of the secondary focal point.
(don't forget the ± sign and the units!)

Practice Questions:

3.10.1 Two thin lenses of powers −4.00D and +10.00D are separated by a distance of 5 cm. If an object is placed 25 cm in front of the primary focal point of the system, where will the image form?

3.10.2 Two thin lenses of powers +3.25D and +2.00D are separated by a distance of 14 cm. If an object is placed 16 cm in front of the primary focal point of the system, where will the image form?

3.10.3 A multiple lens system has a secondary equivalent focal length of +23.25 cm. If an object is placed 10 cm in front of the primary focal point of the system, where will the image form?

Magnification Using Newton's Formulae

Now that we know how to use Newton's formulae to calculate image distance, it's also possible to determine the relative image size (h′) and orientation of the image by calculating the **linear magnification (m)** with Equation 3.16.

Equation 3.16 $\quad m = -\dfrac{f_e}{x} = -\dfrac{x'}{f_e'} = -x'F_e$

Equation 3.16 (explained)

$$mag. = -\frac{primary\ equiv.\ focal\ length}{obj\ dist.} =$$
$$-\frac{img\ dist.}{secondary\ equiv.\ focal\ length} = -img\ dist. \times equiv.\ power$$

DEMO QUESTION 3.11

Two thin lenses of powers +5.50D and +1.00D are separated by a distance of 2 cm. If an object is placed 20 cm in front of the primary focal point of the system, what is the linear magnification of the image?

Step 1: Determine what we need to calculate
linear magnification, m
   Step 2: Define variables
F_1 = +5.50D
F_2 = +1.00D
d = 0.02m *(we need to convert to metres)*
x = −0.20m *(negative distance and we need to convert to metres)*
n = 1.00 *(nothing is specifically mentioned, so we assume the primary medium is air)*
n′ = 1.00 *(nothing is specifically mentioned, so we assume the secondary medium is air)*

DEMO QUESTION 3.11—cont'd

Step 3: Determine necessary equation(s)
$F_e = F_1 + F_2 - (dF_1F_2)$ *(Equation 3.10)*
$f_e' = n / F_e$ *(Equation 3.11)*
$(f_e')^2 = -xx'$ *(Equation 3.12)*
$m = -x'F_e'$ *(Equation 3.16)*
   Step 4: Calculate
$F_e = F_1 + F_2 - (dF_1F_2)$
$F_e = (+5.5) + (+1) - (0.02 \times (+5.5) \times (+1))$
$F_e = +6.39$
$f_e' = n / F_e$
$f_e' = 1 / +6.39$
$f_e' = +0.1565...m$
$(f_e')^2 = -xx'$
$(0.1565...)^2 = -(-0.20)x'$
$0.0244.. = -(-0.20)x'$
$0.0244.. / -0.20 = -x'$
$-0.1225.. = -x'$
$x' = +0.1225..$
(don't forget to keep all the numbers long in the calculator!)
$m = -x'F_e$
$m = -(-0.1225..) \times (+6.39)$
$m = -0.78$
The image is inverted (real) and 0.78× smaller than the object.
(don't forget the ± sign and the units!)

Practice Questions:

3.11.1 Two thin lenses of powers −2.50D and +3.00D are separated by a distance of 3 cm. If an object is placed 45 cm in front of the primary focal point of the system, what is the linear magnification of the image?

3.11.2 Two thin lenses of powers +3.25D and +7.00D are separated by a distance of 19 cm. If an object is placed 8 cm in front of the primary focal point of the system, what is the linear magnification of the image?

Test Your Knowledge

Try the questions below to see if you need to go over any sections again. All answers are available in the back of the book.

TYK.3.1 What is the definition of a thin lens?
TYK.3.2 What would a magnification of −0.6 tell us about the nature of the image?
TYK.3.3 How would you calculate equivalent power of two thin lenses in contact with one another?
TYK.3.4 What is a principal plane?
TYK.3.5 What is the difference between back vertex focal length and secondary equivalent focal length?
TYK.3.6 What determines whether we use step-along vergence or Newton's formulae to find image distance with a multiple lens system?

Reference

1. Tunnacliffe AH, Hirst JG. *Optics*. 2nd ed. UK: Association of British Dispensing Opticians; 1996.

4

Thick Lenses

OBJECTIVES

After working through this chapter, you should be able to:

Define what a 'thick lens' is, and calculate how to measure thickness

Understand the relationship between thickness, curvature of the surfaces, refractive index and how these contribute to the power of the lens

Calculate image position using the virtual object equations or the step-along vergence equations

Define what a 'Fresnel lens' is

Introduction

Up to this point, we have considered lenses with such negligible thickness that it is possible to ignore the refractive index of the material and still reach reasonable estimates of image location and magnification, etc.; these are called thin lenses. However, it is more accurate to take both the thickness and the refractive index into account when performing these calculations. If the thickness is considered, the lens is referred to as a **thick lens**, and in these circumstances the individual lens surfaces need to be considered.

This chapter will cover some of the fundamentals of thick lens theory and calculations.

Lens Thickness

To measure the thickness of a lens, usually corresponding to the central point of the lens (**centre thickness**), it is first important to be able to determine the **sagitta (sag)** and the **edge thickness**. The sag is defined as the height of a segment of a circle (or sphere) from arc to base, whereas the edge thickness is the physical thickness at the edges of the lens. Fig. 4.1 shows a diagram to explain these concepts visually. It is important to know the thickness of the lens

because this, in combination with the curvature and refractive index, helps to understand the power of the lens.

To start calculating the thickness, we need to calculate the sag (s) of a spherical lens, but in order to do this, we need to know the radius of curvature (r) of the surface and the value that equates to half the lens diameter (y). Fig. 4.2 shows these variables labelled on an example lens.

Sag can be calculated using Equation 4.1.

Equation 4.1 $s = r - \sqrt{(r^2 - y^2)}$

Equation 4.1 (explained)

$$sag = radius - \sqrt{(radius^2 - half\ lens\ diameter^2)}$$

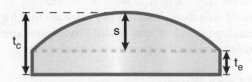

• **Fig. 4.1** Illustration showing a planoconvex lens with centre thickness (t_c), edge thickness (t_e) and sag (s) labelled.

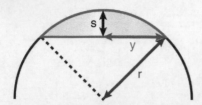

• **Fig. 4.2** Illustration showing a planoconvex lens with sag (s), radius of curvature (r) and half the diameter of the lens (y) labelled.

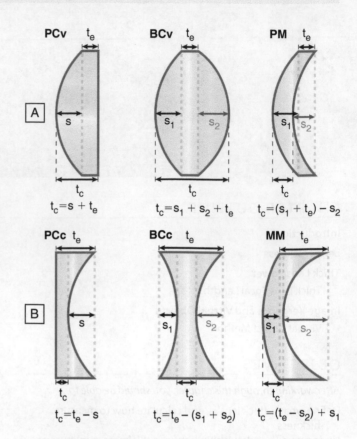

• **Fig. 4.3** Illustration showing sag (s), centre thickness (t_c) and edge thickness (t_e) for positively powered (A) planoconvex (PCv), biconvex (BCv) and plus meniscus (PM) lenses, and negatively powered (B) planoconcave (PCc), biconcave (BCc) and minus meniscus (MM) lenses. Each lens type utilises a slightly different equation for calculating centre thickness.

The centre thickness (t_c) can only be calculated if you know the sag (s) and the edge thickness (t_e), and the equation for this will change depending on the type of lens. As shown in Fig. 4.3, the relationship between the front and back surface of the lens, and whether those surfaces are convex or concave, will affect the equation for centre thickness. Another important point to note here is that the sag is determined by the curvature of the surface, which helps to contribute to the power of the lens. That means that for high powered lenses, the thickness can increase so much that the lenses become heavy. In an optical imaging system this would be ok, but if you're a person who needs glasses, heavy lenses are not ideal! Luckily, the thickness can be reduced (whilst maintaining the same power) by changing the material of the lens to something of a higher refractive index. Remember that higher refractive indices indicate that light is slowing more, leading to higher amounts of refraction. This ultimately means that higher index lenses won't need to be as curved (leading to a smaller sag and smaller thickness) to produce the same power.

Thick Lens Power

In general terms, any lens in which the thickness exceeds an amount that is acceptable for thin-lens assumptions is classed as a thick lens. However, in some cases, lenses that are physically very thin are classed as thick lenses if their front vertex and back vertex powers are substantially different, for example, contact lenses (lenses that sit on the front surface of the eye).

The key thing to note for thick lenses is that you need to take into account the refractive index of the material, so it is a little like having two thin lenses separated by a distance, with a refractive index change in the middle. Importantly, with thick lenses, we can't assume that incident light rays will only refract once as they pass through; instead, we think of them as refracting at each individual surface of the lens. Fig. 4.4 depicts an example thick lens to show that the light will refract twice as it passes through the lens; once at the front surface, and again at the back surface.

To determine the overall power of a thick lens, we need to calculate the power of the front (F_1) and back (F_2) surfaces individually, and we need to know how thick (t) the lens is. To start with then, to calculate the power of each surface, we can use a familiar calculation from chapter 2 which has been updated in Equation 4.2. This will involve using what we know about the radius of curvature of each surface (r_1 and r_2) and the refractive index of the lens and surrounding material (n) in order to calculate the respective powers. However, we need to be careful to remember that we

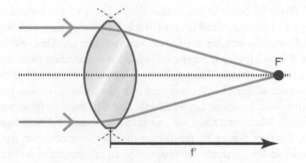

• **Fig. 4.4** Illustration showing parallel light entering a convex thick lens. Notice that the light refracts at both the first and second surface before coming to a focus at the secondary focal point.

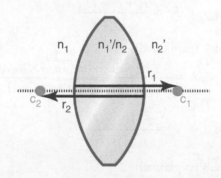

• **Fig. 4.5** Illustration showing relationship between radius of curvature for the front (r_1) and back (r_2) surface of the lens, along with the refractive index variables. The diagram also shows the centre of curvature of the front surface (C_1) and the back surface (C_2).

always assume light travels from left to right, meaning that at the first surface (F_1), the primary refractive index (n_1) will be air, and the secondary refractive index (n_1') will be the lens; however at the back surface (F_2) this will be swapped as the light will travel from the lens (n_2) to the air (n_2'). Fig. 4.5 explains the relationship between the radius of curvature values and the refractive index values.

Equation 4.2 $F_1 = \dfrac{n_1' - n_1}{r_1}$ $F_2 = \dfrac{n_2' - n_2}{r_2}$

Equation 4.2 (explained)

$$power = \frac{secondary\ refr.index - primary\ refr.index}{radius\ of\ curvature}$$

It's key here to make sure we know whether the radius of curvature will be positive or negative – remember that measurements always start *from* the relevant surface *to* the point of measurement (in this case the centre of curvature, C). As we learned in chapter 2, if the radius distance is measured from left to right (in the same direction as light) then it will be positive; otherwise, it will be negative. The trick is to remember that if the front surface is convex, it will have a positive radius of curvature, whereas if it's concave, it will have a negative radius of curvature. Similarly, if the back surface is convex, it will have a negative radius of curvature, and if the back surface is concave, it will have a positive radius of curvature (Fig. 4.6).

In order to determine how the thickness of the lens and the refractive index work together to refract the light, we need to calculate the reduced thickness ($\bar{t}$; pronounced tee-reduced or tee-bar). We do this by dividing the measured thickness (t) by the refractive index of the material (n_g), as shown in Equation 4.3.

Equation 4.3 $\bar{t} = \dfrac{t}{n_g}$

Equation 4.3 (explained)

$$\overline{reduced\ thickness} = \frac{thickness}{refractive\ index\ of\ lens}$$

Once we have all the information needed, we can utilise and modify a familiar equation from chapter 3 to calculate the equivalent power of the lens (Equation 4.4).

Equation 4.4 $F_e = F_1 + F_2 - \bar{t}F_1F_2$

Equation 4.4 (explained)

$$equivalent\ power = lens1 + lens2$$
$$-(reduced\ thickness \times lens1 \times lens2)$$

DEMO QUESTION 4.2

A 3-cm thick biconvex lens (refractive index 1.523) has a front surface with a radius of curvature of 15 cm and a back surface with a radius of curvature of 20 cm. What is the power of the lens?

   Step 1: Determine what we need to calculate equivalent power, F_e

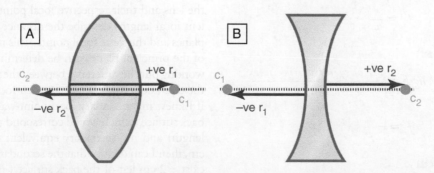

• **Fig. 4.6** Illustration showing relationship between convex (A) and concave (B) surfaces and whether they possess a positive (+ve) or negative (−ve) radius of curvature.

DEMO QUESTION 4.2—cont'd

Step 2: Define variables

$t = 0.03$ m *(we need to convert to metres)*

$n_g = 1.523$ *(refractive index of lens)*

$r_1 = +0.15$ m *(because the front surface is convex the radius is positive and in metres)*

$r_2 = -0.20$ m *(because the back surface is convex the radius is negative and in metres)*

$n = 1.00$ *(nothing is specifically mentioned so we assume the primary medium is air)*

Step 3: Determine necessary equation

$F_1 = (n_1' - n_1) / r_1$ *(Equation 4.2)*

$F_2 = (n_2' - n_2) / r_2$ *(Equation 4.2)*

$\bar{t} = t / n_g$ *(Equation 4.3)*

$F_e = F_1 + F_2 - \bar{t} F_1 F_2$ *(Equation 4.4)*

Step 4: Calculate

$F_1 = (n_1' - n_1) / r_1$

$F_1 = (1.523 - 1.00) / 0.15$

$F_1 = +3.49...D$ *(remember to keep the number long in the calculator)*

$F_2 = (n_2' - n_2) / r_2$

$F_2 = (1.00 - 1.523) / -0.20$

$F_2 = +2.615D$

$\bar{t} = t / n_g$

$\bar{t} = 0.03 / 1.523$

$\bar{t} = 0.0197...$ *(remember to keep the number long in the calculator)*

$F_e = F_1 + F_2 - \bar{t} F_1 F_2$

$F_e = 3.49... + 2.615 - (0.0197... \times 3.49 \times 2.615)$

$F_e = +5.92D$

(don't forget the $\pm$ sign and the units!)

Practice Questions:

4.2.1 A thick lens (refractive index 1.523) has a convex front surface with a radius of curvature of 25 cm. What is the power of the front surface?

4.2.2 A thick lens (refractive index 1.523) has a concave back surface with a radius of curvature of 25 cm. What is the power of the back surface?

4.2.3 A 5-cm thick lens (refractive index 1.523) has a front surface power of -2.00D and a back surface power of $+4.00$D. What is the power of the lens?

Thick Lens Focal Length

If it's possible to calculate the equivalent power of a thick lens, then it is also possible to calculate the **secondary (f_e') and primary (f_e) equivalent focal lengths** (Equations 4.5 and 4.6). Remember that the equation for the primary equivalent focal length requires you to include a minus sign.

Equation 4.5 $$f_e' = \frac{n}{F_e}$$

Equation 4.5 (explained)

$$secondary\ equiv.\ focal\ length = \frac{primary\ refractive\ index}{equivalent\ power}$$

Equation 4.6 $$f_e = -\frac{n}{F_e}$$

Equation 4.6 (explained)

$$primary\ equiv.\ focal\ length = -\frac{primary\ refractive\ index}{equivalent\ power}$$

Now, in order to determine the location of the secondary (F′) and primary focal points (F) relative to the front and back surface of the lens, we need to calculate the front and back vertex focal lengths, which means we first need to calculate front and back vertex power. Remember that vertex power describes the vergence of light leaving a system in a particular direction, providing the incident (approaching) light is parallel (zero vergence). Mathematically, we can calculate **front (F_v) and back (F_v') vertex power** by modifying the thin lens equation for a multiple lens system (see chapter 3) to consider the reduced thickness instead of the distance between the lenses (Equations 4.7 and 4.8). Once we have those values we can calculate **front (f_v) and back (f_v') vertex focal length** (Equations 4.9 and 4.10).

Equation 4.7 $$F_v' = \frac{F_1 + F_2 - \bar{t} F_1 F_2}{1 - \bar{t} F_1}$$

Equation 4.7 (explained)

$$back\ vertex\ power = \frac{lens1 + lens2 - (\overline{thickness} \times lens1 \times lens2)}{1 - (\overline{thickness} \times lens1)}$$

Equation 4.8 $$F_v = \frac{F_1 + F_2 - \bar{t} F_1 F_2}{1 - \bar{t} F_2}$$

Equation 4.8 (explained)

$$front\ vertex\ power = \frac{lens1 + lens2 - (\overline{thickness} \times lens1 \times lens2)}{1 - (\overline{thickness} \times lens2)}$$

Equation 4.9 $$f_v' = \frac{n}{F_v'}$$

Equation 4.9 (explained)

$$back\ vertex\ focal\ length = \frac{surrounding\ refractive\ index}{back\ vertex\ power}$$

Equation 4.10 $$f_v = -\frac{n}{F_v}$$

Equation 4.10 (explained)

$$front\ vertex\ focal\ length = -\frac{surrounding\ refractive\ index}{front\ vertex\ power}$$

Now, thinking about this logically, we know both that vertex focal lengths describe the distance between the surfaces of the lens and their respective focal points and that the equivalent focal lengths describe the distance between the principal planes and the same focal points. This means that the location of the principal planes can be determined mathematically by working out the difference between the vertex focal length and the equivalent focal length for each focal point. For example, if I knew my secondary focal point was $+10$ cm right of the back surface (which would correspond to the back vertex focal length) and my secondary equivalent focal length was $+12$ cm, then I can deduce that the secondary principal plane must exist -2 cm left of the back surface ($+10$ cm $- +12$ cm $= -2$ cm). This is highlighted in Equations 4.11 and 4.12, where we can calculate the distance between the primary principal plane and the first surface of the lens (e), and the distance between the secondary principal plane and the back surface of the lens (e').

Equation 4.11 $\quad A_1P = e = f_v - f_e$

Equation 4.11 (explained)

$A_1P = e =$

front vertex focal length − primary equivalent focal length

Equation 4.12 $\quad A_2P' = e' = f_v' - f_e'$

Equation 4.12 (explained)

$A_2P' = e' =$

back vertex focal length − secondary equivalent focal length

DEMO QUESTION 4.3

Imagine a 2.5-cm thick biconvex lens (surface powers +5.00D and +2.00D; refractive index 1.523). Where is the secondary principal plane, relative to the back surface of the lens?

Step 1: Determine what we need to calculate secondary principal plane location, A_2P'

Step 2: Define variables

$F_1 = +5.00D$
$F_2 = +2.00D$
$t = 0.025$ m *(we need to convert to metres)*
$n = 1.00$ *(nothing is specifically mentioned so we assume the primary medium is air)*
$n' = 1.523$ *(refractive index of lens)*

Step 3: Determine necessary equation(s)

$\bar{t} = t / n_g$ *(Equation 4.3)*
$F_v' = (F_1 + F_2 - \bar{t}F_1F_2) / (1 - \bar{t}F_1)$ *(Equation 4.7)*
$f_v' = n / F_v'$ *(Equation 4.9)*
$F_e = F_1 + F_2 - \bar{t}F_1F_2$ *(Equation 4.4)*
$f_e' = n / F_e$ *(Equation 4.5)*
$A_2P' = e' = f_v' - f_e'$ *(Equation 4.12)*

Step 4: Calculate

$\bar{t} = t / n_g$
$\bar{t} = 0.025 / 1.523$
$\bar{t} = 0.0164...$
$F_v' = (F_1 + F_2 - \bar{t}F_1F_2) / (1 - \bar{t}F_1)$
$F_v' = (5 + 2 - 0.0164.. \times 5 \times 2) / (1 - (0.0164.. \times 5))$
$F_v' = +7.45...$
$f_v' = n / F_v'$
$f_v' = 1.00 / +7.45..$
$f_v' = +0.1343..$
$F_e = F_1 + F_2 - \bar{t}F_1F_2$
$F_e = 5 + 2 - 0.0164.. \times 5 \times 2$
$F_e = +6.84..$
$f_e' = n / F_e$
$f_e' = 1.00 / +6.84..$
$f_e' = +0.1463..$
$A_2P' = e' = f_v' - f_e'$
$A_2P' = e' = +0.1343.. - +0.1463..$
$A_2P' = e' = -0.0120$

The secondary principal plane for this lens exists 1.20 cm left of the back surface of the lens.

(don't forget the ± sign and the units!)

Practice Questions:

4.3.1 Imagine an 0.8-cm thick biconvex lens (surface powers +1.00D and +3.50D; refractive index 1.523).

DEMO QUESTION 4.3—cont'd

Where is the secondary principal plane, relative to the back surface of the lens?

4.3.2 Imagine a 1-cm thick biconvex lens (surface powers +2.00D and +6.25D; refractive index 1.523). Where is the primary principal plane, relative to the back surface of the lens?

Image Vergence and Virtual Objects

Once we know the power of each surface, it's possible to calculate image location (l') by determining the vergence approaching and leaving each surface of the lens. There are two possible methods for this, and so in order to be thorough (and for extra maths practice!), I'll go through them both.

Virtual Object Method

The first method we'll go over is called the 'virtual object' method, because it assumes that the image formed at the first surface will become the new (virtual) object for the second surface. The equations used for is method will be extremely familiar as we've already seen them in chapters 2 and 3, but I have included them here with updated descriptions. As we have two surfaces to consider, we will also be utilising our handy subscript numbers to help us work out which surface we're dealing with.

Equation 4.13 $\qquad L = \dfrac{n}{l}$

Equation 4.13 (explained)

$$object\ vergence = \frac{primary\ refractive\ index}{object\ distance\ from\ surface}$$

Equation 4.14 $\qquad L' = L + F$

Equation 4.14 (explained)

$$image\ vergence = object\ vergence + power$$

Equation 4.15 $\quad L' = \dfrac{n'}{l'} \quad l' = \dfrac{n'}{L'}$

Equation 4.15 (explained)

$$image\ distance = \frac{secondary\ refr.\ index}{image\ vergence}$$

Look at the example diagram shown in Fig. 4.7, where a biconvex thick lens (refractive index 1.523) is located in air. Remember that the primary refractive index will represent air when light is entering the lens (at the front surface), but it will also represent the lens when light is leaving the lens again (at the back surface), so be careful to check your numbers here. Another thing to think about is the presence of the virtual object. This describes the location of the image that would be formed by the first surface (F_1) if the second surface didn't exist. It's referred to as a *virtual* object because this hypothetical image then acts as the object for the second surface. The only problem is that we'll have initially

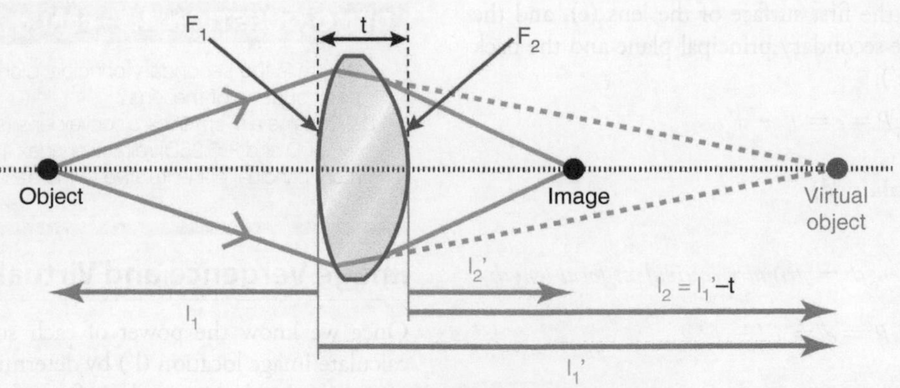

• **Fig. 4.7** Diagram using example biconvex lens to highlight the relationship between surface powers (F_1 and F_2), lens thickness (t), object distance from the apex of the first surface (l_1), virtual object distance from the apex of the second surface ($l_2 = l_1' - t$) and final image distance relative to the second surface (l_2').

calculated its distance relative to the first surface (F_1), and so we'll need to account for the thickness of the lens (t) when we perform our calculations for the back surface (F_2). Please note that when using the virtual object method, we use the genuine thickness of the lens and not the reduced thickness.

DEMO QUESTION 4.4

An object is placed 20 cm in front of a 2-cm thick biconvex lens (refractive index 1.523) with a front surface power of +8.00D and a back surface power of +10.00D. Where does the image form relative to the back surface of the lens?

Step 1: Determine what we need to calculate
image distance relative to the back surface, l_2'

Step 2: Define variables
$l_1 = -0.20$ m *(negative distance and we need to convert to metres)*
$F_1 = +8.00$D
$F_2 = +10.00$D
$t = 0.02$ m *(we need to convert to metres)*
$n = 1.00$ *(nothing is specifically mentioned so we assume the primary medium is air)*
$n' = 1.523$ *(refractive index of lens)*

Step 3: Determine necessary equation(s)
$L = n / l$ *(Equation 4.13)*
$L' = L + F$ *(Equation 4.14)*
$L' = n' / l'$ *(Equation 4.15)*

Step 4: Calculate
$L_1 = n_1 / l_1$
$L_1 = 1.00 / -0.20$
$L_1 = -5.00$
$L_1' = L_1 + F_1$
$L_1' = -5.00 + 8.00$
$L_1' = +3.00$
$L_1' = n_1' / l_1'$
$l_1' = n_1' / L_1'$ *(rearrange to get l_1')*
$l_1' = 1.523 / 3.00$
$l_1' = +0.5077...$ *(this is the distance of the virtual object from the front surface)*
$l_2 = l_1' - t$ *(need the distance of the virtual object from the back surface)*
$l_2 = +0.5077... - 0.02$
$l_2 = +0.4877...$
$L_2 = n_2 / l_2$
$L_2 = 1.523 / +0.4877...$ *(the primary refractive index is now the lens)*

DEMO QUESTION 4.4—cont'd

$L_2 = +3.123...$
$L_2' = L_2 + F_2$
$L_2' = 3.123... + 10.00$
$L_2' = +13.123...$
$L_2' = n_2' / l_2'$
$l_2' = n_2' / L_2'$ *(rearrange to get l')*
$l_2' = 1.00 / 13,123...$
$l_2' = +0.0762$ m
The image forms 7.62 cm right of the back surface of the lens.
(don't forget the ± sign and the units!)

Practice Questions:

4.4.1 An object is placed 10 cm in front of a 4-cm thick biconvex lens (refractive index 1.523) with a front surface power of +4.00D and a back surface power of +5.00D. Where does the image form relative to the back surface of the lens?

4.4.2 An object is placed 20 cm in front of a 1.5-cm thick biconcave lens (refractive index 1.523) with a front surface power of −2.50D and a back surface power of −3.00D. Where does the image form relative to the back surface of the lens?

Step-Along Method

The equations used for the 'step-along method' will also be extremely familiar, as we've already seen them in chapter 3 in relation to thin lenses. The only difference is that instead of two thin lenses separated by a distance, we have two surfaces of a lens of a certain thickness. All we need to do is replace the distance (d) variable with one for reduced thickness ($\bar{t}$) which takes into account the distance and the refractive index, as shown in Equation 4.16.

Equation 4.16
$$L_2 = \frac{L_1'}{1 - \bar{t}L_1'}$$

Equation 4.16 (explained)
$$verg.\,at\,F_2 = \frac{verg.\,leaving\,F_1}{1 - (\textbf{\textit{thickness}} \times verg.\,leaving\,F_1)}$$

To show that this method is equivalent to the virtual object method, I have used exactly the same question in the demo – you can check it yourself at home!

DEMO QUESTION 4.5

An object is placed 20 cm in front of a 2-cm thick biconvex lens (refractive index 1.523) with a front surface power of +8.00D and a back surface power of +10.00D. Where does the image form relative to the back surface of the lens?

Step 1: Determine what we need to calculate
image distance relative to the back surface, l_2'

Step 2: Define variables
$l_1 = -0.20$ m *(negative distance and we need to convert to metres)*
$F_1 = +8.00D$
$F_2 = +10.00D$
$t = 0.02$ m *(we need to convert to metres)*
$n = 1.00$ *(nothing is specifically mentioned so we assume the primary medium is air)*
$n' = 1.523$ *(refractive index of lens)*

Step 3: Determine necessary equation(s)
$L = n / l$ *(Equation 4.13)*
$L' = L + F$ *(Equation 4.14)*
$\bar{t} = t / n_0$ *(Equation 4.3)*
$L_2 = L_1' / (1 - \bar{t}L_1')$ *(Equation 4.16)*
$L' = n' / l'$ *(Equation 4.15)*

Step 4: Calculate
$L_1 = n_1 / l_1$
$L_1 = 1.00 / -0.20$
$L_1 = -5.00$
$L_1' = L_1 + F_1$
$L_1' = -5.00 + 8.00$
$L_1' = +3.00$
$\bar{t} = t / n_0$
$\bar{t} = 0.02 / 1.523$
$\bar{t} = 0.0131...$ *(remember to keep the number long in the calculator)*
$L_2 = L_1' / (1 - \bar{t}L_1')$
$L_2 = 3.00 / (1 - (0.0131... \times 3.00))$
$L_2 = +3.123...$ *(remember to keep the number long in the calculator)*
$L_2' = L_2 + F_2$
$L_2' = 3.123... + 10.00$
$L_2' = +13.123...$
$L_2' = n_2' / l_2'$
$l_2' = n_2' / L_2'$ *(rearrange to get l')*
$l_2' = 1.00 / 13.123...$
$l_2' = +0.0762$ m
The image forms 7.62 cm right of the back surface of the lens. (don't forget the ± sign and the units!)

Practice Questions:

4.5.1 An object is placed 11 cm in front of a 4-cm thick biconvex lens (refractive index 1.523) with a front surface power of +2.00D and a back surface power of +5.00D.

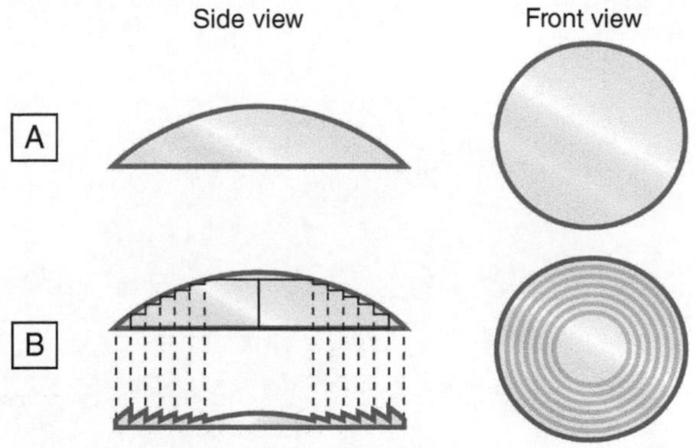

• **Fig. 4.8** Diagram showing side and front views of a biconvex lens (A) and the Fresnel equivalent (B).

DEMO QUESTION 4.5—cont'd

Where does the image form relative to the back surface of the lens?
4.5.2 An object is placed 25 cm in front of a 3-cm thick biconcave lens (refractive index 1.523) with a front surface power of −1.50D and a back surface power of −5.00D. Where does the image form relative to the back surface of the lens?

Fresnel Lenses

As we discussed briefly earlier in the chapter, one thing that is true about lenses is that as the power increases, usually the thickness and the curvature also increases. This naturally increases the weight (and size) of the lens, which can sometimes be a problem when applied to real-world optical problems. For example, I wear a −6.75D lens in my glasses, which can be so thick and heavy (in relative terms) that I usually have to purchase high index lenses, but I actually prefer to wear contact lenses (for ease). An alternative solution to this lens problem, however, is to utilise **Fresnel** (*pronounced Freh-nel*) **lenses**,[1] which are lenses divided up into concentric rings, as illustrated in Fig. 4.8. Here you can see that each small section of the Fresnel lens (B) possesses the equivalent curvature of the planoconvex lens (A), but with a dramatically reduced thickness. This leads to thinner, lighter lenses, but one of the limitations of this type of lens is that image quality will be slightly reduced due to **diffraction** (see chapter 10) occurring at the ridges between each curved ring.

Test Your Knowledge

Try the questions below to see if you need to review any sections again. All answers are available in the back of the book.

TYK.4.1 What is the definition of a thick lens (relative to a thin lens)?

TYK.4.2 What is the difference between the sag and the edge thickness?

TYK.4.3 In an equiconcave lens, does the back surface have a positive or negative radius of curvature?

TYK.4.4 What is a virtual object?

TYK.4.5 What causes the resolution of a Fresnel lens to be reduced relative to a 'regular' lens?

Reference

1. Davis A, Kühnlenz F. Optical design using Fresnel lenses: basic principles and some practical examples. *Optik & Photonik.* 2007;2(4):52-55.

5

The Reduced Eye and Spherical and Cylindrical Lenses

CHAPTER OUTLINE

OBJECTIVES

After working through this chapter, you should be able to:

Outline all the important features of a reduced eye

Outline the difference between a spherical refractive error
   and a cylindrical refractive error

Explain what the far point of the eye is and be able to calculate it

Understand how power of a lens will need to be altered as its
   distance from the eye increases

Interpret a power cross

Introduction

Now that we know the basics of thin and thick lenses, we need to spend a little bit of time focusing on clinical examples of corrective lenses. However, in order to do that effectively, we need to first consider the power of the human eye.

The Human Eye

As you will no doubt be aware, the human eye is a particularly complex anatomical structure, and one of its many functions is to focus light onto the back of the eye (the retina). Interestingly for us, the human eye is able to focus light by adding **convergence** to the incoming light. This means it must be positively powered, which (if we think back to chapter 2) suggests that its front surface must be curved and, in particular, convex. Now, given that it's likely that you have at least one eye, this probably comes as no surprise to you because we know that the front surface (the cornea) is domed and pokes outwards in a convex way from the front surface of the eye (Fig. 5.1).

Importantly, we can imagine that if light travelled from one section of air into another section of air that was curved but had the same refractive index, it probably wouldn't do very much to the path of the light (we can even confirm this mathematically using Equation 2.4 from chapter 2 ($F = (n' - n) / r$ – here we can see that if the primary (n) and secondary refractive indices (n') are identical then no matter the curvature, the power will always be zero). This means that a key feature of the human eye focusing light is that the cornea has a different refractive index to the air, and this has been measured to be roughly 1.376. This means that the human eye can focus light because (1) it is curved, and (2) it is a different refractive index to air (please see chapter 22 for a do-it-yourself demonstration of this). This also explains why your vision is blurry if you try to open your eyes underwater – the refractive index difference between water (1.333) and the cornea (1.376) is much smaller than that of air (1.00) and the cornea (1.376), so the light doesn't focus properly.

As one final fact about the human eye before we get into the depths of chapter 5: light can enter the eye through the convex cornea because the cornea is completely transparent (please see biology textbooks for a cool explanation of how this is possible), which means the light will then travel

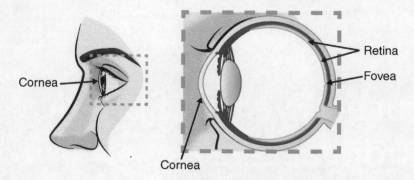

• **Fig. 5.1** An illustration of the side view (profile) of a person's face. The box outlined with a blue dashed line indicates that the image on the right is a zoomed-in cross section of the side view of the eye. In both images, the cornea is labelled as the front convex dome on the front of the eye. In the image on the right, the retina (yellow) and fovea are identified as well.

through the pupil to be focused on the **retina**. The retina is the physiological structure at the back of the inside of the eye that processes the light signal and transduces it into a signal the brain can interpret. The central part of the retina is called the **fovea**, and this is important because this part of the eye provides us with our central vision.

A Reduced Eye

The previous section has briefly covered the complexities of human vision to explain that the human eye has a positive power and that the goal is to focus the incoming light onto the retina at the back of the eye. Now, as we'll remember from chapter 2 (vergence), the amount of power of a surface will greatly affect where the image forms. In the human eye, we need the image to form on the back of the eye, which is approximately 22.22 mm behind the front surface of the eye, and this means there's little room for error. However, this distance (from the front of the eye to the back) will vary depending on individual factors such as height and age, etc.

Providing the incoming light is focused with the right power for the distance of the retina from the cornea, then the eye is appropriately proportioned and the image will be in focus (**emmetropic eye**). If, however, the light focuses too far in front of the retina (**myopic**) or too far behind the retina

(**hyperopic**), then this is called a **refractive error**, meaning the eye has refracted the light inappropriately. Fig. 5.2 shows examples of this in a simple diagram of an eye.

The important thing to remember here is that because the emmetropic eye (in general terms) is powered to focus light from infinity (zero vergence) at the retina, this means the distance between the cornea and the retina is the secondary focal length of the eye, and the fovea corresponds to the **secondary focal point (F′)**.

However, if we wanted to calculate how light travels through the eye mathematically, there would be a lot to consider – the power of the cornea, the refractive index changes (cornea, aqueous, lens and vitreous), the power of the lens and the relative distances of all the front and back surfaces of the structures. Luckily for us, we can use a simplified model of an eye in order to make this easier; this simplified model is referred to as a **reduced eye**.

The reduced eye assumes a dioptric corneal power of +60.00D, meaning the convex corneal radius of curvature is +5.55 mm. This also then assumes an axial length (length of the eye from cornea to retina) of +22.22 mm. Importantly, the eye also possesses a different refractive index (n′ = 1.333) relative to the air outside. Fig. 5.3 shows how the reduced eye can be drawn and Box 5.1 **shows** how this can be calculated.

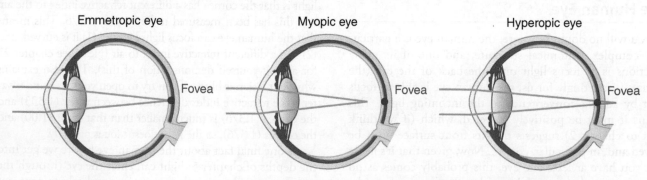

• **Fig. 5.2** Simple diagram of refractive errors. The fovea is the central part of the retina. Emmetropic eyes focus light (shown as blue lines) at the fovea on the retina, whilst myopic eyes focus light in front of the fovea and hyperopic eyes focus light behind the fovea.

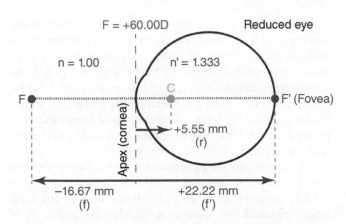

F = +60.00D   Reduced eye

n = 1.00   n' = 1.333

• **Fig. 5.3** Reduced model eye with power, distances and refractive indices labelled appropriately.

Now, we know that not all objects in the world will be an 'infinite' distance away from us, but we are able to account for changes in distance by using our lens (accommodation). This book will not discuss accommodation, but it is good to be aware that we are only discussing distant objects as examples.

Spherical Refractive Error

As discussed previously, in nature not all eyes are appropriately powered for their length, which can lead to myopia or hyperopia, both of which are examples of a spherical refractive error (measured in dioptres; **DS** or **D**). A spherical error is defined by a refractive error that is the same in all meridians, so for example, if an eye had a spherical error of −2.00D, the error would be −2.00D along all possible axes, as shown in Fig. 5.4.

Myopia

Myopia (shortsightedness) is characterised by the eye either being too powerful or the axial length of the eye being too long – both of which result in an image that forms in front of the retina (Fig. 5.5). The result is that people with myopia will see blurry images of objects at far-away distances. However, they will still be able to see objects closer to them (although, how close will depend on how large the refractive error is). For example, I am myopic, and I can only see clearly (without my lenses) to about 14.81 cm away from my eye before things start to get a little blurry, meaning that 14.81 cm corresponds to the **far point** of my eye. However, as I can still see objects clearly at 14.81 cm, the vergence of an object at that location will be focused on my retina, and we can use that information to calculate my refractive error.

$$L = n / l$$
$$L = 1.00 / -0.1481$$
$$L = -6.75$$

Equation 2.1 (from chapter 2) helps us to determine that an object 14.81 cm in front of my eye will have a **far point vergence** of −6.75 at my cornea, which is then focused neatly onto the retina of my eye. This means that my eye needs −6.75 of vergence removed from the visual signal in order to focus correctly, so we can therefore refer to the refractive error of my eye as −6.75D. If we assume that my cornea is appropriately powered at +60.00D, we can calculate the image vergence and then the image distance (which will equate to the axial length of the model eye).

$$L' = L + F$$
$$L' = -6.75 + 60.00$$
$$L' = +53.25$$
$$l' = n' / L'$$
$$l' = 1.333 / +53.25$$
$$l' = +0.02503m$$
$$l' = +25.03mm \text{ (converted to mm)}$$

These equations show that, assuming a 'typical' corneal power (and the refractive index of the reduced eye), my eye would be estimated to be nearly 3 mm *longer* than the model, reduced eye (22.22 mm).

Taken together, this means that in order to allow me to see farther than a measly 14.81 cm, I need corrective, spherical lenses. These lenses could be contact lenses, resting on the front surface of my eye, or lenses in a pair of glasses frames, sitting slightly in front of my eye.

• BOX 5.1   How Can We Calculate the Reduced Eye?

As discussed in the main text, the reduced eye assumes a refractive index of 1.333 and a corneal curvature of 5.55 mm. As our model cornea would be a convex spherical surface relative to the light entering the eye, we know the centre of curvature needs to be positioned to the right of the cornea (within the eye) and that it will therefore have a positive distance.

We can then use Equation 2.4 from chapter 2 to determine the power of the cornea, whilst being careful to remember to convert to metres:
F = n' − n / r
F = 1.333 − 1.00 / +0.00555
F = +60.00D

We can then use the power of the cornea to calculate the emmetropically appropriate distance of the retina, whilst being careful to remember that the refractive index of the eye is not the same as air:
f = n' / F
f = 1.3333 / +60.00
f = +0.022216 m
f = +22.22 mm (converted to mm)

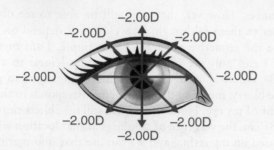

• **Fig. 5.4** A diagram to show that spherical error is the same along all axes/meridians of the eye.

Now, in simple terms, if my eye has a refractive error of −6.75D, as we've determined, then there is −6.75D of vergence that needs correcting at my cornea, so I could prescribe myself a contact lens of the matching power in order to correct my vision. This is because with contact lenses, we need the secondary focal point (F′) of the lens to correspond to the far point of the eye, and there aren't any complicated gaps between the lens and my cornea to think about. However, I usually like to be over-corrected, so I'll always ask for a −7.00D lens, but that's because I'm an awkward patient!

In contrast to this, when prescribing glasses (where the lens sits in a frame) there is a small amount of air between the back surface of the lens and the front of the eye that will affect the vergence of light as it approaches the eye. This means this distance needs to be taken into account when we prescribe lenses, and this distance between the lens and the cornea is referred to as the **back vertex distance** (Fig. 5.6 for an example).

The trick to determining the appropriate power of the lens required is by measuring the back vertex distance on the patient's chosen frames and then taking that distance away from the far point distance. In the example in Fig. 5.7, the back vertex distance (BVD) is −1.5 cm relative to the far point, which is −14.81 cm, meaning the lens placed within the frames needs to have a secondary focal length that corresponds to the distance between the back surface of the lens and the far point.

We can calculate this by subtracting the back vertex distance from the far point, for example (−14.81 cm) − (−1.5 cm) = −13.31 cm. We can then use this distance as our focal length (f) which will allow us to calculate the power (F) of the lens. This can be achieved using the power calculation as shown below:

$$F = n \,/\, f$$
$$F = 1.00 \,/\, -0.1331 \text{ (converted to metres)}$$
$$F = -7.51D$$

This suggests I would need a −7.51D lens if it were to sit 1.5 cm in front of my eye and also shows that the further away from my eye it is, the stronger the lens will need to be, because decreasing the focal length will increase the power respectively.

Hyperopia

Now, hyperopia (also known as long-sightedness) is characterised by the refractive power of the eye being too weak or the axial length of the eye being too short – both of which result in an image that forms behind the retina (see Fig. 5.2). The result of this is that people with hyperopia will see

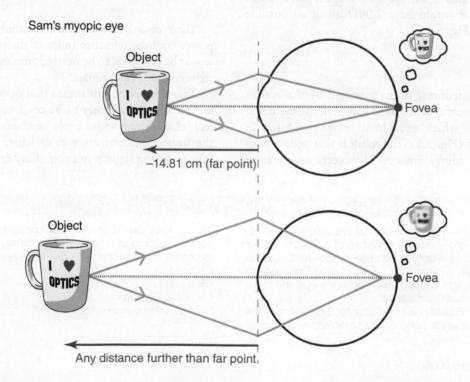

• **Fig. 5.5** A reduced eye showing my brain's interpretation (shown as thought bubbles) of an object if it was at the far point (top) relative to being farther away (bottom).

Frames

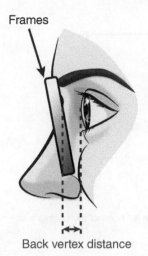

Back vertex distance

• **Fig. 5.6** A diagram showing the back vertex distance.

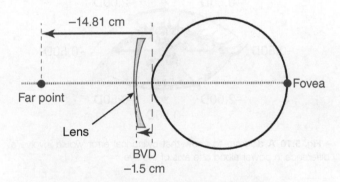

• **Fig. 5.7** A diagram showing the back vertex distance (BVD) relative to the far point of my example myopic eye.

blurry images of objects placed at close-up (near) distances. However, they will still be able to see objects far away (although how well they see them will depend on how large the refractive error is). For example, my partner is hyperopic by approximately +1.00D. This means that if left uncorrected (and ignoring the contribution of the accommodative system), light will only focus correctly on his retina if it has +1.00D of vergence at the cornea of his eye. However,

to slightly complicate things, the light needs to be converging as it approaches his cornea and will therefore be producing a virtual object behind the front surface of the eye (with a positive distance for the corresponding **far point**). Mathematically, we can determine the distance of this virtual object by using the vergence:

$$l = n / L$$
$$l = 1.00 / +1.00$$
$$l = +1.00 \text{ m}$$
$$l = +100.00 \text{ cm}$$

Here we can see that, to focus on the retina, the virtual object will need to be 100 cm behind the front surface of the eye, as shown in Fig. 5.8.

If we assume, then, that my partner's cornea is appropriately powered at +60.00D, we can calculate the image distance (which will equate to the axial length of the model eye).

$$L' = L + F$$
$$L' = +1.00 + +60.00$$
$$L' = +61.00$$
$$l' = n' / L'$$
$$l' = 1.333 / +61.00$$
$$l' = +0.02185 \text{ m}$$
$$l' = +21.85 \text{ mm (converted to mm)}$$

These equations show that, assuming a 'typical' corneal power, my partner's eye would be estimated to be approximately 0.3 mm *shorter* than the model, reduced eye.

Taken together, this means that in order to allow my partner to be able to see completely clearly, he would need corrective, spherical lenses. Again, these lenses could be contact lenses, resting on the front surface of his eyes, or lenses in a pair of glasses frames, sitting slightly in front of his eye.

Just as with myopia, a refractive error of +1.00D means there is +1.00D of vergence that needs correcting at his cornea, so my partner could wear a contact lens of the matching power. This is because with contact lenses, we still need the secondary focal point (F′) to correspond to the far point of the eye (without troubling ourselves with any pesky back vertex distances), which in this example is +100.00 cm behind the front surface of the eye.

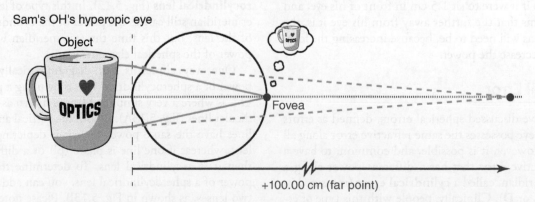

• **Fig. 5.8** A reduced eye showing my partner's, or other half's (OH), brain's interpretation (shown as a thought bubble) if light is producing a virtual object at the far point behind the front surface of the eye.

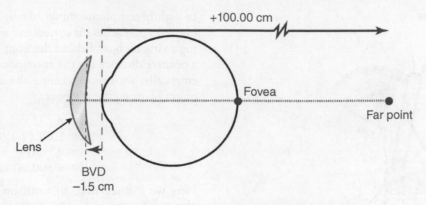

+100.00 cm

Fovea

Far point

Lens

BVD
−1.5 cm

• **Fig. 5.9** A diagram showing the back vertex distance (BVD) relative to the far point of my partner's example hyperopic eye.

However, when prescribing *glasses*, we again need to consider the **back vertex distance**. The difference is that with myopia the increasing back vertex distance reduces the required focal length and therefore strengthens the required lens the further away from the eye it gets. With hyperopia, the increasing back vertex distance will be increasing the focal length, which will, in turn, require a lower-strength lens relative to the contact lens. Again, to calculate this, we must measure the back vertex distance on the patient's chosen frames and then take that distance away from the far point distance. In the example in Fig. 5.9 the BVD is −1.5 cm relative to the far point, which is +100.00 cm, meaning the lens placed within the frames needs to have a secondary focal length that corresponds to the distance between the back surface of the lens and the far point.

We can calculate this by subtracting the back vertex distance from the far point, for example (+100.00 cm) − (−1.5cm) = +101.50 cm. We can then use this distance as our focal length (f) which will allow us to calculate the power (F) of the lens we would need to use. This can be achieved using the power calculation as shown below:

$$F = n / f$$
$$F = 1.00 / +1.015 \text{ (converted to metres)}$$
$$F = +0.99D$$

This suggests that my partner would benefit from a +0.99D lens if it were to sit 1.5 cm in front of his eye, and it also confirms that the further away from his eye it is, the weaker the lens will need to be, because increasing the focal length will decrease the power.

Cylindrical Error

So far, we have discussed spherical errors, defined as errors in which the eye possesses the same refractive error along all meridians. However, it is possible, and common, to have a type of refractive error that has a different power along a particular meridian, called a **cylindrical error** (measured in dioptres; **DC** or **D**). Clinically, people with this type of error are described as having **astigmatism**. Fig. 5.10 shows a simplified demonstration of this.

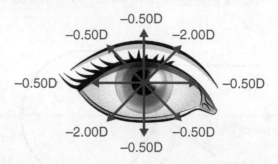

−0.50D

−0.50D   −2.00D

−0.50D   −0.50D

−2.00D   −0.50D

−0.50D

• **Fig. 5.10** A diagram to show that cylindrical error would involve a difference in power along one axis of the eye.

To correct for astigmatism, it's necessary to utilise a type of cylindrical lens. The simplest cylindrical lens is a **planocylindrical lens**, shown in Fig. 5.11. This type of lens only possesses power along one axis, called the **power meridian**. The perpendicular axis (**axis meridian** or **cylinder axis**) will not possess any power (0.00D). With a planocylindrical lens, the optical axis would exist perpendicular to both the front and back surface of the lens. If appropriately powered and angled along the astigmatic axis of the eye, it can correct the incoming light and help it remain in focus at the retina.

It is possible, however, to have a lens that corrects for both spherical and cylindrical refractive error, called a **spherocylindrical lens** (Fig. 5.12). In this type of lens, the power meridian still carries the power of the cylindrical element of the lens, but this time the axis meridian will carry the power of the spherical element.

One way clinicians can diagrammatically depict the power of a spherocylindrical lens is by using a **power cross**. This is where a very simplified lens is drawn as two perpendicular lines (Fig. 5.13A). If both the vertical and horizontal lines have the same power then it is depicting a spherical lens, whereas if one line is plano (pl) or a different power, then it is a cylindrical lens. To determine the combined power of a spherocylindrical lens, you can add together the two lenses, as shown in Fig. 5.13B. Please note that the example in Fig. 5.13B shows **minus-cylinder form** (where the cylindrical power is depicted as negative), but some people

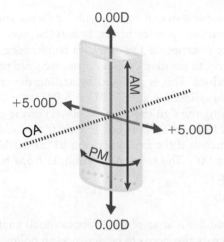

• **Fig. 5.11** A diagram showing a planocylindrical lens. Here, you can see that the power of the lens exists along the power meridian (PM; the curved surface), whilst there is zero power along the axis meridian (AM; the plane surface). The optical axis (OA) is shown perpendicular to both front and back surfaces of the lens.

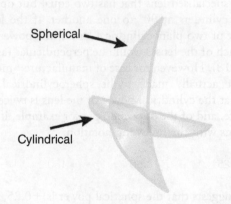

• **Fig. 5.12** A diagram showing a cross section of an example spherocylindrical lens, comprising planocylindrical (cylindrical) and positive meniscus (spherical) components.

use **positive-cylinder form** (where the cylindrical power is positive).

Now, as we've mentioned, the cylindrical power will likely sit along a particular axis of the eye, and so when writing the prescription of a patient with astigmatism, clinicians need to report the spherical power, the cylindrical power and then the **axis** of the cylinder. Importantly, the axis of the cylinder will correspond to the orientation where the cylinder lens has no power (the axis meridian), which is perpendicular to the power meridian – and this is something that often causes errors because it feels counterintuitive to describe the cylinder by its nonpowered axis! I find it helps to think of it as a rotating cylinder – for example, if asked to describe the image in Fig. 5.14, although we know the power exists along the power meridian (PM), we'd probably describe the lens as being oriented vertically, which corresponds to the nonpowered meridian (AM).

However, when describing the orientation of the axis meridian in a cylindrical lens, we need to understand the standard notation for orientation. As a general rule, we measure the angle by using the 3 o'clock position (right, middle) as 0°, and then measure the angle in an anticlockwise direction from that point (Fig. 5.15). This is the same no matter which eye is being refracted. Now, we also only need to consider angles between 0° and 180°, as anything between 181° and 360° has a corresponding angle between 0° and 180°. Importantly, the horizontal line is considered 180°, not 0°.

This means in our example in Fig. 5.14B, the lens would be described as having an axis of 90°.

To describe the power of a lens in a way that's easy for people to understand, the typical lens notation is written as:

Spherical power   *Cylindrical power*   x-axis

Make sure to include the sign of the powers (+ / −). In Fig. 5.16 we have an example spherocylindrical lens comprising +5.00DS spherical power and −7.50DC cylindrical power at an angle of 90°, leading to a lens notation of:

+5.00   −7.50   x 90

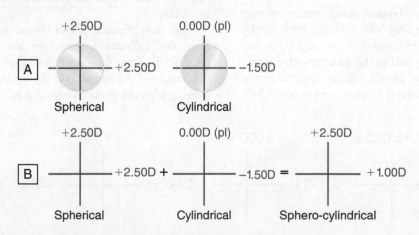

• **Fig. 5.13** A diagram showing power crosses for spherical and cylindrical lenses (A). The combined powers along each axis can produce a power cross for a spherocylindrical lens (B). A zero-power, plano (pl) orientation is depicted as pl.

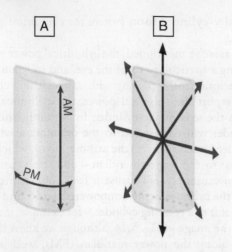

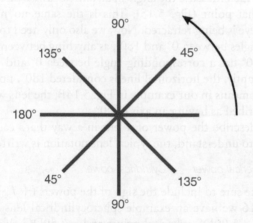

• **Fig. 5.14** Planocylindrical lens with axis meridian (AM) and power meridian (PM) labelled (A), showing that it is sensible to describe its orientation along the AM line (highlighted black arrow) even though it is not the one with the power (B).

• **Fig. 5.15** Diagram showing how to label the orientation of the cylindrical lens. The black arrow indicates the direction of increasing angles.

You can also see in Fig. 5.16 that using minus-cylinder form, we can work out the final lens notation even just by using the combined power cross (on the right), as the spherical power will correspond to the most positive power (+5.00) and the cylindrical power will correspond to the difference between the two final powers (which is −7.50).

As some people work in minus-cylinder forms and some work in positive-cylinder forms, it may be necessary to convert one notation to the other. To convert the minus-cylinder form to positive-cylinder form, we need to **transpose** the values. This is achieved by adding the spherical power to the cylinder (e.g. −7.50D + 5.00D = −2.50D), then changing the sign (but not the power) of the cylinder (+7.50D). If the axis is between 1° and 90°, we add 90° to the axis, whereas if the axis is between 91° and 180°, then we subtract 90°. The transposed example from before is shown here.

$$-2.50 \qquad +7.50 \qquad \times 180$$

If the cylinder is at an oblique (noncardinal) angle, then the power cross also needs to be drawn at an oblique angle, as shown in Fig. 5.17.

Cross-Cylinder Technique

To help quantify the power and direction of astigmatism, clinicians can use a technique called the **cross-cylinder technique**, also called **Jackson cross-cylinder (JCC)**. This utilises a specialised lens that has two equal but oppositely powered cylinders at 90° to one another. If the lens was made out of two planocylindrical lenses, the power meridians of each of the lenses would be perpendicular (as shown in Fig. 5.18). However, for ease of manufacture,[1] most JCC lenses are actually made to be spherocylindrical, which means that the cylindrical power of the lens is twice that of the sphere, and of the opposite sign, for example, if we had a JCC lens with the following notation:

$$+0.25 \qquad -0.50 \qquad \times 180$$

This suggests that the spherical power is +0.25, and the cylindrical power is −0.50 at 90° (remember the axis tells us the axis meridian, not the power meridian). This means that along the 180° axis there is only the spherical power (+0.25), so to get down to the equal opposite sign at 90°, the lens needs to take −0.50 off +0.25 to achieve −0.25 in that meridian.

The neat feature about these lenses is that, apart from two cylindrical axes, they also possess a 'flip' axis (Fig. 5.19). This 'flip' axis shows that if the clinician turns the handle of the lens so that the lens rotates 180°, then the cylindrical axes would swap places. This allows a direct

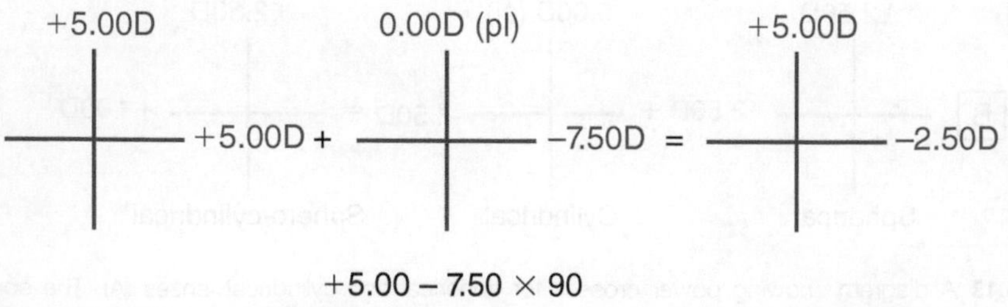

+5.00D   0.00D (pl)   +5.00D

+5.00D +   −7.50D =   −2.50D

+5.00 − 7.50 × 90

• **Fig. 5.16** An example spherocylindrical lens power cross with its corresponding lens notation.

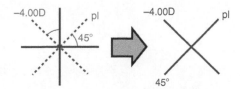

• **Fig. 5.17** An example power cross shown with cylindrical axis along an oblique angle.

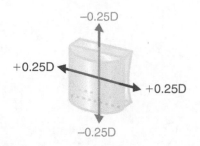

• **Fig. 5.18** A simplified version of a Jackson cross-cylinder (JCC) lens, if made of two planocylindrical lenses. In order to get equal, opposite powers perpendicular to one another, the curved (power) axes need to be perpendicular to one another.

comparison to be made between the positive and negative cylinders, which can inform the final prescription. Similarly, if the clinician changes the orientation of the handle, this will equivalently alter the axes of the JCC, which allows fine-tuning of the axis and power. In clinical practice, clinicians

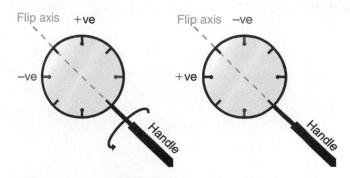

• **Fig. 5.19** Diagram showing a Jackson cross-cylinder (JCC) lens with positive (+ve) and negative (−ve) axes perpendicular to one another. The 'flip' axis is a hypothetical axis that exists in line with the handle. This allows the lens to swap power axes when spun round (rotated 180°, as indicated by the arrow).

will most often use JCC towards the end of an examination to confirm and refine their refraction.

Focimetry

In clinical practice, it's useful to be able to determine a patient's prescription before you begin an eye test, but if it's a new patient then there won't be any records, and the patient is very unlikely to know their refractive error. In these instances, if the patient is wearing a pair of glasses, clinicians can use a **focimeter** to determine the spherical and cylindrical power of the lens before the eye test begins. We will discuss focimetry in more detail in chapter 11.

Test Your Knowledge

Try the questions below to see if you need to review any sections again. All answers are available in the back of the book.

TYK.5.1 What is the presumed power of the reduced eye?
TYK.5.2 What is the difference between spherical and cylindrical refractive error?
TYK.5.3 If the far point of a patient's eye is −25.00cm, what is their refractive error?

TYK.5.4 Which meridian in a cylindrical lens is written as the 'axis'?
TYK.5.5 If you work out that following refraction an image will have a vergence of +4.00D, are the rays converging or diverging?

Reference

1. Rabbetts RB. *Bennett and Rabbetts' Clinical Visual Optics*. 4th ed. Oxford, UK: Butterworth-Heinemann, Elsevier; 2007.

6

Reflection

CHAPTER OUTLINE

OBJECTIVES

After working through this chapter, you should be able to:

Define the laws of reflection

Calculate the angle of reflection

Understand image formation at a plane mirror

Understand how the equations for spherical mirrors differ from those of refractive surfaces and lenses

Determine linear magnification of an image formed by reflection

Introduction

By this point we've covered the basics of refraction, but this is only half the story. Indeed, light can also be reflected by surfaces, and this is an important principle of optical systems. This chapter will focus on **reflection** at plane (flat) and curved surfaces.

What Is Reflection?

When we say something is 'reflected', we mean that it is returned in the plane it originally came from. The principle itself can be likened to bouncing a ball at a wall (providing we pretend gravity isn't a factor) – the ball cannot travel through the wall, so instead it will bounce back as a specified angle depending on the angle it approached the wall (Fig. 6.1). This is the same as the principle of reflection in optics. In some instances, light encounters a material that will reflect the rays back, which, at its core, is the key principle of how we see objects in the real world, as all of our vision depends on light reflecting off objects to reach our eyes (see chapter 1).

Laws of Reflection

In simple terms, there are two laws of reflection to remember, and they apply to both plane and curved surfaces:

First law of reflection: *The incident light ray and the reflected light ray lie in one plane.*

This means that the reflected ray exists along the same line (and on the same side of the reflecting surface) as the incident (approaching) ray.

Second law of reflection: *The angle of incidence (i) is equal to the angle of reflection (i').*

Angles of incidence and reflection are always measured relative to the 'normal' of the surface, with the normal being the hypothetical line that exists perpendicular to the surface at the point where light meets the surface. In Fig. 6.2 you can see that, relative to the normal, the angle of incidence (i) is identical to the angle of reflection (i'). This second law of reflection also leads on to the **reversibility principle,** which means light would reflect back along the same path; in Fig. 6.2 this would mean if the reflected ray became the incident ray, the incident ray would become the reflected ray.

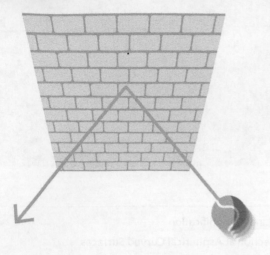

• **Fig. 6.1** Diagram showing tennis ball behaving like a reflected light ray when bounced at a wall.

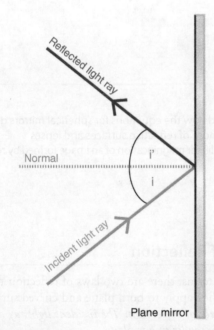

• **Fig. 6.2** Diagram showing an incident light ray reflecting off a plane (flat) mirror. You can see that i = i′ (relative to the normal).

Image Formation – Plane Surfaces

The easiest way to understand a plane mirror (flat reflective surface) is to find a mirror in your house that does not possess magnification or produce distortion. Usually a standard hallway/bathroom/full-length mirror will be a plane mirror, unless it's designed to be curved. If you stand directly in front of a mirror like this, you will see an image of yourself which is the same size as you are in the real, physical world. Importantly, the image of yourself will appear to be standing directly in front of you – this is because the light leaving your body to meet the mirror is travelling along the normal

of the mirror, so it travels back along exactly the same line. It is also interesting to note that the image of you in the mirror will be positioned as far *within* the mirror as you are standing in front of it, so if you're 30 cm in front of the mirror, your alternate dimension mirror self will also be 30 cm *within* the mirror. Another way of saying this might be that the object distance (l) is equal to the image distance (l′) with a plane mirror (Fig. 6.3).

If we now consider a slightly more complex example, let's say we have an object in front of our mirror, like shown in Fig. 6.3. Now you can see that the incident light rays travelling along the normal (labelled 1) produce reflected rays that travel back along the same path. However if we stood in a different position without moving the object, then the image of the object would stay in the same place, but the incident and reflected rays from the object that we utilise to 'see' it will now be travelling along different paths. In Fig. 6.3 this is shown as the labelled rays 1 and 2.

Crucially, what we can also notice about the image of ourselves (or an object) in a plane mirror is that it will be **laterally inversed** (flipped from left to right), so if we raise our right hand, our mirror self appears to raise their left hand. Similarly the image will be **reversed** (flipped front to back), so we see ourself facing the front side of ourselves, indicating our image is facing the opposite way to us. Fig. 6.4 shows an example of this.

To summarise:
1. The image is as far within the mirror as the object is in front.
2. The imaginary line joining the object and the image is perpendicular to the mirror surface (irrespective of the position it is viewed from).
3. The image is the same size as the object.
4. The image is virtual, reversed and laterally inverted.

In summary, if we know the angle of incidence (i) of a ray of light approaching a fixed, plane mirror, then we can also

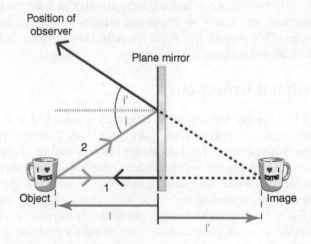

• **Fig. 6.3** Diagram showing that the image of an object remains stationary even if the observer is standing away from the object. The image also shows that the object distance (l) is equal to the image distance (l′).

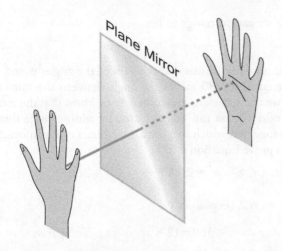

• **Fig. 6.4** Diagram showing that the image of an object in a plane mirror is laterally inversed (left to right) and reversed (front to back).

easily determine the angle of reflection (i′). So what if we complicate things a little by introducing a second plane mirror into the mix?

Multiple Plane Mirrors

Up to this point, we have discussed the angle of reflection (i′) but not the **angle of deviation (d)** – defined as the angle between the original path of the ray and the actual reflected ray. Most of the time this angle isn't necessary with reflection at plane surfaces, but when we have two mirrors it becomes incredibly relevant, so let's start by doing some revision of angles with a single plane mirror. In Fig. 6.5A, you can see that a ray of light is incident upon a plane mirror and is reflected at an angle identical to the angle of incidence (relative to the normal, shown as the orange dashed line). However, in this image, I've also drawn a hypothetical continuation of the incident ray (blue dashed line), into the mirror, to show what the ray

would have done had the mirror not been obstructing its path. The angle of deviation (d), then, will be measured as the angle from the continuation line and the reflected ray. First though, let's determine what we know about the angles – as you can see in Fig. 6.5B, the total angle of deviation (d, shown in green) can be split into two smaller angles which are separated by the mirror. These angles will be equal to one another, and we know that because we can determine that the angle between the incident (blue solid) ray and the mirror will be equal to the angle between the reflected (purple solid) ray and the mirror. Then, we can use the law of opposite angles to determine that the angle between the continuation (blue dashed) ray and the mirror will be the same as the angle between the incident (blue solid) ray and the mirror (for revision on opposite angles, see chapter 2, Box 2.4).

Great, but what has this got to do with two plane mirrors, you ask? Well, in optics, if we have two plane mirrors inclined at an angle towards one another, we can use these principles to determine the total angle of deviation (d), even though it has reflected off two mirrors (Fig. 6.6). In this scenario, two plane mirrors are inclined towards one another at an angle (a) – importantly, this angle must be smaller than 180° because otherwise the light wouldn't be able to reflect off both mirrors. If a ray of light is incident at one of the mirrors and reflects in such a way as to reflect off the second mirror, then the light will reflect back away from the mirrors, at an angle of deviation (d – relative to the original, incident ray). Importantly, both reflected rays (from mirror 1 and mirror 2) obey the laws of reflection (angle of incidence is equal to angle of reflection), and so we also know (thanks to Fig. 6.5B) that the individual angles of deviation can be split into two identical angles. At the first mirror these angles are referred to as α (alpha), and at the second mirror, these angles are referred to as γ (gamma). If you're good at visualising, you might also be able to see that the two α angles and the two γ angles would add together to produce the total angle of deviation. This

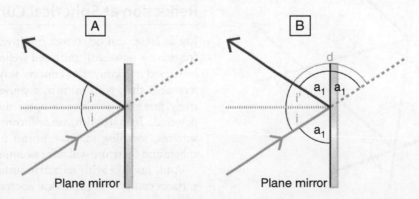

• **Fig. 6.5** Diagram showing how light might have travelled (A) if the mirror had not been in the way (blue dashed line), relative to how it is reflected with the mirror in the way (purple solid line). The diagram also explains how angle of deviation (d) can be determined whether you know the angle between the mirror and the angle of incidence, as this will be equal to the angle between the mirror and the angle of reflection, as well as the angle between the mirror and the original, undeviated (blue dashed) path of light (B).

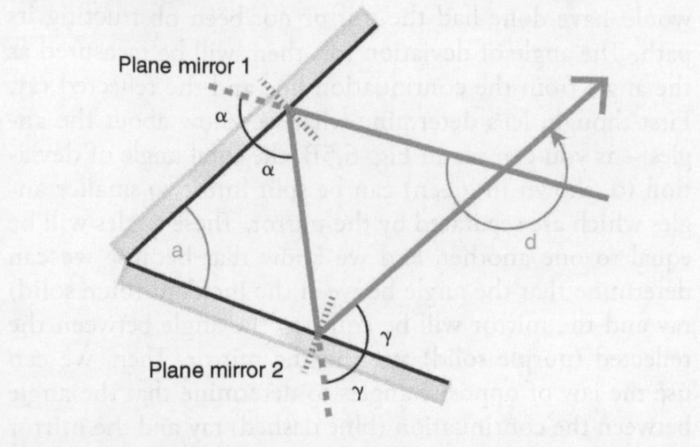

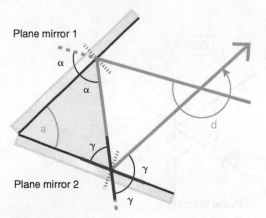

• **Fig. 6.6** If two plane mirrors are inclined towards one another at an angle (a) and light is incident upon one of the mirrors in a way that causes it to reflect off both mirrors (blue solid line), then the total angle of deviation (d) will be equivalent to the deviation at each mirror (2α and 2γ).

means that we can calculate the angle of deviation using Equation 6.1.

Equation 6.1 $d = 2a + 2\gamma \; or \; d = 2(a + \gamma)$

Equation 6.1 (explained)

$$deviation = 2(angle \; 1 + angle \; 2)$$

However, we probably don't actually know the values of α and γ, which could hinder our ability to utilise this equation somewhat. Instead, let's make use of the natural triangle formed by the angle between the mirrors (a) and the first reflected ray of light (shown in yellow in Fig. 6.7). In this triangle, we know that all internal angles need to add up to 180°, and we can also apply our knowledge of opposite angles (shown in Fig. 6.5) to determine that the previously unknown angle within the triangle must be equal to γ – but what does this tell us? Well, it tells us that:

$$a + \alpha + \gamma = 180°$$

• **Fig. 6.7** This is the same diagram as that in Fig. 6.6, but this time a yellow colour is highlighting the triangle that exists between the two mirrors and the first reflected ray of light. Using knowledge of opposite angles, we can determine that the three internal angles of the triangle are a, α and γ.

Which we can rearrange to be:

$$a + \gamma = 180° - a$$

This now informs us that the sum of the angles α and γ will be equal to 180 minus the angle between the mirrors (a). If we think back to Equation 6.1, we know that the total angle of deviation can be calculated by adding twice these values together, which means that we can use this information to prove Equation 6.2.

Equation 6.2 $d = 2(180 - a) \; or \; d = 360 - 2a$

Equation 6.2 (explained)

$$deviation = 360 - (2 \times angle \; between \; mirrors)$$

DEMO QUESTION 6.1

Two plane mirrors are inclined at an angle of 50° towards one another. What is the angle of deviation?
    Step 1: Determine what we need to calculate deviation, d
    Step 2: Define variables
a = 50
    Step 3: Determine necessary equation
d = 360 – 2a *(Equation 6.2)*
    Step 4: Calculate
d = 360 – 2a
d = 360 – 2(50)
d = 360 – 100
d = 260°
    (don't forget the units)

Practice Questions:

6.1.1 Two plane mirrors are inclined at an angle of 35° towards one another. What is the angle of deviation?
6.1.2 Two plane mirrors are inclined at an angle of 41.5° towards one another. What is the angle of deviation?

OK now let's make it interesting – what happens if the reflective surface is curved instead of flat?

Reflection at Spherical Curved Surfaces

Just as lenses can be convex (positively powered) or concave (negatively powered), mirrored (reflective) surfaces can also be curved in a convex or concave way. However, the key difference is that, with mirrors, a convex surface will be negatively powered, whilst a concave surface will be positively powered. To start with, we will consider spherical reflective surfaces, meaning that the mirror forms a small part of a sphere and therefore will have a centre of curvature (Fig. 6.8).

And, just like with refractive surfaces, spherical reflective surfaces can produce spherical aberrations if a wide aperture of light approaches the surface. As with lenses, light will focus along the optical axis, instead of in a single location, and the light rays will follow what's called a 'caustic curve' (see Fig. 6.9 and chapter 2, section titled 'Limiting Spherical Aberration'). This means the quality of the image will be poor

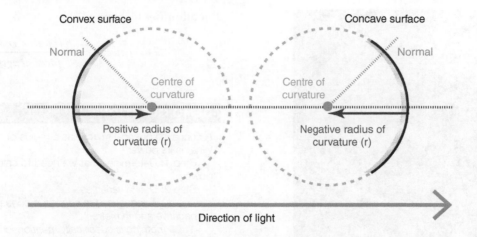

Direction of light

• **Fig. 6.8** Diagram showing relationship between convex and concave surfaces and their centre of curvature.

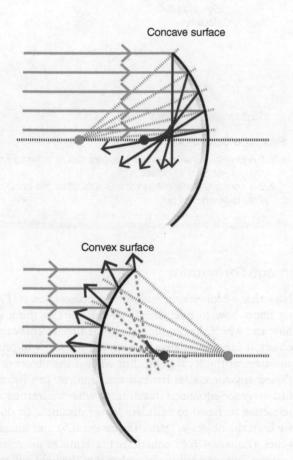

• **Fig. 6.9** Diagram showing a wide pencil of parallel rays will fail to focus at a single point instead producing a caustic curve and spherical aberration (blurring).

because it will be blurred along this section of the optical axis (we will discuss aberrations in more detail in chapter 16). As before, paraxial rays are hardly affected by these aberrations, and so we will assume paraxial rays in our equations.

For a real-world example of reflective spherical aberration, if you have a ring handy, you can place it on the table and shine a torch at it. You'll see the light produces a strange, curved pattern within the ring (Fig. 6.10) – this is spherical

aberration. If you take the image of the caustic curve produced by the concave mirror in Fig. 6.9 (top) and imagine the light incident on both sides of the optical axis, you can see that the aberration would form a pinched shape, curving towards the focal point, just like the reflection in the ring example in Fig. 6.10. Give it a go!

Focal Length and Focal Points

As discussed previously in chapters 2 and 3, the **power** (F) of a surface indicates the degree of vergence it will add to or remove from incoming light rays. For lenses, we can calculate the focal length (f) to give us the lens's primary (F) and secondary (F′) focal points, indicating where light will focus if originating from infinity. However, with spherical mirrors, there will only be one **focal point (F)** and one associated **focal length (f)**, which makes things slightly easier.

Importantly for spherical mirrors, the focal length is equal to half the radius of curvature (r) (see Equation 6.3). Incidentally, this means that the radius of curvature is also equal to twice the focal length, so if you know one, you can easily calculate the other.

Equation 6.3 $f = \dfrac{r}{2}$

Equation 6.3 (explained)

$$focal\ length = \frac{radius\ of\ curvature}{2}$$

Remember, all distances relating to power need to be measured in metres, and they will have a positive or negative sign, depending on their location relative to the surface (because we always measure *from* the surface). In the example in Fig. 6.11, the radius of curvature is left of the reflective surface because it is concave (see Fig. 6.11 for an explanation of this). As our optics convention dictates that we always measure from the surface to the point of interest (in this case centre of

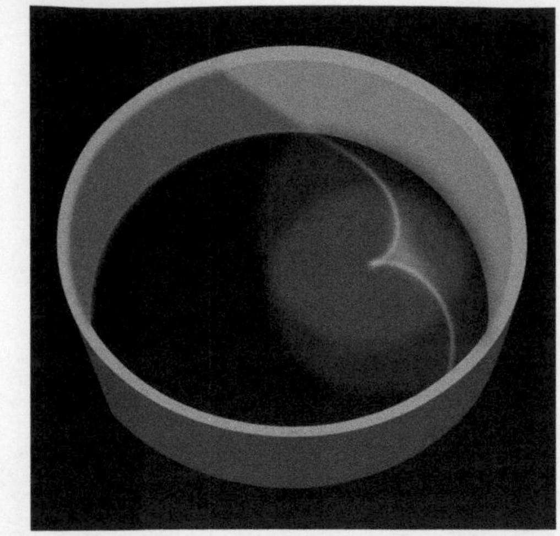

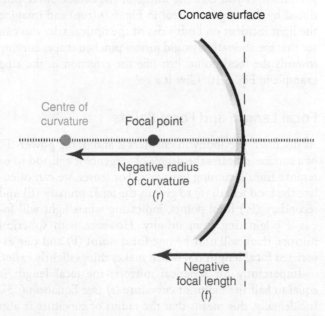

• **Fig. 6.10** Illustration of spherical aberration demo you can do at home.

Concave surface

Centre of curvature

Focal point

Negative radius of curvature (r)

Negative focal length (f)

• **Fig. 6.11** Diagram showing relationship between radius of curvature and focal length for a concave spherical mirror.

curvature and the focal point), we measure from right to left, which is the opposite direction to that of light (which we always assume goes left to right), so in this example, both the radius of curvature (r) and the focal length (f) are negative. If the surface was convex, both distances would be positive.

Just as we have previously seen for refractive surfaces, the focal point of a system is the point at which light from infinity will focus, so once we have determined the focal length, we can use equation 6.4 to calculate power (F). Notice that it's a similar equation to the one we use to calculate power of a refracting surface, but it has a negative sign in order to account for the fact that with reflective surfaces the rays exist within one plane (first law of reflection) instead of passing through the surface.

Equation 6.4 $F = -\dfrac{n}{f}$

Equation 6.4 (explained)

$$power = -\frac{refractive\ index}{focal\ length}$$

DEMO QUESTION 6.2

A concave spherical mirror has a radius of curvature of 50 cm. What is its power?
   Step 1: Determine what we need to calculate power, F
   Step 2: Define variables
r = −0.50 m *(because the surface is concave the radius is negative and in metres)*
n = 1.00 *(nothing is specifically mentioned so we assume the primary medium is air)*
   Step 3: Determine necessary equation
f = r / 2 *(Equation 6.3)*
F = − (n / f) *(Equation 6.4)*
   Step 4: Calculate
f = r / 2
f = −0.50 / 2
f = −0.25 m
F = − (n / f)
F = − (1.00 / − 0.25)
F = +4.00D
   (don't forget the ± sign)

Practice Questions:

6.2.1 A convex spherical mirror has a radius of curvature of 100 cm. What is its power?
6.2.2 A concave spherical mirror has a focal length of 50 cm. What is its power?

Image Formation

Now that we know spherical mirrors possess power (F), and we know how to calculate it, we can start to think about how and where they form images. We already know that an object at infinity (relative to a curved mirror) will produce an image at the focal point, but what if the object is positioned anywhere else? For this situation, we can use modified vergence equations (taken from what we learned about refractive surfaces) to calculate image distance. To do this, we keep the object vergence (Equation 6.5) and image vergence (Equation 6.6) equations the same as for refractive surfaces, but we need to remember that the light will reverse direction when reflected, and so we need to adjust our final image distance equation (Equation 6.7) in order to ensure we calculate the correct direction of light.

Equation 6.5 $L = \dfrac{n}{l}$

Equation 6.5 (explained)

$$object\ vergence = \frac{refractive\ index\ of\ medium}{object\ distance\ from\ surface}$$

Equation 6.6 $L' = L + F$

Equation 6.6 (explained)

$$image\ vergence = object\ vergence + power$$

Equation 6.7 $L' = -\dfrac{n'}{l'}$ $l' = -\dfrac{n'}{L'}$

Equation 6.7 (explained)

$$image\ distance = -\dfrac{secondary\ refr.index}{image\ vergence}$$

DEMO QUESTION 6.3

An object is placed 15 cm in front of a concave spherical mirror with a radius of curvature of 10 cm. Where does the image form?

Step 1: Determine what we need to calculate
image distance, l'

Step 2: Define variables

l = −0.15 m *(the object is 15 cm 'in front of', meaning it's to the left of the surface which gives it a negative distance – and we need to convert to metres)*

r = −0.10 m *(because the surface is concave the radius is negative and in metres)*

n = 1.00 *(nothing is specifically mentioned so we assume the primary medium is air)*

Step 3: Determine necessary equation(s)

f = r / 2 *(Equation 6.3)*
F = − (n / f) *(Equation 6.4)*
L = n / l *(Equation 6.5)*
L' = L + F *(Equation 6.6)*
L' = − (n' / l') *(Equation 6.7)*

Step 4: Calculate

f = r / 2
f = −0.10 / 2
f = −0.05 m
F = − (n / f)
F = − (1.00 / −0.05)
F = +20.00D
L = n / l
L = 1.00 / −0.15
L = −6.67 *(remember to keep the number long in the calculator)*
L' = L + F
L' = −6.67 + 20
L' = +13.33
L' = − (n' / l')
l' = − (n' / L') *(rearrange to get l')*
l' = − (1.00 / 13.33)
l' = −0.075 m

The image forms 7.50 cm left of the surface.
(don't forget the ± sign and the units!)
We know the image forms to the left of the surface because the distance is negative.

Practice Questions:

6.3.1 An object is placed 10 cm in front of a convex spherical mirror with a radius of curvature of 20 cm. Where does the image form?

6.3.2 An object is placed 30 cm in front of a concave spherical mirror with a power of +5.00D. Where does the image form?

Another (slightly quicker but more challenging) way to calculate image distance is to use Equation 6.8, which utilises the known relationship between the object and image distance, relative to the focal length and power of the surface. Remember, if an equation has multiple equals signs (=) in it, then you can choose the two elements you want to use. So, for example, if I am given the focal length (f) and the object distance (l), then I can ignore the part of the equation that uses the radius of curvature (r).

Equation 6.8 $\dfrac{1}{l'} + \dfrac{1}{l} = \dfrac{2}{r} = \dfrac{1}{f}$

Equation 6.8 (explained)

$$\dfrac{1}{image\ dist.} + \dfrac{1}{object\ dist.} = \dfrac{2}{radius} = \dfrac{1}{focal\ length}$$

DEMO QUESTION 6.4

We'll use the same question as in demo 6.2, to show that it's an equivalent process. An object is placed 15 cm in front of a concave spherical mirror with a radius of curvature of 10 cm. Where does the image form?

Step 1: Determine what we need to calculate
image distance, l'

Step 2: Define variables

l = −0.15 m *(the object is 15 cm 'in front of', meaning it's to the left of the surface which gives it a negative distance – and we need to convert to metres)*

r = −0.10 m *(because the surface is concave the radius is negative and in metres)*

n = 1.00 *(nothing is specifically mentioned so we assume the primary medium is air)*

Step 3: Determine necessary equation(s)

(1 / l') + (1 / l) = (2 / r) *(Equation 6.8)*

Step 4: Calculate

(1 / l') + (1 / l) = (2 / r)
(1 / l') + (1 / −0.15) = (2 / −0.10) *(Substitute in our values)*
(1 / l') = (2 / −0.10) − (1 / −0.15) *(Rearrange)*
(1 / l') = −13.33 *(Solve the right side)*
l' = 1 / −13.33
l' = −0.075 m

The image forms 7.50 cm left of the surface.
(don't forget the ± sign and the units!)

Practice Questions:

6.4.1 An object is placed 20 cm in front of a convex spherical mirror with a radius of curvature of 30 cm. Where does the image form?

6.4.2 An object is placed 25 cm in front of a concave spherical mirror with a power of +5.00D. Where does the image form?

Linear Magnification

As you'll recall from our chapter about thin lenses (see chapter 3), 'linear magnification' refers to the size of an image relative to the *original* object. We can use Equation 6.9 to calculate magnification of an image produced by a spherical mirror, providing we know the object (l) and image distances (l'). However, please be very careful when using this equation as, again, you'll notice that it is different from the one we use for refractive surfaces as it includes a minus sign. Also I would always recommend using the object (l) and image (l′) distances to calculate magnification, rather than the vergence values. This is because it's easy to get confused about the image vergence as everything is flipped relative to a lens. For example, a converging image (positive vergence) will have a negative distance.

Equation 6.9 $m = \dfrac{h'}{h} = -\dfrac{l'}{l} = \dfrac{L}{L'}$

Equation 6.9 (explained)

$$mag. = \frac{image\ height}{object\ height} = -\frac{image\ dist.}{object\ dist.} = \frac{object\ verg.}{image\ verg.}$$

However, one thing that remains the same is how useful the magnification value is – it can tell us whether an image is virtual or real, and magnified or minified. See chapter 3, Fig. 3.5, for revision on this if necessary.

DEMO QUESTION 6.5

An object is placed 45 cm in front of a concave spherical mirror with a radius of curvature of 20 cm. What is the magnification of the image?

  Step 1: Determine what we need to calculate magnification, m
  Step 2: Define variables
l = −0.25 m *(the object is 25 cm 'in front of' meaning it's to the left of the surface, which gives it a negative distance – and we need to convert to metres)*
r = −0.20 m *(because the surface is concave the radius is negative and in metres)*
n = 1.00 *(nothing is specifically mentioned so we assume the primary medium is air)*
  Step 3: Determine necessary equation
You can choose which equation to use to determine image distance here – I'll use 6.8
(1 / l′) + (1 / l) = (2 / r) *(Equation 6.8)*
m = (h′ / h) = − (l′ / l) = (L / L′) *(Equation 6.9)*
  Step 4: Calculate
(1 / l′) + (1 / l) = (2 / r)
(1 / l′) + (1 / −0.25) = (2 / −0.20) *(Substitute in our values)*
(1 / l′) = (2 / −0.20) − (1 / −0.25) *(Rearrange)*
(1 / l′) = −6.00 *(Solve the right side)*
l′ = 1 / −6.00
l′ = −0.1667 m *(remember to keep the number long in the calculator)*
m = (h′ / h) = −(l′ / l) = (L / L′)
m = −(l′ / l) *(choose which part we can use)*

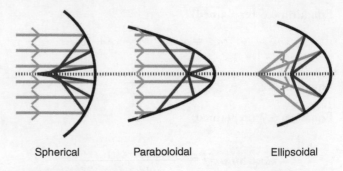

Spherical   Paraboloidal   Ellipsoidal

• **Fig. 6.12** Illustration showing how light focuses with three types of mirror: spherical, paraboloidal (aspherical) and ellipsoidal (aspherical).

DEMO QUESTION 6.5—cont'd

m = −(−0.1667 / −0.25)
m = −0.67X (minified, inverted, real)
  (don't forget the ± sign, and the X represents the units for magnification)

Practice Questions:

6.5.1 An object is placed 20 cm in front of a concave spherical mirror with a radius of curvature of 60 cm. What is the magnification of the image?
6.5.2 An object is placed 30 cm in front of a concave spherical mirror of power +10.00D. What is the magnification of the image?

Reflection at Aspherical Curved Surfaces

In this brief, final section we will consider curved reflective surfaces that fail to fall along a sphere. These types of surfaces are called **aspherical mirrors**. These types of mirrors are capable of producing high-quality images because they do not suffer from spherical aberration, which means that they can produce clear images even with a wide pencil of light. For example, we can use paraboloidal mirrors to focus light from infinity, and we can use ellipsoidal mirrors to focus light from a distance closer than infinity, as shown in Fig. 6.12.

These mirrors can be utilised as wing mirrors on cars to dramatically increase the field of view available to the driver; however, in order to increase the field of view (how much space you can see behind you), these mirrors also minify the image, meaning that other cars, pedestrians and objects may seem farther away than they actually are.

Test Your Knowledge

Try the questions below to see if you need to review any sections again. All answers are available in the back of the book.

TYK.6.1 What are the two laws of reflection?
TYK.6.2 If an object is 50 cm in front of a plane mirror, where will the image form?

TYK.6.3 Describe the nature of an image formed in a plane mirror.
TYK.6.4 Explain why the formula for calculating the focal length (f) of a spherical mirror has a 'minus sign' in it.
TYK.6.4 If a spherical mirror has a radius of curvature of +20 cm, what is the focal length (f)?

7

Ray Tracing

OBJECTIVES

After working through this chapter, you should be able to:

Explain what a ray diagram is

Draw an accurate ray diagram for a convex lens

Draw an accurate diagram for a concave lens

Draw an accurate ray diagram for a convex mirror

Draw an accurate ray diagram for a concave mirror

Introduction

By this point in the textbook you might have become a bona fide maths wizard, but there's also a chance that you might be sick of looking at equations, so let's take a short break to learn how to understand image formation using line drawings.

Yes, you heard me correctly, *line drawings*.

In the optics business, we refer to this as **ray tracing** because we can use scale line drawings to trace the path of the rays from the object to the image, and my best advice is to read this chapter with a pad of paper, a pencil and a ruler so that you can learn to apply the principles as you go.

What Is a Ray Diagram?

A **ray diagram** is a carefully measured line drawing that traces the path light takes from an object to its image formed by an optical system. These diagrams can be produced successfully for both thin lenses and spherical mirrors, but in all cases, we are assuming that we are using **paraxial rays** (rays that lie close to the optical axis).

Ray Tracing – Single Thin Lens

Remember that with a thin lens, the effect of the refractive index of the material is considered so negligible that it is ignored completely. This means that with a thin lens in air, we can assume that the primary refractive index (n) and the secondary refractive index (n′) are identical (both = 1.00). If we think back to the equations from chapter 3, we know that the focal length of a thin lens is determined by the power (F) of the lens and the refractive index in which it resides. To that end, given that the refractive index is identical on either side of the lens, we can assume that the focal length would be the same distance away from the lens in either direction. Now, for our equations we always assume that light is travelling from left to right, meaning that for a positively powered lens that *converges* light, the **secondary focal length** (f′) will exist to the right of the lens to form the **secondary focal point** (F′). However, for ray tracing, we can start to consider what happens if the light were to change direction and travel from right to left. Theoretically, because we're assuming a thin lens, the light should behave identically in either direction, so if made to travel backwards through the system, it will produce a focus at the **primary focal point** (F). The distance between the lens and the primary focal point is called **the primary focal length** (f) and should be equivalent to the negative of the secondary focal length (Equation 7.1 and Fig. 7.1). For example, a +5.00 D lens will have a secondary focal length of +0.2 m (to the right of the lens) and a primary focal length of −0.2 m (to the left of the lens).

Equation 7.1
$$f = -f'$$

Equation 7.1 (explained)

primary focal length = −secondary focal length

For a negatively powered lens that *diverges* light, light originating from infinity will diverge after refracting through the lens, which means we have to draw the rays back to see where they appear to originate from. As Fig. 7.2A shows, this produces a negative **secondary focal length** (f') to the left of the lens to form the **secondary focal point** (F'), which is the exact opposite to that of a positive lens. If the light then travelled backwards through the system (Fig. 7.2B), it would diverge on the opposite side of the lens, meaning the rays would appear to originate from **primary focal point** (F) on the right of the lens. The distance between the lens and the primary focal point is called **the primary focal length** (f) and, again, should be equivalent to the negative of the secondary focal length. For example, a −5.00 D lens will have a secondary focal length

of −0.2 m (to the left of the lens) and a primary focal length of +0.2 m (to the right of the lens).

In these diagrams, you'll also probably notice that we've added points referred to as 2f and 2f'. These are important points for ray diagrams and correspond to twice the secondary focal length (2f') and twice the primary focal length (2f). However, as a word of warning, when we're learning this content it can be very easy to mix up 2f with f' as the description "twice the focal length" for 2f sounds like a similar idea to the "secondary focal length" (f') as they both relate to the number 2. My best advice here is to make sure you understand what they each relate to, which may involve going back over chapter 3 for some revision on secondary focal lengths if necessary.

Drawing Lenses

One of the key aspects of a ray diagram is that the person who views it should know whether it's a positively powered or negatively powered lens. This can be achieved through looking at the behaviour of the rays, but the easiest way to do this is to draw the lens in line with the set specification. The guidelines state that all lenses are drawn as straight, vertical lines, but positively powered lenses are drawn with outward facing arrows (as in Fig. 7.1) whilst negatively powered lenses are drawn with inward facing arrows (as in Fig. 7.2).

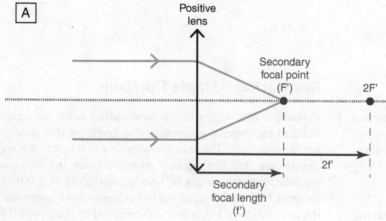

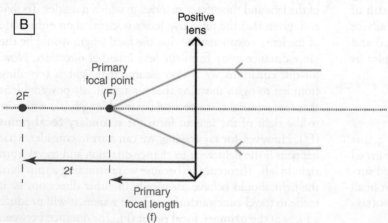

• **Fig. 7.1** Basic principles of ray tracing with a **positive** lens. When light originates from infinity and travels from left to right (A), it produces a focus at the secondary focal point (F') with a positive focal length. If the direction of light is reversed (B) then light will focus at the primary focal point (F) and will have a negative (but equivalent) focal length.

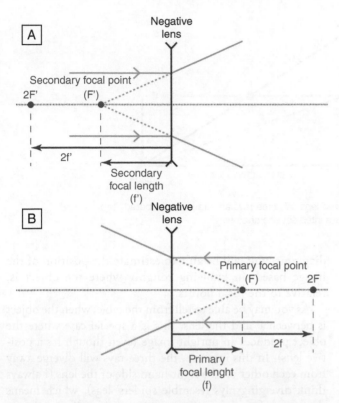

• **Fig. 7.2** Basic principles of ray tracing with a **negative** lens. When light originates from infinity and travels from left to right (A), it diverges as if originating from the secondary focal point (F′) with a negative focal length. If the direction of light is reversed (B) then light will diverge as if originating from the primary focal point (F) and will have a positive (but equivalent) focal length.

Drawing Objects and Images

In ray diagrams, we will learn to draw our objects as upward-pointing arrows, the base of which starts at the optical axis – the idea is that it helps to make the diagram easy to interpret, but I do agree that it's not very imaginative. Then, once we have our arrow-shaped object, we need to think about how we'll draw the light rays. Technically, an object is an extended source with light rays emanating from every part of it (Fig. 7.3A), but it is simpler (and quicker) to limit our drawings to the light emanating from the **tip of the object** (Fig. 7.3B). This helps us to use ray tracing to determine the location of the **tip of the image** after refraction or reflection,

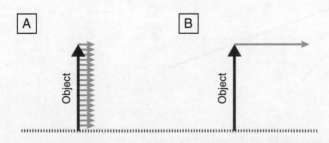

• **Fig. 7.3** Objects drawn as upward-pointing arrows. Although objects are 'extended' sources (A), we only use the tip of the object for our rays (B).

which allows us to assume the distance of the tip of the image relative to the optical axis (which gives us the image height).

When we come to draw our image, this will also be depicted as an arrow with the base starting at the optical axis, but the image will be upright or inverted, depending on the type of lens and where the object is positioned.

Rules for a Positively Powered Lens

Now we're ready to learn how to draw the rays in our ray diagrams. For positive- and negative-powered lenses there are three rays that we need to learn, but they're drawn slightly differently for each lens type, so I'll start with positively powered lenses in this section and then move onto negatively powered lenses in the next section.

The rays are outlined below and demonstrated in Fig. 7.4:

P-ray – drawn from the tip of the object, parallel to the optical axis; refracts through F′

C-ray – drawn from the tip of the object, undeviated through the optical centre (intersection of lens and optical axis)

F-ray – drawn from the tip of the object, through F; refracts parallel to the optical axis

In the example in Fig. 7.4 you can see that the rays all come to a neat little intersection on the right side of the lens, which is the point corresponding to the tip of the image! Importantly, light traveling along the normal (optical axis) through the optical centre will just travel in a straight line, so we know the base of the object and the base of the image both form along the optical axis. We can draw our image by connecting the intersection of the rays to the optical axis (with a very straight, vertical line). In this example, the diagram shows that with this lens and object distance, the image forms slightly to the right of 2F′, and it's inverted (upside-down) and slightly magnified.

Now, if drawn to scale (with the correct focal length and object distance, and even object height when specified), this diagram can tell you the *exact* image distance and *exact* image height for the height of the object. (You can try this for yourself at home with a ruler and a pencil.)

We can also do a quick mathematical confidence check to prove that our ray tracing makes sense. For this, we can just use sensible estimates; for example, if we assume the lens in Fig. 7.4 is +5.00D (a power that for this example has been chosen at random), then our secondary focal length (f′) would be +0.20 m and our primary focal length (f) would be −0.20 m (see chapter 3 for revision on this if needed). This means our 2F point on the left corresponds to −0.40 m (twice the primary focal length). The object itself looks to be slightly closer to the lens than 2F, so let's estimate its distance (l) as −0.375 m. Using our vergence equations from chapter 2, we can then determine that the object vergence (L) for our estimated object distance would be −2.67, which would make our image vergence (L′) +2.33. This means mathematically, the image (l′) *should* form +0.429 m right of the lens, which would

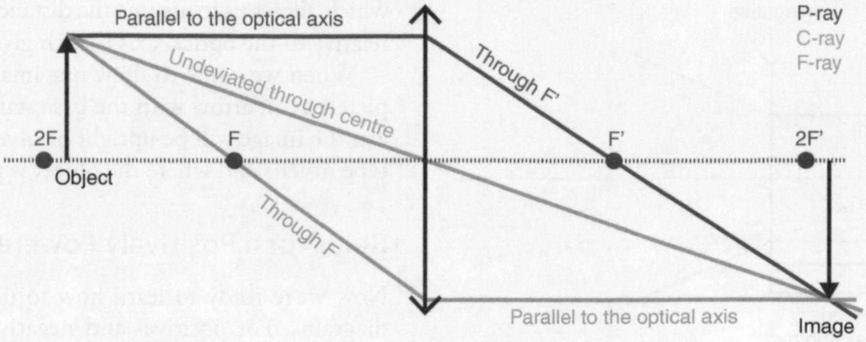

Parallel to the optical axis

Undeviated through centre

Through F'

P-ray
C-ray
F-ray

2F   F   F'   2F'
Object

Through F

Parallel to the optical axis

Image

• **Fig. 7.4** Example ray diagram for a positively powered lens. All three rays are drawn and labelled. The tip of the image is identified as the point where the rays intersect one another.

correspond to slightly right of 2F′... Which looks pretty spot-on in Fig. 7.4 to me!

For positive lenses, the position of the image relative to the object can be determined by learning the contents of Table 7.1, but the highlights are that:

• An object at infinity will form an image at F′
• An object at F will produce an image at infinity
• An object at 2F will produce an inverted image the same size at 2F′
• An object between F and the lens will produce an upright image left of the lens

Importantly, you can also see that as the object moves from infinity towards F, the image moves from F′ towards infinity, so when you become more experienced with ray

diagrams, you will be able to estimate the position of the image based on knowing roughly where the object is, relative to the focal points.

As you may be able to tell from the table, when the object is between F and the lens, this is a special case where the object produces an upright image (even though it's a positive lens). In this instance, the three rays will diverge away from each other on the right-hand side of the lens (I always think diverging rays resemble spiders' legs), which means they won't form a neat intersection to identify our image position. Instead, when the rays diverge like this, we need to draw the refracted rays backwards to see where they *appear* to originate from (as seen in Fig. 7.5), which is also a key principle of ray tracing for negative lenses.

TABLE 7.1	Table Showing Relationship Between Object Position and Associated Image Characteristics with Positive Lenses			
Object Distance (l)	**Image Location**	**Image Distance (l′)**	**Inverted/Upright**	**Image Size**
>2F	Right of lens	>F′ & <2F′	I	<O
2F	Right of lens	2F′	I	= O
>F & <2F	Right of lens	>2F′	I	>O
infinity	Right of lens	F′	I	
F	~	Infinity	~	
<F	Left of lens	>l	U	>O

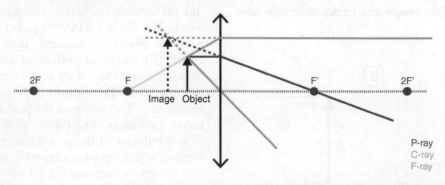

2F   F   F'   2F'
Image Object

P-ray
C-ray
F-ray

• **Fig. 7.5** Ray diagram showing how to draw the rays (and identify the location of the image) when an object is between F and the lens in front of a positively powered lens. You can see it forms a virtual, upright, magnified image.

Rules for a Negatively Powered Lens

The rays for negatively powered lenses are outlined below and demonstrated in Fig. 7.6:

P-ray – drawn from the tip of the object, parallel to the optical axis; refracts as if originated from F′ and drawn backwards on the left of the lens

C-ray – drawn from the tip of the object, undeviated through the optical centre (intersection of lens and optical axis)

F-ray – drawn from the tip of the object, aiming for F; when it meets the lens, refracts parallel to the optical axis and draws backwards on the left of the lens

Unlike with a positively powered lens, negatively powered lenses diverge the rays away from one another on the right of the lens, meaning they will never form an intersection (think spiders' legs again). Instead, we draw the refracted rays backwards and look for an intersection on the left to identify where the rays appear to originate from. This produces an upright image, as shown in Fig. 7.6.

For negative lenses, the position of the image relative to the object can be determined by learning the contents of Table 7.2, but the highlights are that:

• An object at infinity will produce an image at F′
• An object anywhere other than infinity will produce a minified, upright image on the left, between F′ and the lens (and closer to the lens than the object)

Ray Tracing – Equivalent Lenses

OK, but what do we do if there is more than one lens in a system? In chapter 3, we learned about multiple lens systems and **equivalent lenses**, and in this section we will learn how to draw a ray diagram for a lens system with two lenses. It may be useful to refer back to some of the equations in chapter 3 to help you understand some of the steps.

Importantly, for these equivalent lens ray diagrams to be drawn successfully, you need to know the positions of six **cardinal points**. These points include the two **focal points (F, F′)**, the two **principal planes (HP, H′P′)** and two points called the **nodal points (N, N′)**. The first step would be to draw the lenses separated by their distance (d) – this can be scaled down as long as all other distances are scaled down by the same amount. Then you need to draw in the focal points, which you can determine by calculating the back vertex focal length (f_v') (distance between second lens and secondary focal point) and the front vertex focal length (f_v) (distance between the first lens and the primary focal point). Remember to make a note of whether the distances are positive or negative, as this will tell you whether the focal point is to the right of a lens (if positive) or to the left of a lens (if negative). Next, we can determine the location of the principal planes by calculating the secondary equivalent focal length (f_e') (distance between secondary focal point and secondary principal plane) and the primary equivalent focal length (f_e) (distance between primary focal point and primary principal plane) – see Fig. 7.7.

Finally, then, we can calculate the location of our nodal points. Nodal points are present in all optical systems and exist in a location that means an incident (approaching) ray of light heading towards the first nodal point (N) would leave the system along exactly the same angle, but shifted to emerge from the second nodal point (N′). This means that the incident and emergent rays are parallel to one another. If you've ever played any of the portal-creating-based game series then this will make complete sense, but if not then

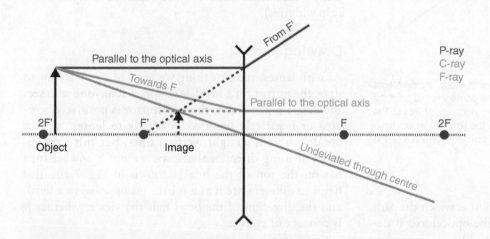

• **Fig. 7.6** Example ray diagram for a negatively powered lens. All three rays are drawn and labelled. The tip of the image is identified as the point where the rays appear to originate from.

TABLE 7.2	Table Showing Relationship Between Object Position and Associated Image Characteristics With Negative Lenses				
Object Distance (l)	Image Location		Image Distance (l′)	Inverted/Upright	Image Size
Infinity	Left of lens		F′	U	<O
~	Left of lens		<l	U	<O

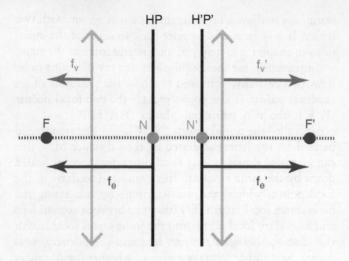

• **Fig. 7.7** Illustration to remind us of the difference between the back vertex focal length (f_v') and front vertex focal length (f_v) relative to the secondary equivalent focal length (f_e') and the primary equivalent focal length (f_e).

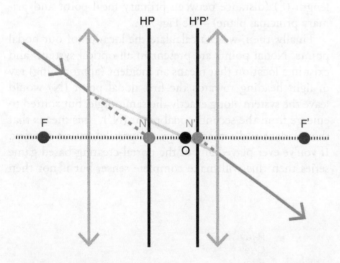

• **Fig. 7.8** Illustration showing how nodal points work. Incident light (shown in blue) enters the system aiming at the primary nodal point (N) and then leaves the system at the secondary nodal point (N′) at the same angle it entered N. The point at which the light ray would have crossed the optical axis is identified as the optical centre (O) of the system.

please see Fig. 7.8. Importantly, the point at which the path of light crosses (or appears to cross) the optical axis is defined as the optical centre of the system (O).

The good news for us is that when the object and image exist within a medium comprising the same refractive index as each other (for example, if the object and image are both in air) then the primary nodal point (N) will correspond to the point where the primary principal plane (HP) intersects the optical axis, and the secondary nodal point (N′) will correspond to the point where the secondary principal plane (H′P′) intersects the optical axis – so now we're all set!

Rules for Equivalent Lenses

The rays for equivalent lenses are outlined below and demonstrated in Fig. 7.9:

P-ray – drawn from the tip of the object, parallel to the optical axis, runs all the way to H′P′; refracts through F′

N-ray – drawn from the tip of the object, towards N, leaves system from N′ at parallel angle to incident ray

F-ray – drawn from the tip of the object, through F; when it meets HP, refracts parallel to the optical axis

An easy way to remember whether the rays need to travel to H′P′ or HP is to think about whether the ray is going to intersect F′ or F – remember that primes (′) always link together!

Ray Tracing – Spherical Mirrors

For the final section of this chapter, we need to consider ray diagrams for positively powered (concave) and negatively powered (convex) spherical mirrors. Importantly, in order to draw an accurately scaled ray diagram for a spherical mirror, we would need to know the focal length (f) and the radius of curvature (r); however, the good news is that if you know one then you can calculate the other using the equations we learned in chapter 6 (Equations 6.3 and 6.4). For example, if we have a concave mirror with a power of +5.00 D, we know the focal length is −0.20 m and so the radius of curvature will be −0.40 m.

When practising drawing the rays, you can draw the focal length and radius of curvature any length you like to fit on the page providing you make sure that the radius is twice the focal length (and remember to scale your answers correctly – see section titled "How to Scale Your Diagrams" for help with this).

Drawing Mirrors

As with lenses, the first thing we need to know is how to draw the mirror for a ray diagram so that anyone who sees the diagram knows whether the mirror is positively powered or negatively powered. Similarly to lenses, mirrors are drawn with straight, vertical lines, but this time instead of using directional arrows, we put a bowl-shaped hat on the top of the line as shown in Fig. 7.10. This helps to differentiate it as a mirror (as opposed to a lens), and the direction of the bowl tells the viewer whether it is concave or convex.

Rules for a Positively Powered (Concave) Spherical Mirror

For positive- and negative-powered mirrors there are four rays that we need to learn, but they're drawn slightly differently, so just like before I'll start with positively powered mirrors in this section and then move onto negatively powered mirrors in the next section.

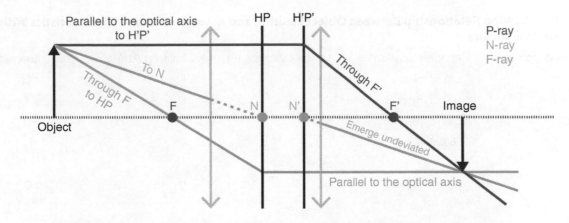

• **Fig. 7.9** Example ray diagram for an equivalent lens system compsising two positively powered lenses (greyed out). All three rays are drawn and labelled. The tip of the image is identified as the point where the rays intersect.

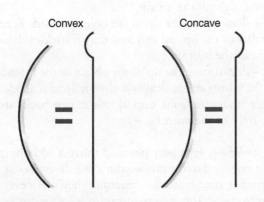

• **Fig. 7.10** Diagram showing the ray diagram convention for convex (left) and concave (right) spherical mirrors.

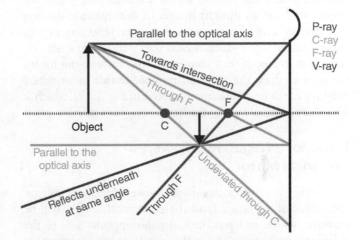

• **Fig. 7.11** Example ray diagram for a positively powered concave mirror. All four rays are drawn and labelled. The tip of the image is identified as the point where the rays intersect one another.

The rays are outlined below and demonstrated in Fig. 7.11:

P-ray – drawn from the tip of the object, parallel to the optical axis; reflects through F
C-ray – drawn from the tip of the object, undeviated through the centre of curvature; reflects back along the same line
F-ray – drawn from the tip of the object, through F; reflects parallel to the optical axis
V-ray – drawn from the tip of the object to the intersection of the mirror and optical axis; then reflects at an identical angle underneath the optical axis

In the example in Fig. 7.11, you can see that the rays all come to a neat little intersection on the left side of the mirror, which is the point corresponding to the tip of the image! Again, light traveling along the optical axis will reflect back along a straight line, so we know the base of the object and the base of the image both form along the optical axis. This means we can draw our image by connecting the intersection of the rays to the optical axis (with a very straight, vertical line). In this example, the diagram shows that with this mirror and object distance, the image forms between C and F, left of the mirror, and it's inverted (real) and minified. Please note, as a little word of warning here, that unless you

are a wizard with a protractor (or drawing the diagram digitally), I would never recommend drawing the V-ray. It will almost certainly lead your diagram astray, as even a very tiny error in the angle of the second line underneath the optical axis will lead to increasingly large errors as the line gets longer. Therefore if it was me, I'd only ever use the other three rays as they are much more reliable.

Just like with lenses, if drawn to scale (with the correct focal length and object distance), this diagram can tell you the *exact* image distance and *exact* image height for the height of the object. (You can try this for yourself at home with a ruler and a pencil.)

For positive spherical mirrors, the position of the image relative to the object can be determined by learning the contents of Table 7.3, but the highlights are that:
• An object at infinity will produce an image at F
• An object at F will produce an image at infinity
• An object at C will produce an inverted image the same size at C
• An object between F and the mirror will produce an upright image right of the mirror

TABLE 7.3	Table Showing Relationship Between Object Position and Associated Image Characteristics With Positive Spherical Mirrors				
Object Distance (l)	Image Location	Image Distance (l′)	Inverted/Upright	Image Size
>C	Left of mirror	>F & <C	I	<O
C	Left of mirror	C	I	= O
>F & <C	Left of mirror	>C	I	>O
Infinity	Left of mirror	F	I	
F	~	Infinity	~	
<F	Right of mirror	>l	U	>O

Again, just like with positive lenses, when the object is between F and the mirror, this is a special case where the object produces an upright image. In this instance, the rays will diverge away from each other after reflecting (again, think spiders' legs), which means they won't form a neat intersection to identify our image position. Instead, this means we need to draw the reflected rays backwards to see where they appear to originate from (as seen in Fig. 7.12), which is also a key principle of ray tracing for negative mirrors.

Rules for a Negatively Powered Spherical Mirror

Remember that for a negatively powered, convex mirror, the radius of curvature (and therefore focal length) will be positive, which will put them on the opposite side of the mirror to the object – this makes ray diagrams slightly more complicated. The rays for negatively powered spherical mirrors are outlined below and demonstrated in Fig. 7.13:

P-ray – drawn from the tip of the object, parallel to the optical axis; reflects as if originating from F and drawn backwards on the right of the mirror

C-ray – drawn from the tip of the object towards the centre of curvature; drawn as if to continue along the same line on the right of the mirror

F-ray – drawn from the tip of the object towards F; reflects parallel to the optical axis and drawn backwards on the right of the mirror

V-ray – drawn from the tip of the object to the intersection of the mirror and optical axis; then reflects at an identical angle underneath the optical axis drawn backwards on the right of the mirror

As we know, negatively powered mirrors add divergence to light rays, and so the rays we draw will diverge away from one another after reflection, meaning they will never form an intersection. This means to find our image we need to draw the reflected rays backwards and look for an intersection on the right to identify where the rays appear to originate from. This will always produce an upright image, as shown in Fig. 7.13. I will also offer the same advice here as I did previously for positively powered mirrors: do not use the V-ray unless absolutely necessary as it is notoriously unreliable.

For negative spherical mirrors, the position of the image relative to the object can be determined by learning the contents of Table 7.4, but the highlights are that:
- An object at infinity will produce an image at F
- An object anywhere other than infinity will produce a minified, upright image between F and the mirror on the right-hand side (and closer to the mirror than the object)

How to Scale Your Diagrams

Now that we've learned how to draw these ray diagrams, it's important to learn another key skill – how to scale them down to fit onto a piece of paper. Let's say that we want to produce a ray diagram to show how an image forms when an object is placed 40 cm in front of a +4.00 D lens.
- Object distance −40 cm
- Lens power +4.00 D

A distance of 40 cm is already too large to fit on an A4 piece of paper, and that's only considering the left side of the

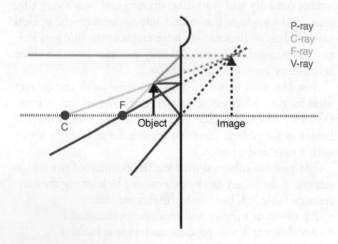

• **Fig. 7.12** Ray diagram showing how to draw the rays (and identify the location of the image) when an object is between F and the mirror in front of a positively powered mirror. You can see it forms a virtual, upright, magnified image behind the mirror itself.

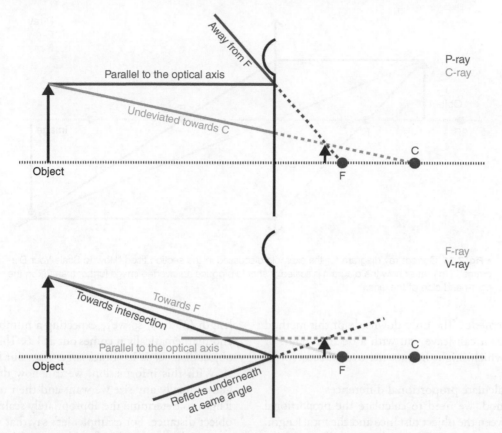

• **Fig. 7.13** Example ray diagram for a negatively powered mirror. All four rays are drawn and labelled, but they have been split across two diagrams for clarity. The P-ray and C-ray are illustrated in the top image, whereas the F-ray and V-ray are illustrated in the bottom image. The tip of the image is identified as the point where the rays intersect one another.

TABLE 7.4	Table Showing Relationship Between Object Position and Associated Image Characteristics With Negative Spherical Mirrors				
Object Distance (l)	Image Location	Image Distance (l′)	Inverted/Upright	Image Size
Infinity	Right of mirror	F	U	<O
~	Right of mirror	<l	U	<O

lens! If we calculate the focal length ($f = n/F = 1/4 = +0.25$ m), we can see that in order to draw our P-ray (which goes through the secondary focal point (F′)), we'd also need 25 cm right of the lens too. This is already totalling a fairly massive 65 cm and is getting out of hand.

Instead of sticking lots of pieces of paper together and digging out our metre ruler, we can scale the drawing down to make it smaller. When done correctly, scaling the diagrams down will be like resizing a digital photograph – as long as all the proportions are sensibly maintained, then it will look identical (just smaller). There is also the added benefit that smaller diagrams are less prone to errors, which is a nice bonus. This scaling down can be done in one of two possible ways.

• Option 1: Divide all the numbers by a set number

For this method, we calculate all our distances (using the same example numbers from before):

−40 cm for object distance
+25 cm for focal length (f)
+50 cm for 2f

Then we divide them all by any number we like. For example, if we divide all our values here by 10 (a nice, easy number), then the distances become:

− 4 cm for object distance
+2.5 cm for focal length (f)
+5 cm for 2f

This easily fits on the page. Importantly, this method works beautifully providing you remember to apply it to all

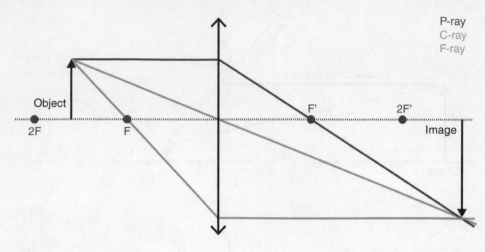

P-ray
C-ray
F-ray

• **Fig. 7.14** Correct ray diagram for the example discussed in the section titled "How to Scale Your Diagrams". No matter how the diagram is scaled, it should produce an inverted image further than 2f' on the right-hand side of the lens.

distance measurements. The only downside of this method is that sometimes it can leave you with a decimal point or two (or three), which might impact the overall accuracy of the diagram.

• Option 2: Calculate proportional differences

For this method, we need to calculate the proportional relationship between the object distance and the focal length. Proportions tell us (numerically) how big or small something is relative to something else. In our case, we would want to know how big or small our object distance is relative to our focal length, so all we need to do is divide one by the other (proportion = object distance / focal length). This will give us a number, so a proportion <1 suggests the object distance is smaller than the focal length, a proportion of 1 suggests they are identical and a proportion >1 suggests the object distance is larger than the focal length. In our example, we know the object distance (40 cm) is larger than the focal

length (25 cm), so we're expecting a number larger than 1, and mathematically it comes out as 1.6. This means that our object distance is 1.6 times larger than our focal length.

With this information, we can now draw our ray diagram literally any size we want and then use our new focal length to determine the appropriately scaled (proportional) object distance. For example, let's say that we want to draw our ray diagram with a focal length of 2.5 cm (chosen because it's small enough to fit on a page). We know our object distance needs to be 1.6 times larger so we can multiply the new focal length (2.5 cm) by our proportion (1.6) to discern that our new, scaled object distance needs to be 4 cm. If you're keen, you'll have noticed that these are the same numbers I used in the previous example from Option 1, which were chosen deliberately to prove that it's a valid method. Try it yourself at home and see how it works out! The final ray diagram should look something like Fig. 7.14.

Test Your Knowledge

Try the questions below to see if you need to review any sections again. All answers are available in the back of the book.

TYK.7.1 Using your knowledge of optical systems, can you explain why a P-ray will pass through F'?

TYK.7.2 Explain how you could use a ray diagram to decide whether an image distance would be positive or negative.

TYK.7.3 In the diagram below, which image is drawn correctly? Explain your answer.

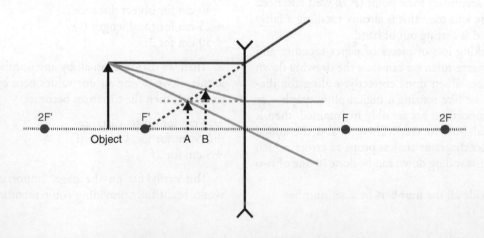

TYK.7.4 Draw a ray diagram to show where an image would form if an object was placed at 2F in front of a positively powered lens.

TYK.7.5 Draw a ray diagram to show where an image would form if an object was placed between F′ and the lens in front of a negatively powered lens.

TYK.7.6 Draw a ray diagram to show where an image would form if an object was placed left of C in front of a positively powered mirror.

TYK.7.7 Draw a ray diagram to show where an image would form if an object was placed at any location in front of a negatively powered mirror.

TYK.7.8 To get an inverted, minified image, what kind of lens would be needed (positive or negative) and where would the object need to be placed?

8

Dispersion and Chromatic Aberration

CHAPTER OUTLINE

OBJECTIVES

After working through this chapter, you should be able to:

Explain what dispersion is

Understand how dispersion occurs

Explain how rainbows are produced

Explain what chromatic aberration is

Discuss the relevance of chromatic aberration in the human eye

Introduction

In this chapter we will start to think about the constituent wavelengths that make up 'light' and how white light (e.g. from the sun) can be separated into these wavelengths through a process called **dispersion**.

Dispersion

As discussed in chapter 1, white light can be produced when the light source emits all the wavelengths of visible light (e.g. a continuous spectrum), or when the light source emits a large enough range of wavelengths (e.g. a discrete spectrum) that it appears white-*ish* due to the additive nature of light. For example, sunlight looks white and comprises a continuous spectrum, but if I had a red bulb, a green bulb and a blue bulb, the resultant light would look white but would be classed as a discrete spectrum due to the limited range of wavelengths. However, in some circumstances it is possible for white light to be separated into the individual wavelengths well enough that we can actually see the different colours ascribed to each wavelength (long-red; short-blue). This happens through a process called **dispersion**. Some of you reading this may have heard about dispersion happening as part of the refractive process when light passes through a prism, but I expect all of you will be familiar with a form of dispersion that happens when it rains on a sunny day to produce a rainbow in the sky! To that end, let's explain dispersion using the example of a rainbow to start with, and then we can move on to discuss prisms and lenses.

Rainbows

When we see a rainbow in the sky (Fig. 8.1), we will perceive what appears to be a continuous spectrum from long-wavelength light (red) all the way to short-wavelength light (blue/violet). Now, it is no coincidence that the distribution of colours in a rainbow falls in exactly the same pattern as we would expect if we ordered them by wavelength, as the reason that dispersion occurs is because the amount that the light undergoes refraction is partly dependent on the material and partly dependent on the wavelength of the light itself. Sticking with the rainbow example, we probably know that rainbows only occur when there is water in the air (e.g. when it rains), which indicates that it is the refractive properties of the water droplets (the rain) that produces the effect. Most of the time, white light from the sun (all visible wavelengths) can refract through the water droplets in the sky without any trouble, but as we can see in Table 8.1, the refractive index of materials changes slightly depending on the wavelength of the incident light. For example, shorter wavelengths of light will experience higher refractive indices than longer wavelengths of light. Importantly, this indicates that there can be a difference in the speed each wavelength travels through the material. More specifically, shorter wavelengths are slowed down to a greater extent than the longer wavelengths when they enter these materials, which means that they refract to a greater extent (think back to Snell's law from chapter 2) and therefore will have a greater angle of deviation relative to longer wavelength light. Sometimes we teach this as 'blue bends best' to help students learn that

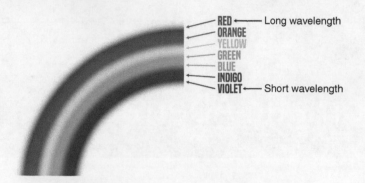

RED ← Long wavelength
ORANGE
YELLOW
GREEN
BLUE
INDIGO
VIOLET ← Short wavelength

• **Fig. 8.1** An illustration showing the colours that can be found in a rainbow. Red wavelengths are longer than violet wavelengths.

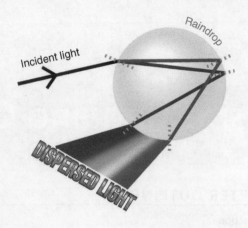

Incident light   Raindrop

DISPERSED LIGHT

• **Fig. 8.2** An illustration showing how a raindrop can split white light into constituent wavelengths through refraction and reflection.

TABLE 8.1	Relationship Between Wavelength (Defined as Visible Colour) and Refractive Index of the Material	
Wavelength	Water (n = ~1.333)	Crown Glass (n = ~1.523)
Red	1.331	1.512
Orange	1.332	1.514
Yellow	1.333	1.518
Green	1.335	1.519
Blue	1.338	1.524
Violet	1.342	1.530

short wavelengths (blue-end of the spectrum) will refract at a greater angle than long wavelengths (red-end of the spectrum), however please remember that this only applies to dispersion and refraction – the opposite is true for diffraction which we will learn about in chapter 10.

However, as we've already discussed, most of the time the white light remains white after refracting through the water droplets, so how does the dispersion produce a rainbow? The answer is that rainbows occur when the sunlight refracts into the droplet, and then reflects back off the farthest surface of the water droplet to make it refract back out of the side it originated from. Fig. 8.2 illustrates what this looks like within a raindrop and how the raindrop can disperse the white light into all the colours of the rainbow. In short, when white light is incident upon a raindrop, each constituent wavelength is refracted by slightly different amounts. The light begins to disperse, but when it reaches the other side of the raindrop, some of the light is reflected back again, and so it is then refracted a second time as it leaves the raindrop. It is the combination of the two refraction opportunities that disperse the light to produce the rainbow – the reflection that occurs on the back surface does not contribute to the dispersion process as reflection does not alter for different wavelengths, bout as the wavelengths will already be slightly dispersed, they will each be reflected slightly differently as they will reflect off different locations of the water droplet. However, now you may be wondering – why doesn't

the whole sky look multicoloured in that case? Why is it restricted to a neat little rainbow shape?, Well, we then perceive this process in the sky as a rainbow as we are only able to perceive the light when it reaches our eyes at a particular angle (which makes the rainbow the characteristic arc shape).

Now, if I asked you what shape a rainbow was, what would you say? I suspect you'd say 'arch', 'bridge', 'semicircle' or something similar to that, and you'd be half right. What if I told you that actually all rainbows are *complete* circles, but we can only see the top half? In fact, we (as observers close to the ground) are only able to see light reflected *above* the horizon, and the position of the rainbow will be dictated by our own position on the ground. This means that if I see a rainbow in the sky outside my office and I text my colleague across campus to demand that they look outside, they will see an entirely different rainbow. Ultimately, the key factor affecting the appearance of the rainbow is the **antisolar point**, defined as the point 180 degrees away from the sun relative to the observer (see Fig. 8.3 for a visual explanation of this). Technically, the central point of the rainbow (*raincircle?*) coincides with the antisolar point, and so logically, in order to see the rainbow you'd have to face away from the sun (which makes sense now that we know rainbows are formed from reflections within raindrops). This also indicates that the height of the sun will directly influence the apparent height of the rainbow,

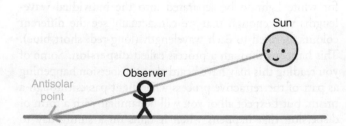

Sun

Observer

Antisolar point

• **Fig. 8.3** Illustration showing that the antisolar point will exist 180 degrees away from the sun, relative to the observer. On a bright, sunny day, it will correspond to the shadow of your head as this highlights the line from the sun to your eyes.

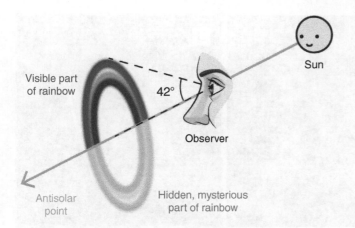

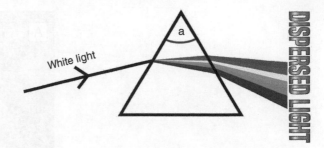

• **Fig. 8.5** The apical angle (a) of a triangular-shaped prism is the angle between the surfaces where the light enters and leaves the prism. White light will be dispersed.

• **Fig. 8.4** Illustration showing how the antisolar point dictates the centre of the rainbow. The radius of the rainbow will be 42 degrees from this point relative to you as the observer.

meaning rainbows produced when the sun is low in the sky will appear to be much larger in appearance than those produced when the sun is up high. Interestingly, rainbows form at a specified 42-degree angle between the observer and the antisolar point (Fig. 8.4), which roughly determines the radius of the rainbow itself. This means if the antisolar point falls below the horizon, the rainbow will be set low down relative to the horizon, whereas if the antisolar point is more level with the horizon, then the rainbow will form 42 degrees above that.

If the light undergoes *two* reflections within a raindrop (caused by interacting with higher raindrops in the sky), then a second (double) rainbow will be produced with the order of the colours reversed, and this sight is occasionally portrayed as very exciting in viral videos on the internet. Importantly this second rainbow should have a radius that roughly corresponds to 52 degrees so it should be larger than the main rainbow.

In summary, rainbows are produced as a feature of refraction that relies on the wavelength properties of light, and they are actually circular – this means it is unlikely (arguably impossible) to find the end of one, and therefore unlikely that there will be an accompanying pot of gold (though never say never).

Prisms

In optical physics, we are most likely to consider dispersion occurring as light travels through a **prism**, as shown in Fig. 8.5. Prisms will be discussed in more detail in chapter 9, but for now all we need to know is that the word 'prism' defines any transparent object that comprises two surfaces that are at an angle towards one another. Most commonly, prisms are thought of in the classic 'triangular' shape such as that in Fig. 8.5, but a glass cube would also be classed as a prism (a square one). However, for the sake of simplicity in this chapter we will only consider triangular prisms. Now, in prisms this process of dispersion is identical to that described with the raindrops before, but this time the prism will be made of plastic or glass (as opposed to water) and so the

refractive index is higher. In the prism example, dispersion occurs when white light refracts at the first surface, and it occurs again when the white light exits the prism at the second surface. The angle between the surfaces where the light enters and exits is called the **apical angle (a)** (see Fig. 8.5).

Importantly, remember that dispersion is defined as the splitting or separating of wavelengths that make up a light source. This means that dispersion can only occur if the light source contains more than one wavelength, so if we used a light source made of only one wavelength (e.g. a red laser), then the light will all refract equally and no dispersion will occur (Fig. 8.6).

If you're interested in the principles of dispersion and feel like it would be beneficial to see it in action, you can follow instructions to make your own prism at home in chapter 20.

Chromatic Aberration

Dispersion itself is a neat example of the relationship between refractive index and wavelength of light, and it produces some beautiful patterns of light in the sky and in the optics lab, however it can cause problems in optical systems. If we think back to chapters 1 and 2, we know that the rectilinear propagation of light states that light must travel in a straight line when in a *homogenous* medium, but we also know that following dispersion, the wavelengths of light will be leaving the material at different angles. This means that the farther the light travels away from the material, the more 'spread out' the wavelengths will be. Similarly, large

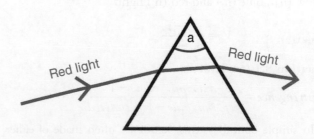

• **Fig. 8.6** The apical angle (a) of a triangular-shaped prism is the angle between the surfaces where the light enters and leaves the prism. Monochromatic (single wavelength) light (e.g. red) will be refracted but cannot disperse.

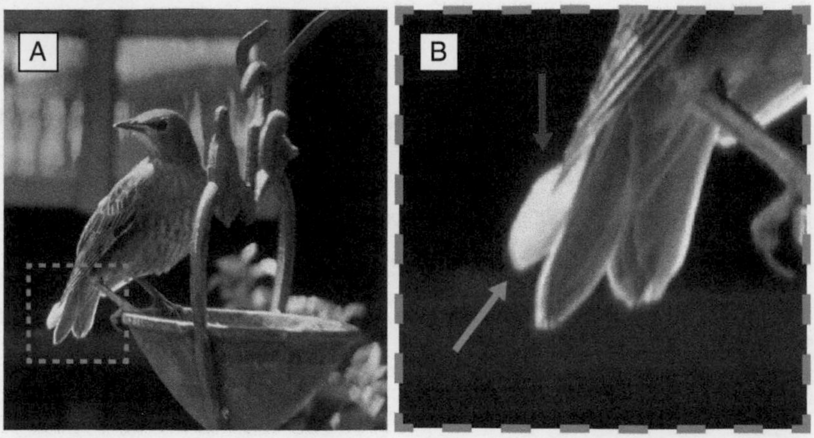

• **Fig. 8.7** A beautiful image of a bird taken through a telephoto lens attached to a mobile phone camera (A). The edges of the lens have introduced a small amount of chromatic aberration into the image, highlighted by the two arrows in the zoomed-in section (B). (Image taken by John Collins.)

amounts of dispersion can occur over shorter distances through the use of high powered lenses, which cause the light to bend a lot. This can cause problems when viewing images, as dispersion can produce varying degrees of distortion in the final image called **aberrations**. A particularly important example of this in optics is **chromatic aberration** (colour-related distortion), which can occur in magnifying optical systems (e.g. telescopes, binoculars, low vision aids) if not carefully considered. This is a term used to describe imperfections in an image related to the splitting of colours, as shown in Fig. 8.7. Interestingly, chromatic aberrations can be categorised across two types: transverse chromatic aberrations (often abbreviated as TCA) and longitudinal chromatic aberrations (often abbreviated as LCA). The key difference is that transverse chromatic aberration is identified when the size of the image changes due to the wavelength of the incident light (see Fig. 8.8A), whereas longitudinal chromatic aberration is identified when individual wavelengths in the incident light focus at different points along the optical axis (see Fig. 8.8B). This chapter will primarily focus on longitudinal chromatic aberration, but please be encouraged to read about the subject if you want to know a little bit more.

The amount of dispersion that a material will produce can be calculated as the **Abbe number** or **constringence number** (two names for the same thing) of the material, denoted by the letter V in Equation 8.1. The n variables in Equation 8.1 are showing the different refractive indices for yellow (n_d), blue (n_f) and red (n_c) light.

Equation 8.1 $\quad V = \dfrac{n_d - 1}{n_f - n_c}$

Equation 8.1 (explained)

$$constringence = \frac{ref.\,ind.\,yellow - 1}{ref.\,ind.\,blue - ref.\,ind.\,red}$$

In simple optical systems, lenses are often made of either crown glass or flint glass. Now, even within the same 'type' of glass, they can possess different constringence numbers depending on their density, but for simplicity in this chapter we will consider common types of crown glass with constringence

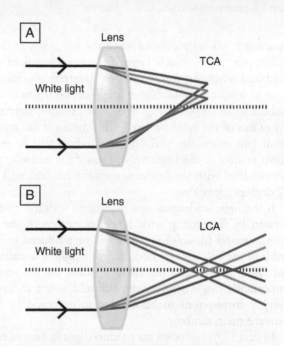

• **Fig. 8.8** Diagram illustrating the difference between transverse chromatic aberration (TCA; A) where size of image is affected by wavelength, relative to longitudinal chromatic aberration (LCA; B) where point of focus on the optical axis is affected by wavelength.

values of ~60, and common types of flint glass with constringence values of ~30. It is important to note here that high constringency indicates low levels of dispersion and low constringency indicates higher levels of dispersion, so if we had two identical lenses, one made of crown glass and one of flint glass, the crown glass lens (V = 60) should disperse light less than the flint glass lens (V = 30).

In optical systems, if this constringency is not accounted for, it can produce the chromatic aberration demonstrated in Fig. 8.7. This chromatic aberration (CA) increases as the power (F) of the lens increases, as indicated in Equation 8.2.

Equation 8.2 $\quad CA = \dfrac{F}{V}$

Equation 8.2 (explained) $chromatic\ abb. = \dfrac{power}{constringence}$

DEMO QUESTION 8.1

What is the chromatic aberration of a crown glass lens with a power of +5.00 D?

Step 1: Determine what we need to calculate chromatic aberration, CA

Step 2: Define variables

V = 60 (the known constringency value for crown glass)

F = +5.00

Step 3: Determine necessary equation(s)

CA = F / V *(Equation 8.2)*

Step 4: Calculate

CA = F / V

CA = 5 / 60

CA = 0.08

(a CA value of 0 would be an 'aberration-free' image)

Practice Questions:

8.1.1 What is the chromatic aberration of a crown glass lens with a power of +20.00 D?

8.1.2 What is the chromatic aberration of a flint glass lens with a power of +10.00 D?

DEMO QUESTION 8.2

What power of flint glass would be required to remove chromatic aberration from a lens made partly of crown glass (+4.00 D)?

Step 1: Determine what we need to calculate power (fl), F_f

Step 2: Define variables

V_c = 60 (the known constringency value for crown glass)

V_f = 30 (the known constringency value for flint glass)

F_c = +4.00

CA = 0 (the question hasn't stated it, but we're aiming to remove all chromatic aberration that would be a value of zero)

Step 3: Determine necessary equation(s)

CA = $(F_c / V_c) + (F_f / V_f)$ *(Equation 8.3)*

Step 4: Calculate

CA = $(F_c / V_c) + (F_f / V_f)$

0 = (4 / 60) + (F_f / 30)

0 = 0.067.. + (F_f / 30)

0 − 0.067.. = F_f / 30

−0.067.. = F_f / 30

−0.067.. × 30 = F_f

−2.00 D = F_f

The flint glass in this achromatic doublet would need to be −2.00 D to remove chromatic aberrations.

Practice Questions:

8.2.1 What power of flint glass would be required to remove chromatic aberration from a lens made partly of crown glass (+8.00 D)?

8.2.2 What power of crown glass would be required to remove chromatic aberration from a lens made partly of flint glass (+2.00 D)?

However, it is possible to design lens systems in such a way to undo the potential for some of the chromatic aberration by utilising a double-material lens called an **achromatic doublet**. We know that different materials possess different constringency values, so it is reasonably logical then to understand that we might be able to use two different materials to bring the chromatic aberration down to zero. A good example would be to use a combination of crown glass and flint glass to produce the power of image that is required whilst also removing all the chromatic aberration (Fig. 8.9).

We can calculate the power of one type of glass lens required to undo the chromatic aberration produced by the lens made of the other type of glass by using a modified version of Equation 8.2 shown as Equation 8.3.

Equation 8.3 $CA = \dfrac{F_c}{V_c} + \dfrac{F_f}{V_f}$

Equation 8.3 (explained)

$chromatic\ abb. = \dfrac{power\ (cr)}{constring.\ (cr)} + \dfrac{power\ (fl)}{constring.(fl)}$

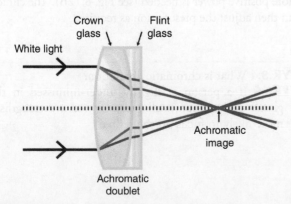

• **Fig. 8.9** When a lens is made of two materials and designed in such a way as to produce a chromatic aberration value of zero, it is called an achromatic doublet.

In conclusion, dispersion occurs when light comprising many wavelengths is refracted through a material. This dispersion can be managed by using a light source comprising only a single wavelength, or by utilising a special lens (achromatic doublet) that removes any impact of dispersion on the final image.

Chromatic Aberration in the Human Eye

Up to this point in the chapter, we've discussed chromatic aberration in optical systems and lenses, but it might interest you to know that longitudinal chromatic aberration is also present in the human eye. This occurs because the shorter wavelengths refract more than the longer wavelengths when transmitting through the optics of the eye (just like in lenses). This means that it is usually assumed that shorter ('blue') wavelengths will focus slightly in front of the retina and longer ('red') wavelengths will focus slightly behind the retina, as illustrated in Fig. 8.10 (remember, 'blue bends best'). However, interestingly, we (as observers) don't usually notice this because (1) it's quite a small effect and (2) the brain is very good at overcoming predictable (frequently experienced), small errors like this.

In optometric practice, optometrists attempt to measure refractive error of the eye (see chapter 5) and then test different corrective spherical or cylindrical lenses to see if they

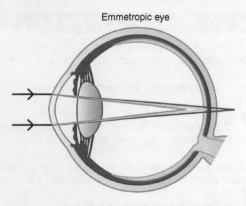

Emmetropic eye

• **Fig. 8.10** Illustration of longitudinal chromatic aberration in the human eye. Longer wavelength light focuses behind the retina (red) whilst shorter wavelength light focuses in front of the retina (blue).

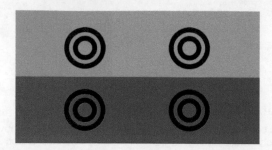

• **Fig. 8.11** Example image of a duochrome test. In clinical practice the wavelengths would need to be carefully calibrated, and so this printed (or digital) example will not work as effectively if you're trying it for yourself at home.

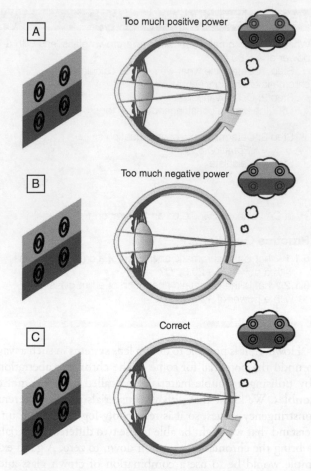

Too much positive power

Too much negative power

Correct

• **Fig. 8.12** A diagram showing the patient's perspective of a duochrome and the associated focusing of the light on the retina when: over-plussed (A), over-minussed (B), and appropriately corrected (C).

can improve visual acuity. This assignment of corrective lenses is referred to as a patient's spectacle **prescription**. Importantly, optometrists can utilise the naturally occurring chromatic aberration in the eye by using a test called a **duochrome** (two-colour test) to check the prescription is accurate. In this test, two sets of targets are presented to the patient, one set on a green background (~535 nm) and one set on a red background (~620 nm)[1] (see Fig. 8.11 for an example). If the prescription is accurate, then the targets should look equally clear on both the green and red backgrounds, indicating that the eye is focused between the red and green (as is appropriate). However, if the patient has been given too much positive power

in the lens ('over-plussed') or too little negative power ('under-minussed'), the target on the red will look clearer – indicating that the combination of the eye and lenses are bending the light too much and more negative power is needed (see Fig. 8.12A). On the other hand, if the patient has been given too much negative power in the lens ('over-minussed'), or too little positive power ('under-plussed'), the target on the green will look clearer – indicating that the combination of the eye and lenses aren't quite bending the light enough and more positive power is needed (see Fig. 8.12B). The clinician can then adjust the prescription as required.

Test Your Knowledge

Try the questions below to see if you need to review any sections again. All answers are available in the back of the book.

TYK.8.1 What wavelength refracts the most – red or blue?

TYK.8.2 Explain how raindrops produce a rainbow.

TYK.8.3 Would dispersion occur if we shone a red laser through a prism? Explain your answer.

TYK.8.4 What is chromatic aberration?

TYK.8.5 If a person is slightly under-minussed in their glasses prescription, will green or red wavelengths be more likely to focus on the retina?

Reference

1. Rabbetts RB. *Bennett and Rabbetts' Clinical Visual Optics*. 4th ed. UK: Butterworth-Heinemann, Elsevier; 2007.

9

Prisms

OBJECTIVES

After working through this chapter, you should be able to:

Describe what a prism is

Explain what the minimum angle of deviation is

Define a 'critical angle'

Discuss how light deviates through a prism (relative to the base and apex)

Calculate prismatic power

Introduction

In the previous chapter, we introduced the topic of prisms and discussed that they are capable of dispersing white light. In this chapter, we will discuss prisms in more detail and learn all about their power, minimum angle of deviation, total internal reflection and critical angle.

What Is a Prism?

When I read the word 'prism', I think of a glass, triangular-shaped object with five sides like the one in Fig. 9.1A. Technically my instinct is correct, and this is a prism, but in optics the true definition of the word 'prism' encompasses *any* object that possesses two flat refracting surfaces inclined at an angle towards each other. This means that all of the glass objects illustrated in Fig. 9.1B are also technically prisms, but this chapter is going to focus on the triangularly shaped prisms.

Deviation of Light

Now, if we take a cross section of a triangular-shaped prism, we can imagine that it would be made of a material other than air – suggesting it will have a different refractive index (n_p) relative to the surrounding air (n_s) (Fig. 9.2). Importantly, prisms also possess an **apical angle** (a), which is defined as the angle that exists between the first and second refracting surface (where the light enters and leaves the prism). This is demonstrated in Fig. 9.2 with a monochromatic (single

wavelength) beam of light (as this prevents dispersion, see chapter 8 for revision on this if necessary).

To start with, let's consider the **deviation** of the light path. If you look at the solid lines in Fig. 9.2, these correspond to the path that the light takes as it travels through the prism. An important feature of prismatic refraction (refraction through a prism) is that **light will always deviate towards the base**, shown by the emergent light ray being angled downwards in this example. For clarity, the 'base' of the prism is the side opposite to the apical angle, so in Fig. 9.2 it is the horizontal line along the bottom of the prism. Now, if you look instead at the dashed lines in Fig. 9.2, you can see that they correspond to the original path the light would have taken if it hadn't been deviated by this pesky prism being in the way. To this end, the angle between the original path of light and the true, deviated path of light is called the **angle of deviation (d)**. It is also crucial to note that this angle of deviation (d) is the sum of the angles of deviation at each surface of the prism (d_1 and d_2) – see Equation 9.1 for an example of this.

Equation 9.1
$$d = d_1 + d_2$$

Equation 9.1 (explained)

$$dev. = dev.\ at\ 1st\ surface + dev.\ at\ 2nd\ surface$$

But, how do we calculate these angles of deviation in the first place? The answer is maths (as always) and **cyclic quadrilaterals**. Now, if you haven't heard of cyclic quadrilaterals

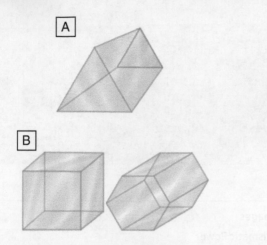

• **Fig. 9.1** Drawing of 'classic' triangular prisms (A) and examples of other types of prism (B).

before, don't worry, you can utilise the information in Box 9.1 to help you learn what they are.

The information provided in Box 9.1 highlights that we can edit Equation 9.1 to look like Equation 9.2 (depending on the information we have at the time):

Equation 9.2 $\quad d = (i_1 + i_2') - a$

Equation 9.2 (explained)

$$dev. = (1st\ ang.\ inc. + 2nd\ ang.\ ref.) - apical\ ang.$$

This shows us that the angle of deviation (d) is directly related to the angle that the light enters the prism (i_1), the angle light leaves the prism (i_2'), and the apical angle (a) of the prism itself – neat.

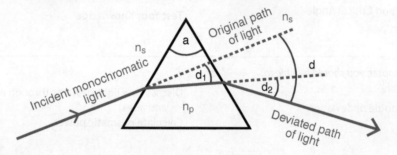

• **Fig. 9.2** Illustration showing refractive index outside the prism (n_s) will differ to the refractive index inside the prism (n_p). If a monochromatic (single wavelength) beam of light is incident upon the surface, the light will refract at both the incident first surface and the emergent second surface, producing two angles of deviation (d_1 and d_2). The overall angle of deviation (d) is the difference between the original path of the light relative to the deviated path of light.

• **BOX 9.1**   **Opposite Angles, Cyclic Quadrilaterals and Prisms**

If we think back to chapter 2, we remember that angles of incidence (the angle at which rays of light approach a refractive surface) are measured relative to the 'normal' of the surface – a hypothetical line that exists at a perpendicular angle to the surface itself (at the point where light intersects the surface). We also learnt all about opposite angles (see Box 2.4 for revision on this), and with understanding deviation in prisms, opposite angles hold the key. For example, in Fig. B9.1, we can see that we can apply the knowledge that vertically opposite angles are equal in order to calculate the deviation at the first surface (d_1), showing that:
$d_1 = i_1 - i_1'$

The same is true for the second angle of deviation (d_2) at the second face of the prism (Fig. B9.2) showing that:
$d_2 = i_2' - i_2$

And as Equation 9.1 taught us, we know that total deviation is equal to $d_1 + d_2$, so that means we can also say that:
$d = (i_1 - i_1') + (i_2' - i_2)$

Now, let's take a moment to think about **cyclic quadrilaterals**. The definition of a cyclic quadrilateral is that it must have four sides, and all four vertices (corners) must connect to a hypothetical circle (see Fig. B9.3B). Cyclic quadrilaterals also require all internal angles to add up to 360°, and opposite angles within the quadrilateral must add up to 180°. Now, you're likely thinking '*Why is Sam telling us all this?*', and the answer is because the 'normal' lines of each surface (at the point where light enters and leaves the prism) form a cyclic quadrilateral (Fig. B9.3A). This means that using our newfound knowledge of cyclic quadrilaterals, we know that

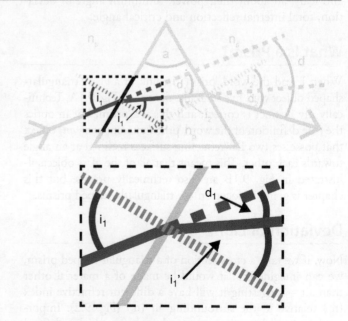

• **Fig. B9.1** Illustration showing how principle of opposite angles applies to the first surface of the prism. Image highlights that $i_1 = d_1 + i_1'$ and therefore $d_1 = i_1 - i_1'$.

• BOX 9.1   Opposite Angles, Cyclic Quadrilaterals and Prisms – cont'd

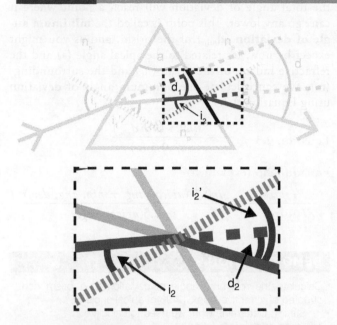

• **Fig. B9.2** Illustration showing how principle of opposite angles applies to the second surface of the prism. Image highlights that $i_2' = d_2 + i_2$ and therefore $d_2 = i_2' - i_2$.

the apical angle (a) and the angle formed by the two normal lines (b) must add up to 180°. However we also know that angles along a straight line equal 180°, which means that this hypothetical angle outside of the cyclic quadrilateral in Fig. B9.3B would also be equal to that of the apical angle.

Another important mathematical fact about triangles is that external angles (along a straight line) will be equal to the sum of the opposite two interior angles (see Fig. B9.3C). This is because the internal angles of a triangle all add up to 180°, and angles along a straight line add up to 180°, so if we consider Fig. B9.3C for a moment, we know that:

$$180° = b + i_1' + i_2$$

and

$$180° = b + a$$

Thereby proving that:

Equation B9.1:

$$a = i_1' + i_2$$

Thus highlighting that we can rearrange our earlier equation to turn:

$$d = (i_1 - i_1') + (i_2' - i_2)$$

into:

$$d = (i_1 + i_2') - a \text{ (see Equation 9.2)}$$

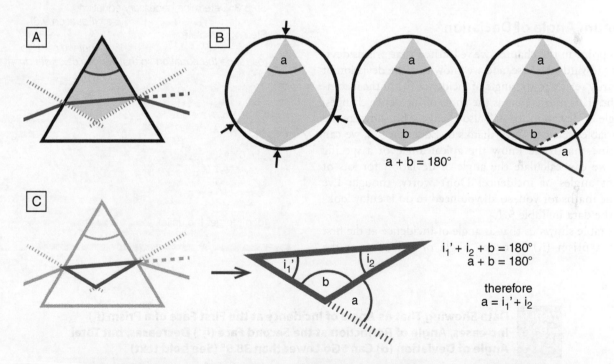

• **Fig. B9.3** (A) Diagram showing how the two 'normal' lines (orange dashed lines) of the prism create a cyclic quadrilateral (blue). (B) Diagram showing properties of cyclic quadrilaterals to prove that the external angle (right) will be equal to the apical angle (a) of the prism. (C) Diagram showing that the apical angle (a) will be equal to the sum of the two internal angles formed by the light ray (i_1' and i_2).

DEMO QUESTION 9.1

A ray of light is incident upon a prism at an angle of 35° and leaves the prism at an angle of 67°. If the prism has an apical angle of 50°, what is the angle of deviation of the light?

Step 1: Determine what we need to calculate
angle of deviation, d
Step 2: Define variables
i_1 = 35° *(angle of incidence at first surface)*
i_2' = 67° *(angle of refraction at second surface)*
a = 50° *(apical angle)*
Step 3: Determine necessary equation
d = $(i_1 + i_2')$ − a *(Equation 9.2)*
Step 4: Calculate
d = $(i_1 + i_2')$ − a
d = (35 + 67) − 50
d = 52°
(don't forget the units!)

Practice Questions:

9.1.1 A ray of light is incident upon a prism at an angle of 20° and leaves the prism at an angle of 40°. If the prism has an apical angle of 55°, what is the angle of deviation of the light?

9.1.2 A ray of light is incident upon a prism at an angle of 21.2° and leaves the prism at an angle of 58.5°. If the prism has an apical angle of 30°, what is the angle of deviation of the light?

Minimum Angle of Deviation

By this point in the chapter, we've learned that prisms deviate light towards the base, and we know that the deviation of light partly relates to the angle of incidence (i_1) of the incoming light. This means that as the angle of incidence changes, the angle of deviation (d) will also change – but how are the two variables related? Well, thanks to Equation 9.2, we can determine that if we know the apical angle of a specific prism, we can calculate the angle of deviation for lots of different angles of incidence. Don't worry, though; I've done the maths for you, so all you need to do is enjoy looking at the data in Table 9.1.

This table shows us that as angle of incidence at the first face of a prism (i_1) increases, angle of refraction at the

second face (i_2') decreases. However, it also shows us that the total angle of deviation will reach a point where it can't go any lower. This point is called the **minimum angle of deviation (d_{min})** of the prism, and as you might expect by now, it's related to the apical angle (a) and the refractive indices of the prism (n_p) and the surroundings (n_s). We can calculate the minimum angle of deviation using Equation 9.3:

Equation 9.3
$$\frac{n_p}{n_s} = \frac{sin0.5\,(a+d_{min})}{sin0.5\,(a)}$$

Equation 9.3 (explained)

$$\frac{RI\ prism}{RI\ surround} = \frac{sin0.5\,(apical\ ang.+min.\ ang.\ dev.)}{sin0.5(apical\ ang.)}$$

DEMO QUESTION 9.2

Calculate the minimum angle of deviation of a prism constructed of refractive index 1.498 of apical angle 55°.

Step 1: Determine what we need to calculate
minimum angle of deviation, d_{min}
Step 2: Define variables
n_p = 1.498
n_s = 1.00 *(not specified so we assume air)*
a = 55 *(apical angle)*
Step 3: Determine necessary equation
$n_p / n_s = (sin0.5(a + d_{min})) / (sin0.5(a))$ *(Equation 9.3)*
Step 4: Calculate
$n_p / n_s = (sin0.5(a + d_{min})) / (sin0.5(a))$ *(but we need to rearrange the equation so that we can calculate dmin)*
$n_s (sin0.5(a + d_{min})) = n_p (sin0.5(a))$
1.00 (sin0.5(55+d_{min})) = 1.498 (sin(0.5 × 55))
sin0.5(55+d_{min}) = 1.498 (sin(27.5))
sin0.5(55+d_{min}) = 0.6917..
0.5(55+d_{min}) = sin⁻¹(0.6917..)
0.5(55+d_{min}) = 43.76..
27.5 + 0.5(d_{min}) = 43.76..
0.5(d_{min}) = 43.76.. − 27.5
0.5(d_{min}) = 16.26..
d_{min} = 16.26.. / 0.5
d_{min} = 32.53°
(don't forget the units!)

TABLE 9.1	Data Showing That as Angle of Incidence at the First Face of a Prism (i_1) Increases, Angle of Refraction at the Second Face (i_2') Decreases, but Total Angle of Deviation (d) Can't Go Lower than 38.9° (See bold text)		
i_1 (deg)		**i_2' (deg)**	**d (deg)**
30		83.3	53.3
40		60.6	40.6
50		48.9	**38.9**
60		40.5	40.5
70		34.4	44.4
80		30.7	50.7

DEMO QUESTION 9.2 – cont'd

Practice Questions:

9.2.1 Calculate the minimum angle of deviation of a prism constructed of refractive index 1.498 of apical angle 60°.
9.2.2 Calculate the minimum angle of deviation of a prism constructed of refractive index 1.65 of apical angle 30°.

Total Internal Reflection and Critical Angle

For this section of the chapter, let's do some quick revision of how light refracts through surfaces. Do you remember in chapter 1, we discussed that when light is incident upon a surface, it can be transmitted through, absorbed, reflected or a combination of all of these things? (If not please see chapter 1 for revision on this.) Well, along that same line of thought, when we discuss light refracting through surfaces, we are over-simplifying the process by assuming that 100% of the light is transmitted through the surface. In reality, some of the light is reflected back, and the *amount* of light reflected and the *angle* of reflection (i′) will depend on the angle of incidence (i). Now, this common, small amount of reflection occurs when light travels from a low-refractive index medium to a higher refractive index medium, and vice versa, but now we are going to discuss a phenomenon called **total internal reflection,** which can *only* occur when light travels from a higher refractive index into a lower one.

In chapter 2, Snell's law (Equation 2.2) taught us that if light travels from a high refractive index medium to a lower refractive index medium, then the angle of refraction (i′) will be larger than the angle of incidence. This is important because, as you can see in Fig. 9.3, if the angle of incidence (i) is large enough, eventually the refracted light will travel along the surface of the material it's leaving (Fig. 9.3B), meaning that its angle of refraction (i′) is equal to 90° (relative to the normal). The specific angle of incidence required for this to

happen is called the **critical angle** (i_c). Importantly, if the angle of incidence increases beyond the critical angle, then all the light will be reflected back into the material it originated in, which is called **total internal reflection** (Fig. 9.3C).

The critical angle itself is entirely reliant upon the refractive index of the material, meaning that, for example, the critical angle of a prism made of diamonds (n = ~2.4) will be different to that of a prism made of perspex (n = ~1.495). With prisms, we can use Equation 9.4 to calculate the critical angle of each specified prism:

Equation 9.4
$$\sin(i_c) = \frac{1}{n_p}$$

Equation 9.4 (explained)

$$\sin(critical\ angle) = \frac{1}{ref.\ index\ prism}$$

Crucially, in normal circumstances in which a prism is likely sitting in a room surrounded by air, the critical angle of the prism can only exist at the second surface, as light is trying to leave the prism. This is because at the first surface, the light isn't moving from a high- to a low-refractive index (as air is the lowest refractive index available to us), whereas as it leaves the prism, it is moving from a high- to a low-refractive index, so total internal reflection can occur. This means that if light leaving the prism leaves at 90° to the normal, then the angle of incidence at the second face (i_2) will be equal to the critical angle (i_c) of the prism (Fig. 9.4).

Now, using a combination of skills we've learnt throughout this textbook so far, if we know the apical angle and the refractive index of a prism, we can calculate the smallest angle of incidence possible before total internal reflection occurs. Or, to phrase it differently, we can calculate the angle of incidence needed to produce the critical angle at the second face of the prism.

To do this, we first need to calculate the critical angle (i_c) of the prism in question (Equation 9.4), which tells us the angle of incidence at the second surface (i_2). We can then calculate the angle of refraction at the first surface (i_1′) using Equation B9.1, which leads us to be able to use Snell's law (see chapter 2, Equation 2.2) to calculate the angle of incidence required at the first face to make it all happen (i_1).

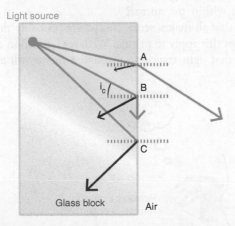

• **Fig. 9.3** Diagram showing that when light travels from a high refractive index glass block (1.523) to air (1.00), the angle of refraction will be larger than the angle of incidence (A), and some light will be reflected back within the glass block. At a specific angle of incidence known as the critical angle (i_c), the light will refract at 90° to the normal and travel along the surface of the glass block (B). If the angle of incidence exceeds the critical angle, then all light will be reflected back – this is called total internal reflection (C).

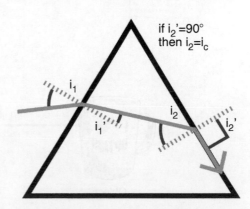

• **Fig. 9.4** Diagram showing that as light emerges at the second face at 90° (i_2′) then the angle of incidence at the second face (i_2) must be equal to the critical angle (i_c).

DEMO QUESTION 9.3

Determine the smallest angle of incidence at the first face of an equilateral triangular prism of refractive index 1.65 for light to just pass through the second face. The apical angle of the prism is 60°.

Step 1: Determine what we need to calculate

angle of incidence, i_1

Step 2: Define variables

$n_p = 1.65$

$n_s = 1.00$ *(not specified so we assume air)*

$a = 60$ *(apical angle)*

Step 3: Determine necessary equation

$\sin(i_c) = 1 / n_p$ *(Equation 9.4)*

$a = i_1' + i_2$ *(Equation B9.1)*

$n (\sin i) = n' (\sin i')$ *(Equation 2.2)*

Step 4: Calculate

$\sin(i_c) = 1 / n_p$

$\sin(i_c) = 1 / 1.65$

$i_c = \sin^{-1} (1 / 1.65)$

$i_c = 37.31..°$

$i_2 = i_c$

$a = i_1' + i_2$

$i_1' = a - i_2$

$i_1' = 60 - 37.31..$

$i_1' = 22.69..°$

$n (\sin i) = n' (\sin i')$

$n_s (\sin i_1) = n_p (\sin i_1')$

$1.00 (\sin i_1) = 1.65 (\sin 22.69..)$

$\sin i_1 = 1.65 (\sin 22.69..) / 1$

$i_1 = \sin^{-1} (1.65 (\sin 22.69..))$

$i_1 = 39.54°$

(don't forget the units!)

Practice Questions:

9.3.1 Determine the smallest angle of incidence at the first face of an equilateral triangular prism of refractive index 1.498 for light to just pass through the second face. The apical angle of the prism is 50°.

9.3.2 Determine the smallest angle of incidence at the first face of an equilateral triangular prism of refractive index 1.523 for light to just pass through the second face. The apical angle of the prism is 55°.

9.3.3 Determine the smallest angle of incidence at the first face of an equilateral triangular prism of refractive index 1.65 for light to just pass through the second face. The apical angle of the prism is 45°.

Images

Hopefully, by this point in the chapter, we're happy to accept that prisms will deviate the path of light, but before we move on, I think it's also important to think about what that means in the real world.

Let's use an example of an object – perhaps our favourite mug (Fig. 9.5). We already know that in order to be able to see the object, we need it to be illuminated (lit up) so that light can reflect off the surface of the object to reach the backs of our eyes – this allows us to perceive an image of the object (see Fig. 9.5). However what we don't often think about is that this means the light will travel along a specified path to your eye, and because light travels in straight lines in a homogenous medium (see chapter 1 for revision on this), providing the light doesn't undergo any refraction (change in direction) then the image of the object will correspond to the point where the object is.

However, what happens if the light ray changes direction before it reaches you? I think the easiest way to illustrate this is to think about plane mirrors (see chapter 6 for revision on this). We can hopefully understand that when we look at an object reflected in a mirror, the image of the object will appear to exist 'within' the mirror itself (Fig. 9.6). This occurs because the light ray is reflected off the mirror at an angle relative to us. This means the light ray reaching our eyes will appear to be coming from within the mirror, which then projects the image of the object to exist 'behind' the mirror! However, thankfully we understand how mirrors work, so we just interpret it as a reflection rather than a magical portal into a parallel, backwards dimension (*although it always surprises me when my cats successfully utilise mirrors to keep an eye on me from across the room – how do they understand how to do that?*). You can demo this principle for yourself at home by looking into a regular mirror and trying to think about where it looks like the image is (instead of what we know is happening) – can you see that it looks like the images are 'within' the mirror?

Ok, that all makes sense, but you're probably thinking – how does this apply to prisms? Well, we learned in an earlier section that light travelling through a prism will always be

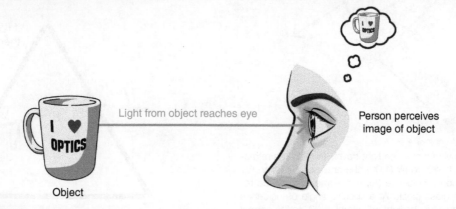

Object

Light from object reaches eye

Person perceives image of object

• **Fig. 9.5** Illustration showing how light travels from an object to our eyes – this allows us to perceive the image of the object.

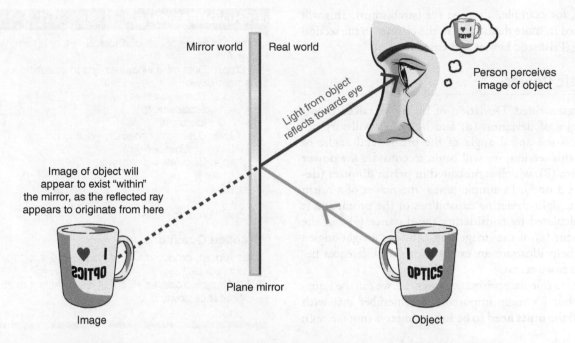

• **Fig. 9.6** Illustration showing how light travels from an object to our eyes if reflecting off a plane mirror – this allows us to perceive the image of the object, but the ray that reaches our eye appears to be coming from within the mirror, and so we perceive the image as being within the mirror.

deviated towards the base of the prism, but we now also know that we perceive images based on where the light appears to be coming from. This means that in order to understand where the image is in a prism, we have to imagine a straight line is projected backwards from the emergent light ray on the right side of the prism (Fig. 9.7). This illustrates another important feature of prisms – the **image is always**

deviated towards the apex. So now we can remember that with prisms:

1. Light will deviate towards the base.
2. The image will deviate towards the apex.

This understanding of how light can be deviated is a very important clinical consideration, as optometrists will sometimes need to prescribe prismatic lenses for patients if

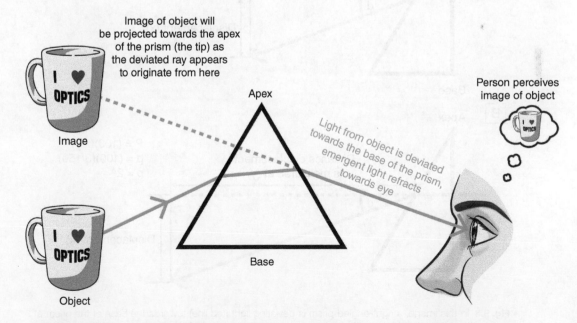

• **Fig. 9.7** Illustration showing how light travels from an object to our eyes if refracting through a prism. This allows us to perceive the image of the object, but the ray that reaches our eye appears to be coming from the apex side of the prism, so we perceive the image as being in a different location to the object itself.

they have, for example, a turned eye (strabismus). This will be discussed in more detail later in the chapter in the section discussing 'Prismatic Lenses and Base Notation.'

Prismatic Power

In the section titled 'Deviation of Light' we talked (a lot) about angles of deviation (d) and how they will vary depending on the apical angle of the prism (and angles of light). In this section, we will begin to consider the **power** of the prism (P), which is measured in **prism dioptres (denoted as pd or $^\Delta$)**. In simple terms, the power of a prism dictates the light-deviating capabilities of the prism, and it can be calculated by considering the distance (y) and the displacement (x) of the image. Fig. 9.8 uses a right-angled prism to help illustrate an example of the differences between these two terms.

In order to calculate prismatic power (P), we can use Equation 9.5, but it's really important to remember that **with prisms, all the units need to be in centimetres** (not metres!):

Equation 9.5

$$P = (100)\left(\frac{x}{y}\right)$$

Equation 9.5 (explained)

$$prismatic\ power = (100) \times \left(\frac{displacement}{distance}\right)$$

Now, if you were a huge fan of maths when you did your secondary school exams, then you may have already realised that because the angle of deviation (d), the distance (y), and the displacement (x) all form part of a right-angled triangle,

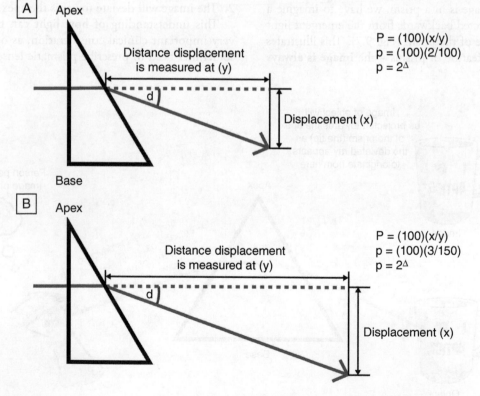

A   Apex

Distance displacement is measured at (y)

d

Displacement (x)

Base

P = (100)(x/y)
p = (100)(2/100)
p = 2$^\Delta$

B   Apex

Distance displacement is measured at (y)

d

Displacement (x)

P = (100)(x/y)
p = (100)(3/150)
p = 2$^\Delta$

• **Fig. 9.8** In this image, a right-angled prism is deviating light (red line) towards the base of the prism at a set angle of deviation (d). In both examples, the prism possesses the same power (2$^\Delta$) but in (A) the displacement (x) is measured at a shorter distance (y), which means the displacement is less than that in (B). This is because the angle of deviation (d) is constant and so trigonometry teaches us that the distance and displacement are intrinsically related.

we can of course use trigonometry to show the relationship between these three numbers. If you revise some trigonometry with me in Fig. 9.9, you'll be able to see that we know the adjacent (distance) and opposite (displacement) sides of the triangle, which means we can use tan to solve for the angle or side lengths.

However, what's cool about this is that we know from Equation 9.5 that the division of the displacement over distance is part of how we calculate prismatic power, which means that we can also substitute in our angle of deviation (d) to calculate prismatic power (P) using Equation 9.6:

Equation 9.6 $P = (100)(\tan d)$

Equation 9.6 (explained)

$$prismatic\ power = (100) \times (\tan\ angle\ of\ dev.)$$

Now we can also determine that the power of the prism is related to the angle of deviation – which makes sense because logic tells us that if prisms deviate light, then the power of the prism should dictate how much deviation occurs. Using Equation 9.6, you can see that large angles of deviation (d) will produce large powers (P), and vice versa.

However, one final link we need to make is between the angle of deviation and the apical angle (a). As we learned in chapter 2, the refractive index of a material will dictate the amount of refraction that occurs at the boundary of the surface of the material. With prisms, this means the refractive index will have a role in determining how light is deviated. We also know from chapter 2 that the distance light travels will determine its vergence as it approaches a surface, and so we can also deduce that the distance between the first and second surfaces of the prism will also have a role in how light is deviated as it leaves the prism. Importantly, this distance between the first and second surface of the prism is intrinsically linked to the size of the apical angle. It should come as no big surprise then to learn that we can use Equation 9.7 to calculate the angle of deviation:

Equation 9.7 $d = (n_p - n_s) \times a$

Equation 9.7 (explained)

$$dev. = (refr.\ index\ prism - \\ refr.\ index\ surround) \times\ pical\ ang.$$

Crucially, the take-home message here is that increasing the apical angle (and thereby increasing the distance between the first and second surface, along with the size of the base of the prism), will also increase the angle of deviation and therefore increase the overall power of the prism.

So, in summary, chunky prisms will have more power and deviate light to a greater extent than their narrow counterparts.

Prismatic Lenses and Base Notation

Clinically, it's important to understand how prisms refract light, because they may be prescribed for patients who experience **diplopia (double vision)**. Diplopia typically arises because the visual axes of the eyes are not exactly aligned, which means that the image of the world falls in two, distinct regions of the retina in each eye (Fig. 9.10).

In some cases, these patients may be able to have their vision corrected, but in cases where the eye is unable to be straightened effectively, one of the ways to reduce the impact of diplopia is to prescribe a prismatic lens to deviate the light to make it fall on the corresponding part of the retina, relative to the other eye (Fig. 9.11).

Remember that in the section titled "Deviation of Light" we learned that light always deviates towards the base of the prism? This means that, in general, it's *relatively* straightforward to determine the direction the prism would need to be oriented in order to deviate the light in the right direction (once we understand the principles of course). In Fig. 9.11,

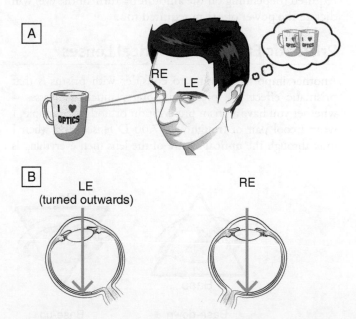

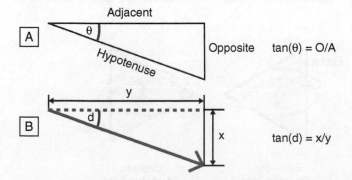

• **Fig. 9.9** Diagram showing revision of right-angled triangles (A) so that we can understand how to apply trigonometry to the distance and displacement from the deviated light leaving the prism (B).

• **Fig. 9.10** Diagram showing diplopia (double vision) affecting a patient whose left eye is turned outwards (A). This causes the light to fall on different parts of the retina of each eye B), producing two images of the object.

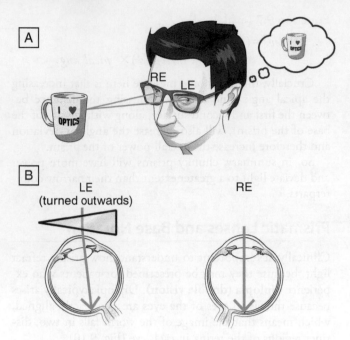

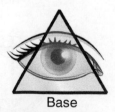 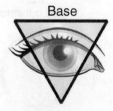 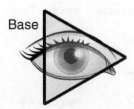 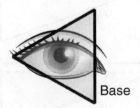

• **Fig. 9.11** Diagram showing diplopia (double vision) can be corrected by prescribing a prismatic lens (A). This causes the light to deviate towards the base, which means the light falls on corresponding parts of the retina of each eye (B).

the left eye (LE) is turned outwards, which means the light needs to be deviated inwards in order to match the right eye (RE). This means we need the base of the prism to be near the inner side of the eye in order to deviate the light in that direction, so we call this a 'base-in' prism. Fig. 9.12 shows the notation for types of base.

It's good to also remember that the amount of deviation required (depending on the amount of 'turn' of the eye) will dictate the power of prism required too.

Prismatic Effects in Spherical Lenses

Another important feature to consider with prisms is that prismatic effects are present in pretty much all glasses – whether you have a prism prescription or not! For example, I wear a cool pair of (roughly) −7.00 D lenses, and when I look through the **optical centre** of the lens then everything is

clear and in focus. However, if my glasses slip down my nose (as is their vocation in life) then my eyeline will stop corresponding to the optical centre and will instead be looking through a different region entirely, which induces **prismatic effects** as it begins to deviate the light inappropriately (Fig. 9.13).

These prismatic effects are present in both positively powered and negatively powered lenses and can be understood simply in terms of the basic shape of the lens. Fig. 9.14 shows the cross-section of two lenses, and highlights that an example positive lens and an example negative lens could be represented (simply) as two prism-shaped lenses instead.

The amount of prismatic power at various distances from the optical centre of a spherical lens can be calculated using **Prentice's rule**, which takes into account the distance **in cm** from the optical centre (**decentration − c**) and the **power of the lens (F)** – see Equation 9.8:

Equation 9.8 $$P = cF$$

Equation 9.8 (explained)

$$prism\ power = decentration \times lens\ power$$

DEMO QUESTION 9.5

How much prism power will be induced if a patient looks through their +5.00 D lens 6 mm left of the optical centre?

Step 1: Determine what we need to calculate prismatic power, P

Step 2: Define variables
F = +5.00 *(lens power)*
c = 0.6 cm *(decentration converted to cm)*

Step 3: Determine necessary equation
P = cF *(Equation 9.8)*

Step 4: Calculate
P = cF
P = 0.6 × 5
P = 3$^\Delta$

(don't forget the units!)

Practice Questions:

9.5.1 How much prism power will be induced if a patient looks through their −2.50 D lens 2 mm left of the optical centre?

9.5.2 How much prism power will be induced if a patient looks through their +4.25 DS lens 1 mm right of the optical centre?

Base-down
(deviates light
downwards)

Base-up
(deviates light
upwards)

Base-out
(deviates light
outwards)

Base-in
(deviates light
inwards)

• **Fig. 9.12** Illustration of notation for prism directions.

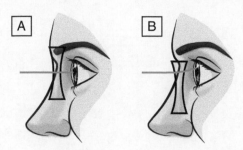

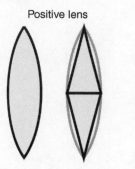

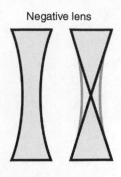

• **Fig. 9.13** Side view of a person wearing negative lenses. When looking through the optical centre, light focuses appropriately (A), but if looking through part of the lens nearer the edge, then prismatic effects can be induced (B).

Positive lens   Negative lens

• **Fig. 9.14** Lenses induce prismatic effects that get greater as you move away from the optical centre of the lens.

Test Your Knowledge

Try the questions below to see if you need to go over any sections again. All answers are available in the back of the book.

TYK.9.1 Will light deviate towards the base or the apex of the prism?

TYK.9.2 What is the 'critical angle'?

TYK.9.3 If a prism were submerged in water, would it deviate light differently from in air? Explain your answer.

TYK.9.4 Would increasing the apical angle increase the power of the prism or decrease it?

Physical Optics

10

Superposition, Interference and Diffraction

CHAPTER OUTLINE

OBJECTIVES

After working through this chapter, you should be able to:

Explain the key features of a wave (wavelength, phase, amplitude)

Explain the difference between phase difference and path difference

Define the terms 'superposition', 'interference' and 'diffraction'

Explain what a diffraction pattern looks like

Explain real-world examples of interference to your friends

Introduction

At this point in the textbook, we have almost exclusively considered light to be travelling in straight lines, and we've been discussing principles of **geometric optics**. However, as we touched on in chapter 1, some phenomena can only be explained by thinking of light as a wave, which is why we consider light to exhibit **wave-particle duality**. This principle highlights that it's important for us to start thinking about the wave-like properties of light (**physical optics**). This chapter aims to take you through the fundamental principles of physical optics and introduce **superposition**, **interference** and **diffraction**.

Features of a Single Wave

To start with, let's review what makes up a wave and some of the key terminologies. Fig. 10.1 shows the **peaks/crests** as the top of the wave, with the **troughs** being the bottom of the wave. It also shows the difference between the **wavelength** (distance between two corresponding points on a wave), **amplitude** (maximum distance from the equilibrium

point (centre line) to the peak or trough of a wave), and **frequency** (number of **cycles** per second).

As a general rule, the energy of a wave is related to the wavelength (λ) and the amplitude (A). As we learned in chapter 1, as wavelength increases, energy decreases, and as wavelength decreases, energy increases (Equation 10.1),

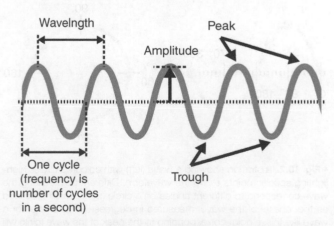

• **Fig. 10.1** Diagram showing key features of a wave.

showing that wavelength and energy have an inverse relationship (as one gets bigger, the other gets smaller).

Equation 10.1 $E = \dfrac{hc}{\lambda}$

Equation 10.1 (explained)

$$energy = \dfrac{Plancks\ constant \times speed\ of\ light}{wavelength\ of\ light}$$

In terms of amplitude, however, the rules are a little more straightforward, because as amplitude increases, energy also increases. In fact, as the amplitude is doubled, the energy of the wave will be quadrupled, as shown by Equation 10.2.

Equation 10.2 $E \propto A^2$

Equation 10.2 (explained)

$$energy\ (is\ proportional\ to)\ amplitude^2$$

The final feature of a wave to discuss is the phase – defined as the location of a point on the wave within a cycle. I find this is made clearer if we imagine the wave is a point rolling on the edge of a wheel, like shown in Fig. 10.2. Here you can see that at the peak of this wave, its phase corresponds to 90°, and as half a wavelength corresponds to half a phase cycle, the bottom of the trough will be 180° further round, making it correspond to a phase of 270°.

Features of Multiple Waves

What happens if more than one wave exists within the same space? We know that white light from the sun, for example, is made up of all the wavelengths of visible light, and we know that we could shine two laser lights at the same spot on a wall (if we felt so inclined) – so what happens to the waves when they meet? Well, when two waves meet each other, they will overlap and interact in a process called **superposition**. This means that the waves will kind of mix together to form a **resultant wave** – and this resultant wave

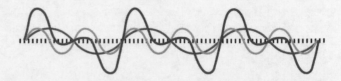

• **Fig. 10.3** Two smaller-amplitude waves (blue) are interacting (superposition) to form a resultant wave (pink).

will have a larger or smaller amplitude than the individual waves, depending on how they interact. Fig. 10.3 shows an example where two smaller-amplitude waves (blue) are interacting to form a resultant wave (pink).

Now, let's go back to think about our extremely common example of shining two lasers at the same spot on a wall. The cool feature of lasers is that they possess only a single wavelength. This means that a red laser, for example, will only output light of a single wavelength in the 'red' end of the spectrum (around 700 nm). If we have two identical lasers then, the waves produced will be identical in their wavelength (and therefore frequency), which would make them **coherent**. If we shine one laser at a point on the wall, depending on the distance, it will arrive at a specified point (phase) of the cycle (Fig. 10.4A). If we add another laser and shine it at the same point on the wall, and if it is the exact same distance away, it will arrive **in phase** (at the same point in the cycle; Fig. 10.4B). However, if the distance of the second laser pointer from the wall is varied, then the second wave will arrive at a different point in the phase and will be **out of phase** with the first wave (Fig. 10.4C).

For waves to be considered to be **in phase** with one another, they either need to have travelled exactly the same distance or have travelled a distance that results in a 0° or 360° separation. If the waves travel any other distance, resulting in any other degree of phase separation, then they can be described as being out of phase, and the amount of separation between the waves is called the **phase difference**.

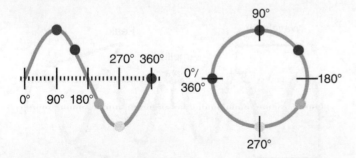

• **Fig. 10.2** Illustration showing a wave (left) with coloured circles highlighting specific points along the waveform. Different points along the wave correspond to different angles on a circle (right) which is defined as the 'phase' of the wave, measured in degrees. For example, for a wave like this, a point corresponding to the peak of the wave (pink) will be at 90° phase.

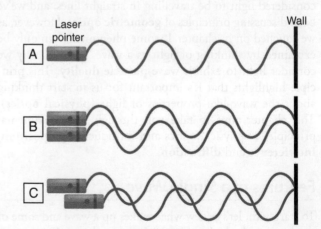

• **Fig. 10.4** If a single laser is shone at a wall, it will produce light (A). However, if several laser pointers are shone at a wall, they may arrive at different points in the phase of the wave. If they arrive at the same point in the phase, they are **in phase** (B), whereas if they arrive at different points in the phase, they are **out of phase** (C). See text for more details.

Importantly, if multiple waves meet and interact with one another, then they produce **interference**, defined as the variation in wave amplitude that occurs when multiple waves interact. Let's consider a hypothetical example in which we have two identical light sources producing two identical waves (like with the laser pointers before). If the two waves are in phase, then the amplitudes will add together to increase the amplitude of the resultant wave, which is considered **complete constructive interference** (I like to remember this by thinking that it 'constructs' a taller amplitude) (Fig. 10.5A) and will produce a bright light (**maxima**). However, if the waves are 180° out of phase (meaning the peaks of one wave line up with the troughs of another wave) then the amplitudes will add together to produce a net amplitude of zero, meaning they cancel each other out. This is called **complete destructive interference** (Fig. 10.5B) and will produce an absence of light (**minima**).

When we talk about waves, we can discuss their phase difference (as before) or their path difference. This means that whilst phase difference can be expressed in degrees of separation in phase, **path difference** is defined as the difference in distance travelled between the two waves and is therefore expressed relative to the wavelength (λ). For constructive interference to occur, we know that we need the waves to be in phase, which means that either they need to travel the same distance (path difference 0λ), or they need to travel a distance that equates to a whole multiple of the wavelength (path difference 1λ, 2λ, 3λ, ... $n\lambda$). However, with destructive interference, we know the waves will be 180° out of phase, meaning that one will have travelled half a wavelength further (path difference 0.5λ) or any multiple

of this that isn't a whole number (path difference 1.5λ, 2.5λ, 3.5λ, ... $n+0.5\lambda$). This means that if you slowly increase the path difference between two waves, it will cycle through constructive interference (0λ), destructive interference (0.5λ), constructive interference (1λ), and so on. The exciting part of this is that it means if we have two coherent light sources (identical wavelength and frequency) then we can utilise the amount of interference to measure small differences in distance.

Utilising Interference to Measure Distances

Let's imagine we have our two hypothetical, identical light sources again, both producing identical waves of light. If we asked someone to shine them at a wall so that they interfered with one another, and then measured the resultant wave at the wall, we would be able to tell whether they were producing constructive or destructive interference and therefore be able to identify whether there was a path difference. In a classic experimental set-up, the 'Michelson interferometer', a single laser light source is shone at a beam splitter to produce two, identical waves. These waves then reflect back off mirrors to meet at a detector which can measure the amount of interference (Fig. 10.6). If you move one of the mirrors by a distance that equates to 0.25 of the wavelength of light, then the wave that reflects off that mirror will have to travel 0.5λ further than the other to reach the detector (0.25λ more to reach the mirror and then 0.25λ more to travel back). This would produce destructive interference at the

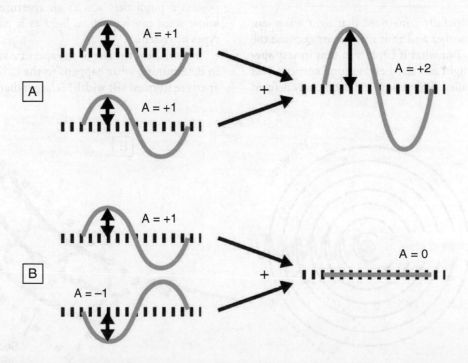

A = +1
A = +1
A = +2

A = +1
A = -1
A = 0

• **Fig. 10.5** Diagram showing two identical waves (left) interacting to produce a resultant wave (right). If the waves are in phase (A) then the amplitude of the resultant wave will increase to the sum of the contributing waves (complete constructive interference). However, if the waves are 180° out of phase (B) then the amplitude of the resultant wave will be cancelled out (complete destructive interference).

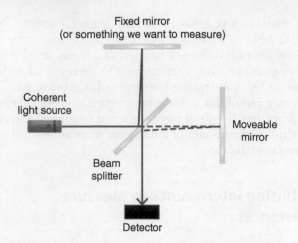

Fixed mirror
(or something we want to measure)

Coherent
light source

Moveable
mirror

Beam
splitter

Detector

• **Fig. 10.6** An example set-up for a Michelson interferometer. The beam splitter allows some light to pass through to the moveable mirror whilst reflecting the rest of the light towards the stationary mirror.

detector. Now, imagine if the stationary mirror in this set-up was at a distance we didn't know – for example, if we were wanting to measure the distance between the front of an eye to the retina (axial length). By moving the second mirror back and forth, the interference pattern at the detector will change relative to the distance the light has travelled to the back of the eye, and hence we can determine the distance (in this case axial length). This (in very simple terms) is the fundamental principle of how optical coherence tomography (OCT) works, which will be discussed in chapter 17.

Diffraction

OK so now we're hopefully convinced that light waves can interfere with one another and thus increase or decrease the resultant amplitude. But what if I told you that in very specific circumstances, light can also bend around corners? This bending of light is called **diffraction** and is officially defined

as: the bending of waves around corners of an obstacle (or edges of an aperture) into regions that should (according to the rectilinear propagation of light) produce shadows.

In order to understand how diffraction occurs, we first need to take a step back to learn a little bit more about the theory of **wavefronts**. We touched on wavefronts in chapter 2 in relation to vergence (remember the more curved the wavefront, the higher the vergence, and so flat wavefronts imply a light source is an infinite distance away). Importantly, the wavefronts can be thought of as corresponding to the peak of a wave, and we can understand how they propagate light by understanding **Huygen's principle** (also called Huygen's construction). This principle asserts that at every point of a wavefront there is a source of secondary waves – a little bit like if we imagine that every single point on a wavefront is a source of a new, smaller wavefront called a **wavelet** (I promise I'm not making this up) (Fig. 10.7B). The envelope (shape) of all of these wavelets will form the secondary wavefront of the main light source.

Now, when these wavefronts are incident upon a corner of an obstacle, it's easy to imagine that light will be stopped by the obstacle and create a shadow, as shown in Fig. 10.8A. However, as Huygen's principle asserts that each wavefront will possess several sweet little wavelets, the envelope of which will determine the next (secondary) wavefront, then this means there will be a small amount of overlap at the edges (Fig. 10.8B), which would then potentially allow the light to bend around the corner.

In terms of optometry and dispensing optics, we care about this because diffraction also occurs when light passes through an **aperture** (a hole or **slit**), and as the human eye possess a pupil that acts as an aperture, it's important to know what can happen to light as it passes through these types of systems.

Importantly, the size of the aperture will play a huge part in determining what happens to the light. If the size of the aperture (termed **slit width**) is larger than the wavelength of

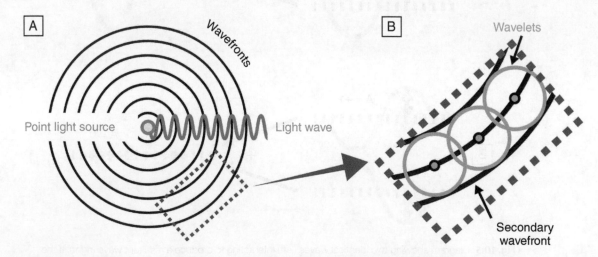

Wavefronts

Point light source

Light wave

Wavelets

Secondary wavefront

• **Fig. 10.7** Diagram showing how each wavefront (see A) will possess wavelets (small sources of secondary wavefronts; see B). The next (secondary wavefront) will correspond to the envelope of the wavelets. Please note that although this diagram only shows three wavelets, you should try to imagine they exist at every single point along the wavefront.

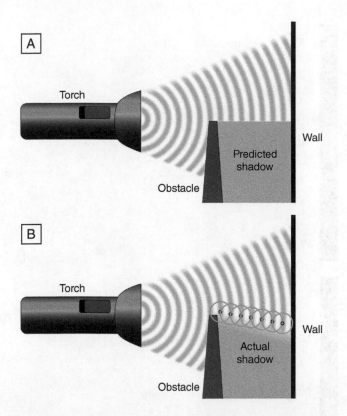

• **Fig. 10.8** Diagram showing difference between shadow predicted by rectilinear propagation of light (A) and actual shadow produced (B) (explained by Huygen's principle).

the light, then light will pass through unimpeded; however, if the slit width is smaller than the wavelength of light then it will produce diffraction (Fig. 10.9).

Single Slit Diffraction

In the previous section, we learned that when light passes through a slit with a slit width smaller than the wavelength of the light, diffraction occurs – but what does this look like? Well, when light is diffracted, it produces a **diffraction pattern** – a mathematically predictable pattern of light that contains bright spots (**maxima**) and dark areas (**minima**) that are produced by different levels of interference on the other side of the slit. In Fig. 10.10, you can see that light of a particular wavelength is passing through a slit (and let's assume it's undergoing diffraction) – as the light only passes through one slit, this is called **single slit diffraction**. Single slit diffraction predicts that at the point on a wall corresponding to the area directly in front of the slit, all the light waves will arrive **in phase** and therefore produce **constructive interference** (bright maxima). However, in the area adjacent to this area, the waves from each edge of the slit will travel slightly different distances which leads to a path difference; when this path difference corresponds to a difference equal to n + 0.5λ, then the light will arrive at the wall **out of phase,** and **destructive interference** will occur (dark minima).

This pattern repeats itself as you get farther away from the central maxima, but intensity and size of the maxima

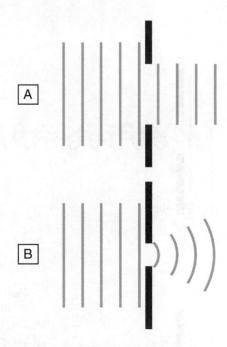

• **Fig. 10.9** Diagram showing that large slit widths do not produce diffraction (A). The slit width must be smaller than the wavelength to produce diffraction (B).

decrease as the path difference becomes increasingly large (Fig. 10.11).

Mathematically, we can calculate the path difference (ΔD) of the light by using trigonometry (I can tell you're getting excited about this – see Fig. 10.12). All we need to know is the angle of diffraction (φ) and the slit width (a). To calculate the angle of diffraction we can use Equation 10.3, and to calculate the path difference we can use Equation 10.4.

Equation 10.3 $\sin \phi = \dfrac{y}{\sqrt{L^2 + y^2}}$

Equation 10.3 (explained)

$$\sin(ang.\,diff.) = \dfrac{dist.\,btw\ maxima}{\sqrt{slit\,/\,wall\ dist.^2 + dist.\,btw\ maxima^2}}$$

Equation 10.4 $\sin \phi = \dfrac{\Delta D}{a}$

Equation 10.4 (explained)

$$\sin(ang.\,diffr.) = \dfrac{path\ diff.}{slit\ width}$$

DEMO QUESTION 10.1

A single slit is placed 20 cm in front of a wall. If the first and second maxima are 10 cm apart from one another, what is the angle of diffraction?

Step 1: Determine what we need to calculate
angle of diffraction, φ

Step 2: Define variables
L = 0.2 m *(converted to metres)*

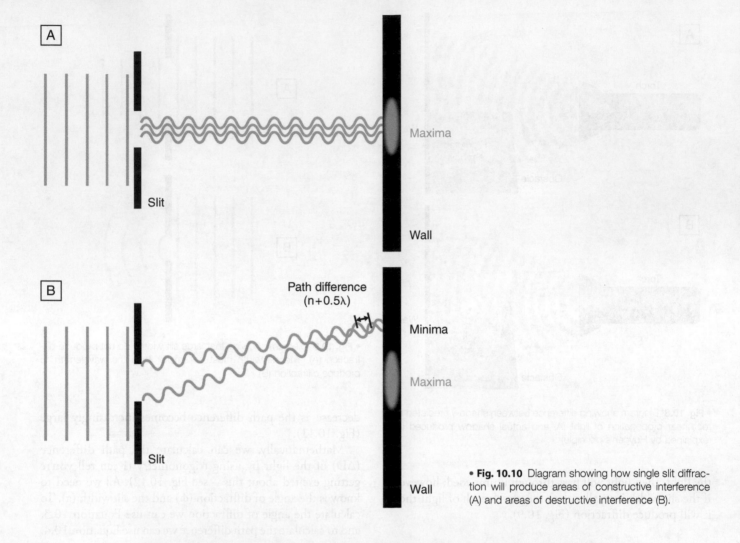

• Fig. 10.10 Diagram showing how single slit diffraction will produce areas of constructive interference (A) and areas of destructive interference (B).

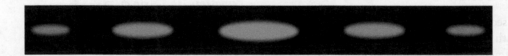

• Fig. 10.11 Example diffraction pattern produced by single slit diffraction.

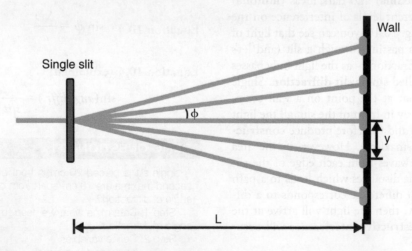

• Fig. 10.12 Diagram showing relationship between maxima distance (y), wall distance (L), and angle of diffraction (φ).

Practice Questions 10.1:

10.1.1 A single slit is placed 40 cm in front of a wall. If the first and second maxima are 8 cm apart from one another, what is the angle of diffraction?

10.1.2 A single slit is placed 55 cm in front of a wall. If the first and second maxima are 18 cm apart from one another, what is the angle of diffraction?

Multiple Slit Diffraction

Now, in the wonderful world of optics, it's possible to diffract one light source through multiple slits[1] (as opposed to just one as outlined in the previous section). The difference is that when we increase the number of slits, we create **interference patterns** at the wall that coincide with the **diffraction pattern** (Fig. 10.13).

This is because the light coming from each slit acts as its own light source (in a way) which adds the interference pattern on top of the diffraction pattern, and these combine to produce the resultant pattern that will have areas of minima within the maxima (Fig. 10.14).

It's also possible to diffract light through an item called a **diffraction grating** – which essentially describes a small film that comprises a number of slits all in a line next to each other. Importantly, for this to work in diffraction terms, these lines need to be *extremely* close together and so often that it's not possible to see the slits in a diffraction grating with your naked eye. These gratings are usually labelled as the number of lines per mm, and as a general rule of thumb, the more lines per mm, the smaller the gap (**slit width**) between them (e.g. 600 lines per mm would have a smaller slit width than 300 lines per mm). Diffraction gratings are used in optical systems to measure and separate wavelengths of light, as different wavelengths will diffract differently through the grating. This is because the slit width plays a huge part in the angle of diffraction (Equation 10.4), and we learned in the section titled 'Diffraction' that the slit must be smaller than the wavelength in order to produce diffraction – thereby indicating that the smaller the width (relative to the wavelength), the greater amount of diffraction. This suggests long wavelength light (e.g. red) will diffract more than short wavelength light (e.g. blue), which is the opposite to what we'd expect for dispersion (see chapter 8).

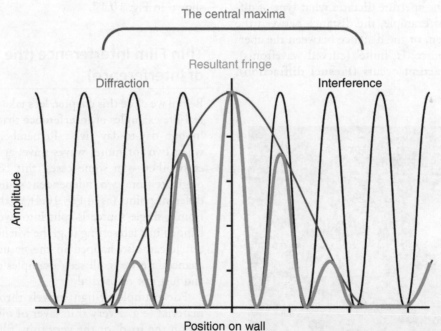

• **Fig. 10.13** A diagrammatic explanation of how multiple slits will add an interference pattern (black) on top of the diffraction pattern (pink) to produce minima within the maxima in the resultant fringe (blue).

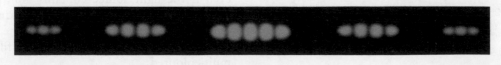

• **Fig. 10.14** Example diffraction pattern produced by double slit diffraction.

Diffraction of white light through a grating can be viewed in a demo in the associated video content on the Elsevier website, a screenshot from which is shown in Fig. 10.15.

Circular Diffraction

The previous examples of diffraction all assume that the slit (or aperture) is a long, thin aperture. For example, if I taped two pieces of card very close together to produce a single (very narrow) slit, I could produce a diffraction pattern if I shone a laser pointer at the slit (and in fact I have done this before, much to the amazement of a handful of students!). The principle of diffraction suggests that light will bend around the corners of the slit, which is why the diffraction pattern spreads out at an angle perpendicular to the angle of the slit. For example, a vertical slit will produce a horizontal diffraction pattern.

However, diffraction can also occur for **circular apertures** (which more easily applies the principles of diffraction to optical systems which possess circular apertures, e.g. cameras and telescopes). In these cases, the circular aperture would need to be very small in diameter (in order to be smaller than the wavelength of light), but this will allow the light to diffract in all directions around the edges of the circle! This means that instead of the flattish, single orientation diffraction pattern we see with the narrow slit (see Fig. 10.11), we get fun circular diffraction patterns as shown in Fig. 10.16. The other cool thing about these types of diffraction patterns is that the distance the light travels on the other side of the aperture dictates what type of diffraction occurs. If, for example, the distance between the aperture and the screen, or the distance between the aperture and the light source, is 'finite' (curved wavefronts), then **near-field diffraction** occurs (**Fresnel diffraction**),

whereas if the screen and light sources are at 'infinite' distances away from the aperture (planar wavefronts), then **far-field diffraction** occurs (**Fraunhofer diffraction**). The pattern produced by Fraunhofer diffraction is called an **airy disc**, and this is important in terms of diffraction because it defines the smallest point at which a light source can be focused, and therefore is associated with the resolvable power of any optical system.

The Resolving Power of a System

As we have just alluded to, diffraction is an important concept because the **resolution** (highest resolving power) of all optical systems will be limited by its aperture size, and this relationship is due to diffraction. Typically, although a smaller aperture will increase the resolution (by removing aberrations – see chapter 16 for more detail on aberrations), at a certain degree of smallness, light will diffract around the edges of the aperture and reduce the resolution again. The point at which resolution is highest but diffraction doesn't occur is called the **diffraction-limit** of the system, and this also applies to the pupil of the human eye. Interestingly, this minimum resolvable power (diffraction-limit) of an imaging system can be determined using the **Rayleigh criterion**. This proposes that two overlapping images (airy discs) will only become distinguishable from one another when separated at a distance such that the centre of the zero-order (central) maxima of one disc lines up with the first minima of the other. This principle is shown in Fig. 10.17.

Thin Film Interference (the Fun Side of Interference)

Before we close this chapter, let's take a moment to think of real-life examples of **interference** that we might experience in our day-to-day lives. Remember, interference occurs when two (or more) waves travel at different distances to each other – in some cases, this could be because they originate from two independent sources that are located at different points (as in Fig. 10.4), or this can happen if light from a single source is split into two (or more). This can happen in a lab setting (e.g. the Michelson interferometer), but it can also happen in the natural environment, and chances are we've all seen examples of interference before and just not realised it!

For example, if light travels through a thin film of a material (e.g. a very thin layer of oil on top of some water on the road, or the very thin 'film' of a soap bubble), then interference can occur. In these circumstances, even if there is only one light source (e.g. from the sun), and even if the light source contains multiple wavelengths (of visible light), something called **thin film interference** takes place, which can make the light reflecting off the front and back surface of the film appear to be multicoloured.

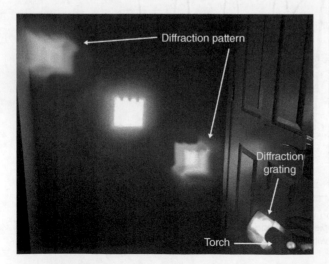

• **Fig. 10.15** Photograph showing white light passing through a diffraction grating. Long wavelength (red) light will diffract at a larger angle relative to shorter (blue) wavelength light, so the diffraction pattern shows the splitting of light from blue-red as we move away from the central maxima.

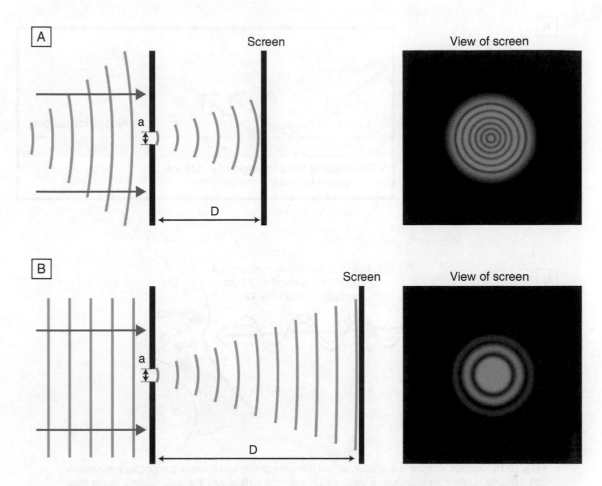

• **Fig. 10.16** Illustration of Fresnel diffraction (A; curved wavefronts) and Fraunhofer diffraction (B; planar wavefronts) with a circular aperture.

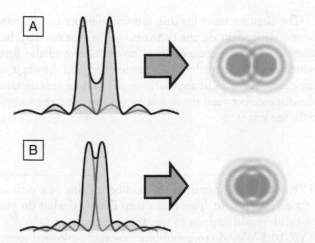

• **Fig. 10.17** Diagram illustrating the Rayleigh criterion. If two images (airy discs) are farther apart than the radii of their central maxima, then they are easily resolvable (A). The smallest distance they can be separated by whilst still being resolvable is determined by the Rayleigh criterion which dictates that this smallest resolvable power occurs when the images are separated at a distance such that the centre of the zero-order (central) maxima of one disc lines up with the first minima of the other (B). In both images, the blue lines indicate the intensity profiles of the individual images, whilst the black lines show the 'visible' profile.

To understand this better, let's stick with the soap bubble example (but the same is true for the oil on the water in the road). Thin film interference occurs because, as the incident white light reaches the 'film' of the bubble, some of the light reflects at the front surface of the film whilst some passes through to the back surface. Then at the back surface, some light transmits through, but some is reflected back again, which means that even though we started with one light source, there will be (in this case) two waves that reflect back towards us (the observer). This means that we'll have two waves reaching us, one of which has now travelled a slightly greater distance than the first as it's been to the back surface of the film (Fig. 10.18A). If the second wave (reflecting off the back surface) travels a whole multiple of the wavelength farther than the first wave (**in phase**), then **constructive interference** is observed (light), whereas if the second wave travels a half multiple of the wavelength farther than the first wave (**out of phase**), then **destructive interference** is observed (no light). Remember, though, with white light (from the sun), the light comprises many wavelengths of light (from violet to red), and so as the white light reflects at both the front and back surfaces of the soap bubble film, sometimes the long wavelengths will be in phase, and other

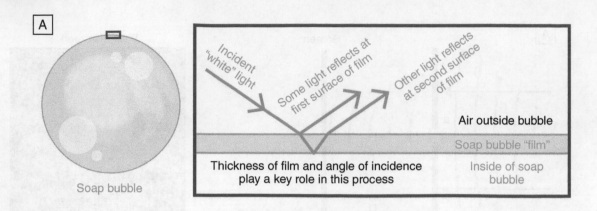

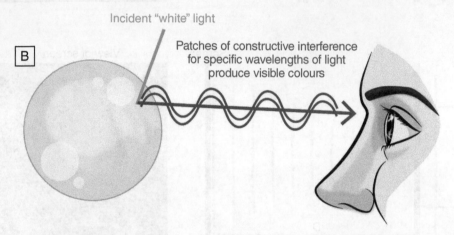

• **Fig. 10.18** Diagram showing explanation of how thin film interference makes soap bubbles look remarkably colourful. Light from a source reflects at both the front surface and the back surface of the soap bubble (A), which produces constructive or destructive interference depending on path difference. Areas of constructive interference produce a reflection that appears to be the colour associated with those wavelengths (B) (e.g. red).

times the shorter wavelengths will be in phase. This produces an interference pattern which splits the white light into its constituent wavelengths and produces a multicoloured appearance on the soap bubble (or the oil on the water) (Fig. 10.18B)! You can also see this for yourself in a demonstration at home if you read the instructions in chapter 23 later in the book.

The circumstances for thin film interference to occur are largely dependent on the thickness of the film (as that dictates how far the second wave travels relative to the first, which in turn determines the interference) and the angle of incidence of the light approaching the film (as this dictates the distance between the first reflected wave and the second reflected wave).

Test Your Knowledge

Try the questions below to see if you need to review any sections. All answers are available in the back of the book.

TYK.10.1 What is the 'phase' of a wave?

TYK.10.2 If two identical waves are 180° 'out of phase', what will happen?

TYK.10.3 What does Huygen's principle predict about light when it gets blocked by an obstacle?

TYK.10.4 If we increased the number of slits in a diffraction experiment from one slit to five slits, what do you think would happen to the diffraction pattern?

TYK.10.5 Why do soap bubbles look multicoloured sometimes?

Reference

1. Young T. The Bakerian lecture. Experiments and calculation relative to physical optics. *Philos Trans R Soc Lond.* 1804;94:1-16.

Clinical Applications

11

Focimetry

OBJECTIVES

After working through this chapter, you should be able to:

Explain what focimetry is

Discuss the principles underlying focimetry

Be able to link focimetry with your understanding of spherical and cylindrical refractive errors (see chapter 5)

Introduction

In this chapter we're going to think about lenses and how we can measure the power of lenses using an instrument called a **focimeter** (internationally it is also known as a lensometer – but they are the same thing). This chapter will be most useful to you if you have access to a focimeter to try out the theory and have a go, but it will still (hopefully) be interesting even if you can't apply it practically.

What Is a Focimeter?

A focimeter is a device that can be used to determine the spherical power, cylindrical power (and corresponding axis), prismatic power and the optical centre of a lens. You may be thinking, why on Earth would we need a device that does that? But in practice this is an important instrument which allows clinicians to measure the power of a patient's glasses, even if the patient themselves doesn't know their prescription. It also allows dispensing opticians to check the power of lenses before dispensing them to patients.

In broad terms, there are three main types of focimeter:
1. Conventional (eyepiece focusing)
2. Projection (screen focused)
3. Automatic electronic (automated)

In this chapter we will focus on the first type – the conventional focimeter – but it's good to be aware that other types exist.

How Does a Focimeter Work?

The focimeter itself requires two main parts – a **focusing system** (collimator, which narrows the beam of light)

and an **observation system** (telescope, which focuses the image for the user); see Fig. 11.1 for a schematic of this. The focusing system itself aims to produce an image of the **target** (illuminated lines) overlaid onto a **graticule** (a pattern of lines in an optical device used as a measuring scale; sometimes called a reticle) and project it to infinity. As the focimeter is used to measure a large range of lens powers, logic tells us that the target (acting as the object) will need to be moveable in order to position the target (acting as an object) at the correct location so as to project it to infinity. However, for the focimeter to work correctly, the eyepiece of the observation system also needs to be focused for your eyes (to account for any uncorrected prescription you might have) before you introduce the lens you're trying to measure. This will mean that the target and graticule are all lovely and in focus (Fig. 11.2).

Assuming that the eyepiece of the focimeter is focused appropriately for the user, the user can place a patient's spectacle lens onto the **lens (frame) rest** (Fig. 11.3). Importantly, the back surface of the lens should be sitting on the lens rest and will need to be clamped into position in order to provide an accurate reading. However, it's also important to note that before clamping the lens, it will need to be moved upwards/downwards and leftwards/rightwards until the target is visibly aligned with the centre of the graticule. At this point, the user will have located the **optical centre** of the lens, and most focimeters have a process for allowing the user to mark this point on the lens (to help later on). It's important to find the optical centre, because this is the point where no prismatic effect will be introduced (see chapter 9 for review on this) and so the power will be able to be accurately determined.

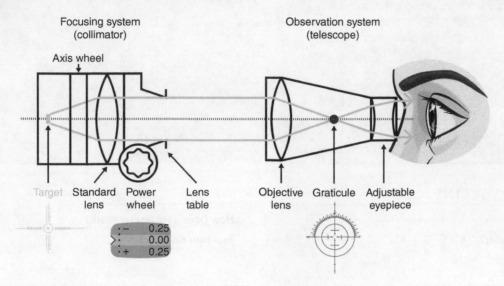

Focusing system (collimator)

Observation system (telescope)

Axis wheel

Target | Standard lens | Power wheel | Lens table | Objective lens | Graticule | Adjustable eyepiece

:−	0.25
>:	0.00
:+	0.25

• **Fig. 11.1** A schematic of a focimeter, with the focusing system (including target) on the left and the observation system (including graticule) on the right. The lens you want to measure would sit on the lens rest, in between the two systems.

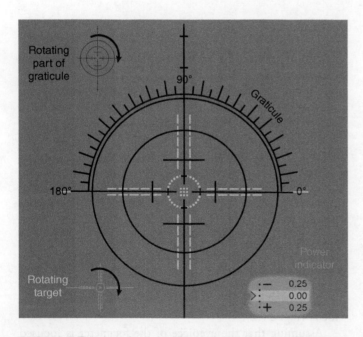

Rotating part of graticule

90°

Graticule

180°

0°

Rotating target

Power indicator

:−	0.25
>:	0.00
:+	0.25

• **Fig. 11.2** The view of an example target (green) and example graticule (black) as seen through a focimeter eyepiece. If in focus, all the lines should be completely clear.

The next step is to determine the spherical power (though this can only be achieved after the lens's optical centre has been identified). At this point (unless the lens has no power), the target will be out of focus (because the power of the lens is adding or removing positive or negative power to the target that was in focus previously). In order to determine **spherical power** and get the target back into focus, the user will need to turn the **power wheel** until the lines of the target become clear. If the lens only possesses spherical power then when the collimator part of the focimeter is correcting for the appropriate amount of power (e.g. −2.00 D), all the target lines will become clear, and the power can be read from the instrument at that point.

In terms of the target itself (the lit-up green bit), the target in our example is made up of nine three-by-three squares, a ring of circles, and then two sets of perpendicular lines. The ring of circles will remain stationary (the fixed target), whilst the squares and the lines will rotate when we turn the axis wheel (the rotating target). If we're using the focimeter to measure a spherical lens, and the focimeter is focused, the fixed target will still look like circles and the rotating part of the target will be in focus wherever it is rotated to. However,

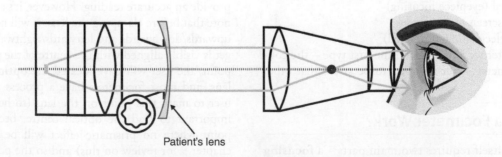

Patient's lens

• **Fig. 11.3** Diagram showing focimeter set up with a patient's lens on the lens rest.

if the lens is **toric** (meaning it has a cylindrical power as well as spherical; see chapter 5 for review on this), then it will only be possible to get some of the lines of the target into focus using the power wheel alone. If this is the case, the clue that **cylindrical power** is present will be that the ring of circles will appear stretched at a particular angle and start to resemble lines (like those shown in Fig. 11.4), even when the maximum and minimum powers are neutralised – which we'll discuss in a moment. The lines formed for these two powers will be orientated at 90° to each other, and the orientation of these lines indicate the axes for the two major power meridians, and so the fixed target allows us to locate these two meridians. The rotating target lines, which are also at 90° to each other, will only be clear when they are aligned with the lines formed by the fixed target – that is, when they are aligned to the two major meridians.

In Fig. 11.4, the target is clearly out of focus, but hopefully you can also see that the target seems to be stretched along an oblique angle. In this case, the first thing to do is to adjust the power wheel until the ring of circles (the fixed target) comes into focus to help us identify the angle of stretch. Then we can rotate the target using the **axis wheel** until the shorter target lines fall along the 'stretch' angle, as shown in Fig. 11.5.

Then, adjust the power wheel until the short lines come into focus (and are straight and unbroken – if they seem more focused but broken you may need to reassess the axis wheel) and make a note of the reading on the power wheel; however, you'll notice that even though the short lines are in focus, the longer target lines will be stretched and blurry. At this point, we need to continue to adjust the power wheel (without adjusting the axis wheel) until the longer lines come into focus (which should also blur the shorter lines

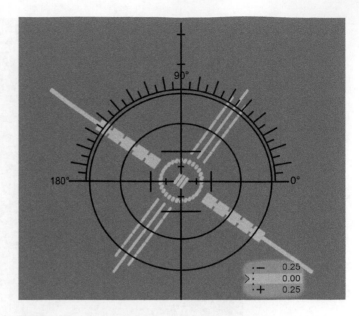

• **Fig. 11.5** The target has now been rotated so that the shorter lines of the target line up along the line of the stretch; this will help us to determine cylindrical power.

again). We then make a note of this new reading from the power wheel.

Let's say that the shorter lines were in focus at −2.50 and the longer lines were in focus at −3.00, with **negative sphere-cylinder form** we assume the most positive of the two powers is the spherical power of the lens, so in this example −2.50 is more positive than −3.00, which means we would say that the spherical power of this lens is −2.50 DS.

The cylindrical power can now be determined as the *difference* between the most positive and least positive powers (e.g. −2.50 D and −3.00 D would indicate a cylindrical power of −0.50 DC). The axis of the cylinder corresponds to the direction of the least positive power, which can be read by seeing where the most negatively powered lines intersect the graticule in degrees. This can be achieved by rotating the long arm of the graticule to align with these target lines to reveal the axis of the cylindrical power. See Fig. 11.6 for an example of this.

To determine whether **vertical prismatic differences** are present between the two lenses, when you switch from one lens to the other you should note whether the second lens is still able to centre the target on the centre of the graticule. If so, then no prismatic differences are present. However, if instead, the second lens has moved the target above or below the centre of the graticule, then vertical prismatic differences exist between the two lenses. The amount of prismatic difference can be determined by reading off the graticule as shown in Fig. 11.7, and if the target falls below the graticule, then there is base-down prism, and if the target falls above the graticule centre, then there is base-up prism (because prisms deviate light towards the base). However, it is still important to note that this method only identifies the total prism difference between both lenses; in order to calculate the amount of vertical prism in each lens, you would

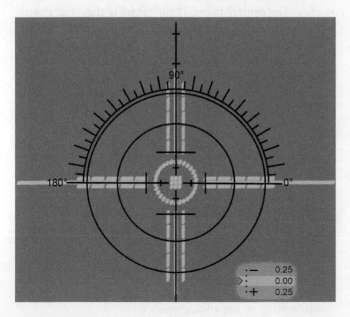

• **Fig. 11.4** Illustration of view down a focimeter. This lens has power (so the target is out of focus), and we can identify the presence of cylindrical power because the target appears to be stretched at an oblique angle.

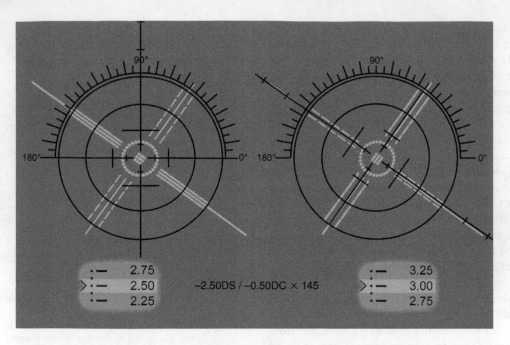

• **Fig. 11.6** A diagram showing the first reading on a focimeter (left) with the most positive power on the power wheel corresponding to the spherical power of the lens, and the second reading (right) showing the least positive power (and the axis). For negative sphere-cylinder form, the difference between the most positive power (−2.50) and the least positive power (−3.00) is taken as the cylindrical power (−0.50).

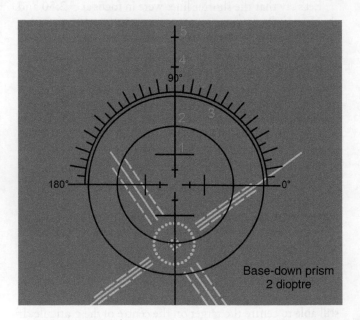

• **Fig. 11.7** A diagram showing a 2-dioptre, base-down prismatic difference between the two lenses. In this diagram, orange text has been added to help show which lines represent which prismatic power.

need to also consider the patient's pupil position relative to the optical centre for each lens.

Horizontal prism can only be determined by taking into account the patient's interpupillary distance (IPD). For example, if a patient has an IPD of 62 mm, then once you have identified the optical centre of the first lens, you can measure from this point across the IPD distance to the other lens and then position the lens on the focimeter using this mark as the central point. If the target is then not central but instead is slightly to one side, then horizontal prismatic differences are present. Again, this method only identifies the total prism difference between both lenses; in order to calculate the amount of horizontal prism in each individual lens, you would need to also consider the patient's pupil position relative to the optical centre of each lens.

Test Your Knowledge

Try the questions below to see if you need to review any sections. All answers are available in the back of the book.

TYK.11.1 What does a focimeter do?
TYK.11.2 What is the graticule?

TYK.11.3 Why is it important to focus the eyepiece before attempting to use a focimeter?
TYK.11.4 If the target falls below the centre of the graticule, would this indicate base-down or base-up prism?

12

Photometry

OBJECTIVES

After working through this chapter, you should be able to:

Explain a solid angle

Explain luminous flux, luminous intensity, illuminance and
   luminance

Describe the two laws of illumination

Explain what colour temperature is and be able to interpret
   Kelvins

Introduction

The word **photometry** can be broken down into photo-
(light) and -metry (measurement), so it should come as no
surprise then to hear that this chapter will be focused on
discussing my cats' favourite toys…

Obviously I'm joking; this chapter will explain how we
can measure light in the real world and will link this to clinical considerations where appropriate.

Angles and Lights

In the introduction, we discussed that the term photometry
means 'measurement of light', but more specifically than
that, it refers to measurement of **visible light** – the part of
the electromagnetic spectrum that is detectable by the human eye. This could include natural light (e.g. from the
sun), but more often we use photometry to discuss artificial
light sources (e.g. from a lamp). For example, if you've ever
bought a lightbulb and spent a while wondering what the
difference between the watts and the lumens are (and what
they mean), then this chapter is for you!

To start with then, let's consider a light bulb (a bog-
standard light bulb), as shown in Fig. 12.1. Here you can
clearly see that the bulb itself is emitting light in all directions
(and although this is a two-dimensional (2D) image, please
imagine it exists in three-dimensional (3D) space), meaning
that we can say it's emitting light *spherically* from its centre.
However, this means that if we want to measure the angle of
light that's being emitted by the light source, we need to be
able to determine the relevant 3D angle.

But how do we measure 3D angles? Well, let's start by
reviewing some prinicples of 2D angles. In a 2D circle, like
the one in Fig. 12.2, any **planar (flat) angle** (θ) measured
from the centre can be represented in **degrees** (°) or **radians**
(rad or r), which is typically expressed relative to pi (π). In
the example in Fig. 12.2, the angle is 90°, which Table 12.1

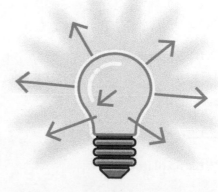

• **Fig. 12.1** Diagram of a light bulb to show that it emits light in all
directions.

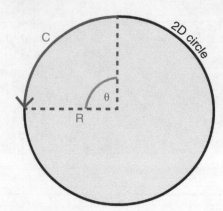

• **Fig. 12.2** Circle showing planar angle from the centre (θ) which corresponds to 90°. The distance from the apex of the angle and the circumference of the circle is equal to the radius of the circle (R). The distance along the circumference required to create the angle is called the arc (c).

TABLE 12.1	Table Showing Conversion Between Turns, Degrees and Radians in a 2D Circle	
Turns (complete revolutions of a circle)	Degrees (°)	Radians (rad)
0	0	0
0.25	90	$\pi/2$
0.5	180	π
0.75	270	$3\pi/2$
1.00	360	2π

shows us would convert to 0.25 turns around the circumference (outside edge) of the circle, or $\pi/2$ radians.

However, what if we don't know the angle? To calculate the angle we can utilise the relationship between the **radius** (R) and the **length of the arc** (c) through Equation 12.1.1 (radians) and Equation 12.1.2 (same but in degrees). Remember that because these equations use SI units, all measure of distance must be in metres (m).

Equation 12.1.1
$$\theta = \frac{c}{R}$$

Equation 12.1.1 (explained)
$$angle\ (rad) = \frac{length\ of\ arc\ (m)}{radius\ of\ circle\ (m)}$$

Equation 12.1.2
$$\theta = \frac{c}{R} \times \frac{180}{\pi}$$

Equation 12.1.2 (explained)
$$angle\ (deg) = \frac{length\ of\ arc}{radius\ of\ circle} \times \frac{180}{\pi}$$

DEMO QUESTION 12.1

Calculate the planar angle shown as '?' in the image below:

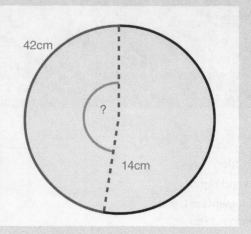

Step 1: Determine what we need to calculate
planar angle, θ
Step 2: Define variables
c = 0.42 m *(we need to convert to metres)*
R = 0.14 m *(we need to convert to metres)*
Step 3: Determine necessary equation
θ = c / R *(Equation 12.1.1)*
Step 4: Calculate
θ = c / R
θ = 0.42 / 0.14
θ = 3 radians
(now we can divide by π to understand how this number relates to π radians (π is 3.14 so it's probably going to be close to 1 π radians...))
θ = 3 / π
θ = 0.95 π rad
(or we could also convert to degrees...)
θ = c / R * (180 / π)
θ = 3 * (180 / π)
θ = 171.89°
(in either case, don't forget the units!)

Practice Questions 12.1:

12.1.1 Calculate the planar angle shown as '?' in the image below:

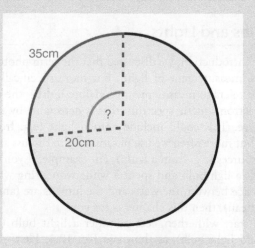

12.1.2 Calculate the planar angle shown as '?' in the image below:

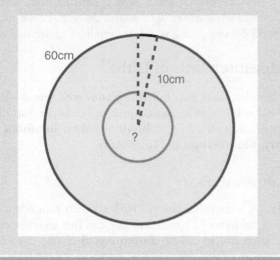

OK, so now (even if we don't like them very much), hopefully we can appreciate the link between degrees and radians for 2D angles, but we know at some point we're going to need to discuss 3D angles.

Three-dimensional angles are tricky. To make them a little less tricky, let's start by considering a 2D circle; however, the 2D circle is so unbelievably tiny that it looks like a dot (Fig. 12.3A). If we put another larger circle in front of the

tiny little circle, closer to us (Fig. 12.3B), we could join the two together by their entire circumferences to make a cone (Fig. 12.3C). We can see from this thought experiment that the shape of the apex (pointy bit) of the cone would be directly related to (1) the distance between the point and the circle (larger distance with same size circle = smaller apex) and (2) the size of the larger circle (larger circle at same distance = larger apex) (Fig. 12.3D). This, in essence, is how we define 3D angles, which are termed **solid angles**.

To this end, the **solid angle** (ω) can be considered the amount of the **field of view** (m²) from a particular point (termed the **apex**). Crucially, the solid angle of the 'cone' (field of view) is measured in **steradians** (sr) which can be thought of as 3D radians. In a real-world example of this, we can imagine the apex as corresponding to an observer's eye, and the amount of space taken up by the page of this book (or the screen of an e-book) as the field of view (Fig. 12.4).

Now, if we turn our example of a solid angle and relate it to a sphere, this can be likened to the 3D version of the 2D planar angles we discussed in Fig. 12.2. For planar angles within a circle, the angle is related to the distance from the centre of the circle to the outside edge (radius) and the amount of the circle that is covered by the angle (the arc). With solid angles, this principle remains the same, but this time we need to consider the relationship between the square of the distance from the centre of the sphere to the outside edge (**radius, R**) and the amount of surface of the sphere that is covered by the angle (**area, A**) (Fig. 12.5). To see this in action, please review Equation 12.2 (steradians)

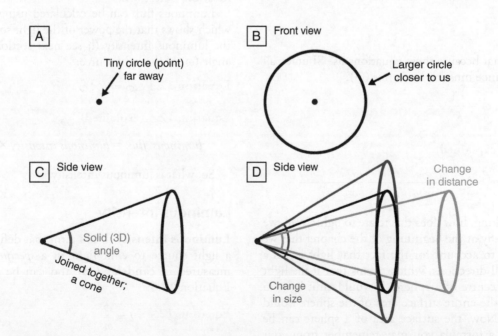

• **Fig. 12.3** Diagram showing concept of solid (3D) angles. We start with a tiny circle far away (A) and we superimpose a larger circle closer to us (B). If we viewed this from the side (C), we could join the two circles from circumference to circumference to make a cone shape. This cone shape defines our solid angle. As we can see, the area of the larger circle (D, pink) and the distance away of the larger circle (D, blue) will have an impact on the solid angle.

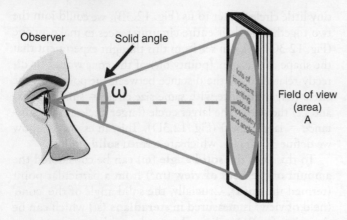

• **Fig. 12.4** Diagram showing real-life example of link between solid angle, field of view and distance of object from the observer.

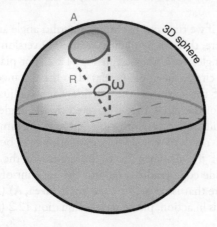

• **Fig. 12.5** Diagram showing a solid angle (ω) in relation to a sphere (3D shape).

and remember that because these equations use SI units, all measures of distance must be in metres (m).

Equation 12.2 $\omega = \dfrac{A}{R^2}$

Equation 12.2 (explained)

$$solid\ angle\ (sr) = \frac{area\ of\ sphere\ surface\ (m^2)}{radius\ of\ sphere^2\ (m)}$$

You may be thinking, how does this relate to light? Well, we did mention briefly at the beginning of the chapter that we want to be able to account for the fact that light leaves a light source in all directions, which means that if the light bulb was at the centre of a sphere, it would emit light in such a way that the entire surface area of the sphere would be illuminated. Now, the surface area of a sphere can be calculated using a formula you may remember from your secondary school days: $4\pi R^2$. If we substitute this into Equation 12.2, we get:

$$\omega = 4\pi R^2 / R^2$$

which can be simplified to:

$$\omega = 4\pi$$

This means that when light is emitted in all directions, the solid angle of the light is considered to be 4π steradians (or 12.57 steradians, which is literally 4 multiplied by π).

Measurements of Light

Now that we're hopefully reasonably well versed with what a 3D solid angle is, this chapter will consider four different measurements of light: **luminous flux**, **luminous intensity**, **illuminance**, and **luminance**.

Luminous Flux

This is a scientific term I love because it reminds me of an integral part of a time-travelling car. But its true definition is slightly less 'sci-fi'. **Luminous flux** (φ) describes the measure of power (or perceived power) emitted by a light source. To put this into context, when you buy a light bulb, it will disclose the wattage and the associated **lumens (lm)**. The lumens are describing the power of the bulb (which is often associated with brightness), which means the higher the lumens, the higher the power and the brighter the bulb. This means that when purchasing a lightbulb for your home, you can review the packaging to see how many lumens are associated with the bulb and how many watts. The difference is that the wattage tells you the amount of energy that the lightbulb *consumes*, whereas the lumens indicate how much power (brightness) the bulb *emits*.

Luminous flux can be calculated using Equation 12.3, which shows that the power of the light source is related to the luminous intensity (l; see next section) and the solid angle (ω) of the light source:

Equation 12.3 $\phi = l \times \omega$

Equation 12.3 (explained)

$luminous\ flux = luminous\ intensity \times solid\ angle$

So, what is luminous intensity?

Luminous Intensity

Luminous intensity (l) is a term that defines the power of a light source to emit light in a *specified* direction. It's measured in **candelas (cd)** and can be calculated using Equation 12.4:

Equation 12.4 $l = \dfrac{\phi}{\omega}$

Equation 12.4 (explained)

$$luminous\ intensity = \frac{luminous\ flux}{solid\ angle}$$

To put this into perspective, let's consider two hypothetical light sources – a spherical light bulb and a torch. Both light sources emit a luminous flux of 500 lumens (φ), but the spherical light bulb emits light in all directions, giving it a solid angle (ω) of 4π steradians, whilst the torch emits light in a given direction which leads to a solid angle of 1π steradians. If we substitute our values into Equation 12.4, we can see that the light bulb emits a luminous intensity of 39.79 candelas, whereas the torch emits a luminous intensity of 159.15 candelas. I think this serves as a nice example, because it makes sense that if both sources emit the same power (luminous flux), and if one has all the power in a smaller space, it should have a higher intensity (which it does).

Illuminance

Moving on then, unless we're afraid of the monsters that hide in the dark, one of the primary reasons we have light sources is to help us see objects in our environment. As discussed in chapter 1, this requires light to light up (illuminate) an object and reflect off the object to our eyes. We can then process the light signal and interpret what it is that we're seeing.

This 'lighting up' of objects is called **illuminance** (E) and more specifically is defined as the luminous flux density at a point on a surface or object – in other words, the amount of light power per unit area of the surface/object. Illuminance is measured in **lux (lx)** and can be calculated using Equation 12.5, which shows us that as the distance from the source increases, the illuminance will decrease, which is called the **inverse square law of illumination**.

Equation 12.5 $E = \dfrac{l}{d^2}$

Equation 12.5 (explained)

$$illuminance = \dfrac{luminous\ intensity}{distance\ from\ source^2}$$

A second law of illumination (the **cosine square law of illumination**) specifies that the angle of the surface/object relative to the source also plays a part in the illuminance (Equation 12.6). With this law, as the angle of the source to the surface gets larger, the illuminance will decrease.

Equation 12.6 $E = \dfrac{l\cos A}{d^2}$

Equation 12.6 (explained)

$$illuminance = \dfrac{luminous\ intensity \times cos \times angle}{distance\ from\ source^2}$$

So the take-home message here is that increasing distance, or increasing the angle of the object away from the light source, will *decrease* the illuminance of an object (Fig. 12.6), which in practical terms means that if light

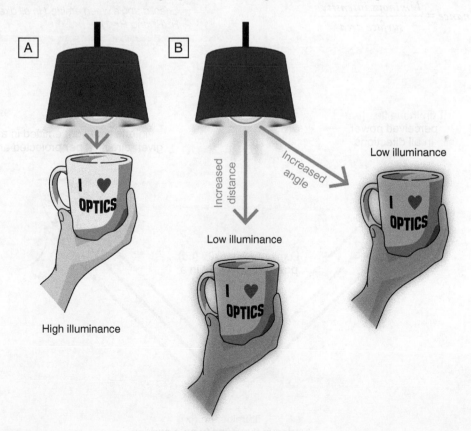

• **Fig. 12.6** Diagram illustrating the laws of illumination. If the object is very close to the light source and at a straight angle, then illumination will be high (A), whereas as the distance from the light source increases, or the angle from the light source increases (B), the illumination will reduce.

levels are making it difficult to see (e.g. a menu in a restaurant), you can either move closer to a light source or hold the object at a more suitable angle for an improved visual experience.

Luminance

OK, so now we know that the light falling onto an object is the illuminance (or illumination), but what do we see? When we look at a well-lit object (like in Fig. 12.7), we can tell that it's well lit because it will appear to be visibly bright. This apparent brightness represents the intensity of light heading from the object to us (which can be described as the intensity of light emitted in a given direction per projected area of a luminous/reflecting surface), which is called **luminance** (L) (not to be confused with illuminance – see Box 12.1). Luminance is measured in **candelas per square metre (cd/m²)** and can be calculated using Equation 12.7, which shows us that as the area (S_A) increases, the luminance will decrease. Please note however that this equation assumes a flat surface (e.g. part of a table).

Equation 12.7 $\quad L = \dfrac{I}{S_A}$

Equation 12.7 (explained)

$$luminance = \frac{luminous\ intensity}{surface\ area}$$

• BOX 12.1 Illuminance or Luminance?

One of the trickier parts of photometry is getting your head around the difference between 'illuminance' and 'luminance', as they describe very similar things and are almost identical in their spelling (just to keep things interesting).

The trick is to think about what happens when we see an object – light will be incident upon the object, some of the light will be absorbed whilst some is reflected (see chapter 1 for revision on this). The reflected light will travel towards us (the observer), and we can process that information and determine what the object is.

The light that falls on the object is the illuminance (hence why we describe objects as being 'illuminated', or when someone helps to explain something, we might use a phrase that suggests they've 'illuminated' the point). However, the light that reflects off the object is the luminance, which means it's partly determined by the illuminance, but also by the surface properties themselves.

DEMO QUESTION 12.2

A spherical light source of diameter 2 m emits 2000 lm uniformly in all directions. What is the average illuminance on a surface 3 m from its centre?

Step 1: Determine what we need to calculate illuminance, E

Step 2: Define variables

$\phi = 2000$

$r = 1\ m$ *(radius is equal to diameter divided by 2)*

$d = 3\ m$

$\omega = 4\pi$ *(solid angle when emitted in all directions as $\omega = 4\pi R^2/R^2$ and R=1)*

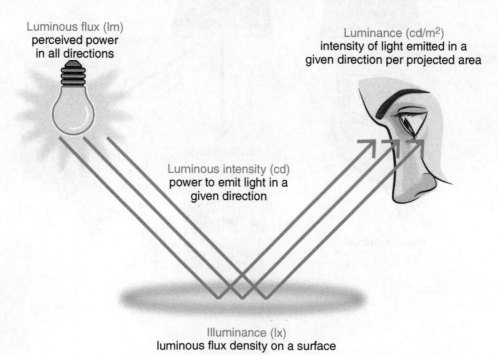

Luminous flux (lm)
**perceived power
in all directions**

Luminance (cd/m²)
**intensity of light emitted in a
given direction per projected area**

Luminous intensity (cd)
**power to emit light in a
given direction**

Illuminance (lx)
luminous flux density on a surface

• Fig. 12.7 Diagram designed to help you remember the difference between luminous flux, luminous intensity, illuminance and luminance.

DEMO QUESTION 12.2 – cont'd

Step 3: Determine necessary equation

$I = \phi / \omega$ *(Equation 12.4)*

$E = I / d^2$ *(Equation 12.5)*

Step 4: Calculate – but remember your calculator needs to be in 'radians'

$I = \phi / \omega$

$I = 2000 / 4\pi$

$I = 159$ cd

$E = I / d^2$

$E = 159 / 3^2$

$E = 159 / 9$

$E = 17.70$ lx

(don't forget the units!)

Practice Questions 12.2:

12.2.1 A spherical light source of diameter 2 m emits 1500 lm uniformly in all directions. What is the average illuminance on a surface 2 m from its centre?

12.2.2 A spherical light source of diameter 2 m emits 300 lm uniformly in all directions. What is the average illuminance on a surface 50 cm from its centre?

A Cool Experiment

If you're interested in learning more about the **inverse square law of illumination**, then you can do a quick and easy experiment at home to see it in action. All you need to do is set up two identically powered light sources at a reasonable distance (60 cm+) from one another, with them both pointed towards one another (as shown in Fig. 12.8). You will also need some oil (the normal kind from the kitchen) and a piece of paper. Importantly, you don't need to know the power of the light sources, as long as they are both the same. Now, the inverse square law of illumination states that as you increase the distance away from these light sources, the illuminance should reduce. As these light sources are facing each other – this means that if we put an object like a piece of paper very close to one of the light sources – the illuminance on the paper from the close source should be higher than from the opposite source. It also means that if we put the paper right in the middle of the two light sources, then illuminance levels should be identical on either side. But how do we prove this?

Well, let's think about a piece of paper. In normal conditions, a standard piece of paper will mostly reflect light (as opposed to letting it transmit through to the other side). However, if the paper is saturated with oil, the patch of oil will reflect much less of the light and will instead transmit more light through to the other side. You can test this for yourself by putting a small (2 cm) dot of oil onto a piece of paper and holding it up to a light source. I'd predict that the oil patch will appear brighter than the rest of the paper because it's letting the light pass through to your eye! This implies that if the light source behind the oil patch is brighter (higher levels of illumination) on one side, then two things will be true: (1) the side of the oil spot facing away from the bright light source will look bright (as it lets the light pass through) and (2) the side of the oil spot facing the light source will look dark, as the patch of oil is letting more light transmit through in that spot than the rest of the paper, meaning it reflects less back in that region relative to the rest of the paper.

Figs 12.8, 12.9 and 12.10 demonstrate this nicely, showing that with two identical light sources, the oil spot will appear bright if the illuminance level is higher behind it (Fig. 12.8), and it will appear dark if the illuminance level is higher in front of it (Fig. 12.9). If the illuminance levels are the same on both sides, then the oil spot will seem to disappear because equal amounts of light are being transmitted through the oil spot and reflected off the paper (Fig. 12.10), and with two identical light sources, the inverse square law of illumination tells us that this can only occur if the paper is positioned exactly halfway between the two light sources. Try it for yourself and see!

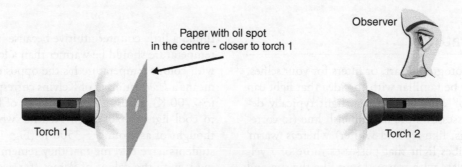

Paper with oil spot in the centre - closer to torch 1

Observer

Torch 1

Torch 2

Bright oil spot, dark paper
Brighter light transmitted through than reaches the paper

• **Fig. 12.8** Illustration of experiment with two identical light sources pointing towards one another and a piece of paper with a spot of oil on the front of it. The oil allows light to transmit through the paper (where it would normally be reflected), so if viewing from the right, when the paper is near torch 1, the light from torch 2 reflecting off the paper will be less bright than the light from torch 1, which is transmitting through the oil. So the oil spot will appear bright, relative to the paper.

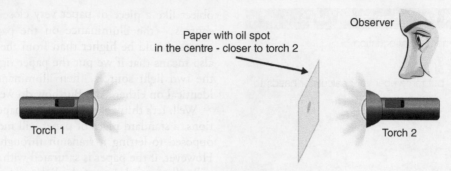

Paper with oil spot
in the centre - closer to torch 2

Observer

Torch 1

Torch 2

Dark oil spot, bright paper
Brighter light reflected than is transmitting from the other side

• **Fig. 12.9** Illustration of experiment with two identical light sources pointing towards one another, and a piece of paper with a spot of oil on the front of it. The oil allows light to transmit through the paper (where it would normally be reflected), so if viewing from the right, when the paper is near torch 2, the light from torch 2 reflecting off the paper will be brighter than the light from torch 1, which is transmitting through the oil. So the oil spot will appear dark, relative to the paper.

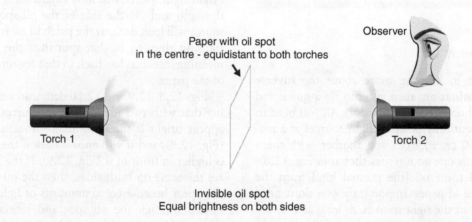

Paper with oil spot
in the centre - equidistant to both torches

Observer

Torch 1

Torch 2

Invisible oil spot
Equal brightness on both sides

• **Fig. 12.10** Illustration of experiment with two identical light sources pointing towards one another, and a piece of paper with a spot of oil on the front of it. The oil allows light to transmit through the paper (where it would normally be reflected), so if viewing from the right, when the paper is exactly halfway between the light sources, the light from torch 2 reflecting off the paper will be as bright as the light from torch 1, which is transmitting through the oil. So the oil spot will become invisible, relative to the paper.

Colour Temperature

If you're big into photography, art, or filters for your selfies, then you'll probably be familiar with the idea that light can be described as 'cool' or 'warm'. 'Cool' light typically describes light that possesses more of a blueish hue (to correlate with cold things, like ice and winter) whereas 'warm' light typically describes light that possesses more of a yellowish hue (to correlate with warm things like the sun and the beach). This means that light sources can be categorised depending on their **colour temperature,** which is measured in **Kelvins (K)**. Now, fair warning here, Kelvins are, I

think, a little counterintuitive because in my brain a higher temperature should be warmer than a low temperature, but with colour temperature it's the opposite way around. This means a *lower* number of Kelvins corresponds to warm light (~2700 K), whilst a *higher* number of Kelvins corresponds to cool light (~7000 K). Neutral 'white' light would be thought of as around ~3500 K (Fig. 12.11). Some of my students have told me that they remember this by associating it with the colour of flames (for example, on a Bunsen burner); in this case the higher temperature flames are blue whilst the lower temperature flames are yellow (just like with Kelvins).

Colour temperature

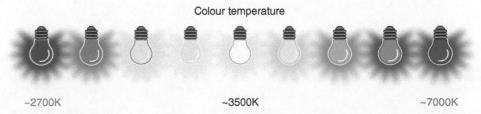

~2700K   ~3500K   ~7000K

• **Fig. 12.11** Colour temperature of light (measured in Kelvins, K) is warm at low levels (left) and cool at high levels (right).

Test Your Knowledge

Try the questions below to see if you need to review any sections again. All answers are available in the back of the book.

TYK.12.1 What does 'photometry' mean?

TYK.12.2 Describe a 'solid angle'.

TYK.12.3 What does 'luminous flux' mean and what is it measured in?

TYK.12.4 Which of the following statements uses photometry terms correctly and why: '*The cup is poorly illuminated*,' or '*The cup is poorly luminated*'?

TYK.12.5 What does a high number of Kelvins (6000 K) suggest about a light source?

13

Optical Instruments and Low Vision Aids

CHAPTER OUTLINE

OBJECTIVES

After working through this chapter, you should be able to:

Explain what an 'optical instrument' is
Explain how cameras work
Explain how Galilean, Keplerian and reflecting telescopes work

Explain how optical instruments can help people with low vision

Introduction

An **optical instrument** can include any device or equipment which can alter an image for enhancement or viewing purposes. This includes **cameras, binoculars, telescopes and monoculars** – some of which are clinically relevant as they're utilised as **low vision aids,** which are devices that help people with low acuity to be able to see. This chapter will explain the principles of these devices and then discuss their use in practical settings.

Cameras

I think it's useful to start this chapter by going over cameras, because we all use cameras on our mobile devices fairly regularly, so we can apply the knowledge that we already have. A **camera**, then, is a device that focuses light onto a screen, digital sensor or a film for the purposes of viewing the image. Historically the term originates from the use of **camera obscuras**, which were dark rooms with a pinhole to let the light in; this pinhole projected an image onto a flat wall which could be viewed by the **observer**[1] (for details on how pinhole cameras work, see Box 13.1 and chapter 18). Since then, cameras have developed significantly to include the use of fancy lenses and digital enhancing software.

If we think about it logically, then, in the most basic of forms, the camera needs to be constructed to allow light into the camera itself, without letting too much in that it will affect the quality of the image, so it needs to be a box with a hole in the front of it. In optics, the hole that lets light into an optical instrument is called the **aperture stop** (or **iris**), and importantly, this hole should not affect the field of view (what the instrument can see). If it helps as an example, the human eye can be thought of as an optical instrument and our iris is the aperture stop. When we're in brightly lit places, our pupils (the hole in our iris) get smaller (to reduce the amount of light entering the eye), but this only helps with the brightness, it doesn't restrict our field of view at all – and the same is true for aperture stops in cameras. Our basic camera will also need a screen (or equivalent) at the back of the box to project the image onto, so in theory it could just be an enclosed box with a pinhole on the front (Fig. 13.1A), or it could be an enclosed box with a slightly larger aperture and a simple lens, to focus the image (Fig. 13.1B).

However, as we've hinted at already with our example of the human eye, sometimes we need to alter the amount of light that can enter the instrument (e.g. if it's very dark, maybe we want our camera to let in more light), or we might want to change the focus (e.g. if we want to take an image of something that's very far away). In this case, we

• BOX 13.1   How Does a Pinhole Camera Work?

A **pinhole camera** (or *camera obscura*) is a name for an imaging device that utilises the theory behind pinhole photography. When light emanating from an object shines through a pinhole, it produces an upside-down image. This is because light rays have to travel in straight lines (to a limit, see chapter 10 to review how light can bend around corners when diffraction occurs). This means that light coming off the tip of the object (e.g. the top of the mug in Fig. B13.1) will travel in a straight line through the pinhole and end up near the floor, whilst light rays from the base of the object travel in a straight line through the pinhole and end up near the ceiling. When these rays form a focus, it necessarily produces an inverted image.

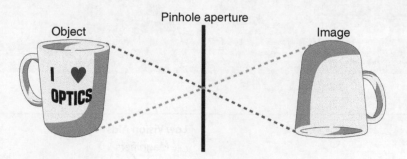

• **Fig. B13.1** Diagram showing the path of light rays from a mug, producing an upside-down image in a pinhole camera. The image is also flipped left to right, so in the image (on the right), the text will be facing the other way (which is why it's missing).

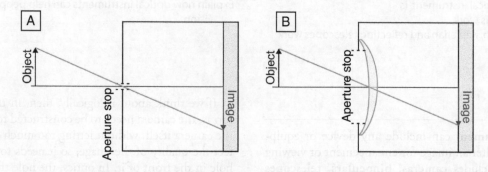

• **Fig. 13.1** Illustration of 'basic' camera constructions for a pinhole camera (A) or a single-lens camera (B).

need our camera to be able to alter the size of the aperture stop (depending on our lighting requirements), and we need to be able to zoom, or replace the lenses to those of different **focal lengths (f)**, which as you probably know is how modern-day cameras work.

The focal length of a camera (usually reported in millimetres (mm)) is determined by where the lens will focus light that enters with zero vergence (from infinity). So, for example, a camera lens with an 18 mm focal length would focus zero vergence light 18 mm behind the lens. This means that as the focal length of the lens changes, the lens will be closer to, or further away from, the sensor at the back of the camera in order to work effectively. This is why some telephoto lenses are so long (e.g. 300 mm focal length). The focal length also determines the **magnification (m)** and the **field of view**. Long focal lengths will have narrow fields of

view and high magnification, whereas short focal lengths will have wide fields of view and lower levels of magnification (Fig. 13.2).

In terms of varying the diameter of the aperture stop to let in more or less light, it's relatively straightforward as we just need a size-changing aperture within the camera. However, photographers describe the diameter (ø) relative to the focal length (f) of the lens – called the *f*-number – as this helps them understand what effect the aperture stop will have on the final image. The equation for calculating the *f*-number is shown in Equation 13.1. Here you can see that if a camera had a lens with a focal length of 100 mm, with an aperture stop 25 mm wide, the *f*-number would be 4 (100/25), and so it would be written as *f*/4, which means the aperture stop in this case has a diameter that equates to a quarter of the focal length. This also highlights that

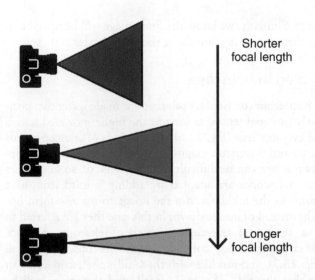

• **Fig. 13.2** Diagram showing the relationship between lens focal length (increasing downwards) and field of view (shown in shades of blue).

changing either the focal length or the diameter of the aperture stop would alter the *f*-number.

Equation 13.1 $N = \dfrac{f}{\varnothing}$

Equation 13.1 (explained)

$$f - number = \frac{focal\ length}{aperture\ diameter}$$

Importantly, smaller aperture stops (which let in less light) might need longer exposure times, which is another thing to take into consideration when planning your shots. In general terms, the smaller the *f*-number, the more light is let into the instrument, and the better the lens will perform in low levels of light. Altering the aperture size (and *f*-number) can also affect something called **depth of field**,

which describes the range in which something can be in focus. For example, let's say I'm taking a photo of my two cats sitting near each other, but one is approximately one metre closer to me than the other. A large depth of field would mean I could take a photo that has both of the cats in focus at the same time, whereas a small depth of field would mean I'd have to focus my camera on one or the other, and the one that wasn't in focus would be blurry (Fig. 13.3). In general, smaller apertures lead to larger depths of field, and larger apertures produce smaller depths of field.

In summary, cameras are very clever, and there's an awful lot to think about when trying to take a photograph!

Telescopes

Telescopes are optical instruments designed with the purpose of helping us see objects that are far away, and they do this by magnifying the far-away object so we can see it more clearly. For example, if we use a telescope to look at the moon, the image of the moon is magnified to help us see it in more detail.

A 'basic' telescope will need to be made of two lenses – an **eyepiece lens** (the one near your eye) and an **objective lens** (the one nearer to the object). These lenses work together just like the multiple lens systems we discussed in chapter 3 to produce an image that is in focus for us as the observer. An interesting thing to learn here is that the image we see through the telescope will be visible through what's called the **exit pupil** of the instrument. An **exit pupil** is the view of the **aperture stop** from the back of the instrument, so it's only possible to see the exit pupil through the eyepiece, which makes sense (the view the other way round would be called the **entrance pupil**, but we're not going to worry about that in this book). The position and size of the exit pupil in a telescope will control the **field of view**, which means it also serves as the **field stop**. A field stop is an aperture in an optical instrument that controls the field of view (how much of the scene is visible at any one time).

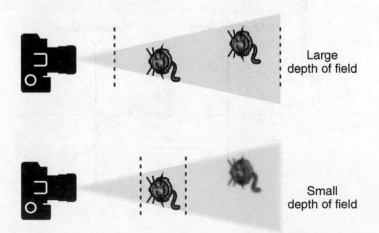

• **Fig. 13.3** Diagram showing visual representation of depth of field. Larger depths of field mean more depth (areas at different distances from the lens) can be in focus at the same time.

There are a few different types of telescopes, so it's helpful to discuss them separately.

Galilean Telescope

A Galilean telescope is made using a negatively powered eyepiece lens and a positively powered objective lens (Fig. 13.4). This produces a virtual (upright), magnified image for the observer. The issue with a Galilean telescope is that the exit pupil doesn't coincide with the pupil of the observer; as you can see in Fig. 13.5, the exit pupil (the clear window that the image forms in) is produced in between the two lenses, meaning it can be likened to looking through a keyhole. The observer will need to line up their own pupil with the exit pupil in order to get the best view. It also means that if the observer is holding the eyepiece lens too far away from their eye, it will restrict what they can see.

Fig. 13.5 also highlights that the field of view will be reduced, as the three rays leaving the telescope are closer together than the three rays entering the telescope. We can also see evidence of the magnification of the image because the angle of the image relative to the optical axis (w') is larger than that of the object (w), suggesting the image is

larger. Similarly, we know the final image will be upright, as the three image rays are above the optical axis.

Keplerian Telescope

A **Keplerian (or Kepler) telescope** is made using two positively powered lenses, as long as the higher-powered lens is the eyepiece lens (Fig. 13.6). These kinds of telescopes produce a real (inverted), magnified image. However, an upside-down image can be difficult to make sense of, so sometimes these telescopes are adapted by adding a third lens (or a prism) in the middle to flip the image to make it form upright instead of upside down; in this case they are referred to as a **terrestrial telescope**. Keplerian telescopes produce an exit pupil that coincides with the observer's pupil (Fig. 13.7), and just like with the Galilean telescope, we can see that the field of view is small, and the image will be magnified. However, this time we can see that the image rays are below the optical axis, indicating an inverted image.

Reflecting Telescope

The problem with refractive telescopes (telescopes that use lenses) is that lots of aberrations can be introduced

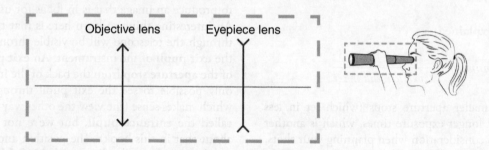

• **Fig. 13.4** Galilean telescopes have a negatively powered eyepiece lens and a positively powered objective lens.

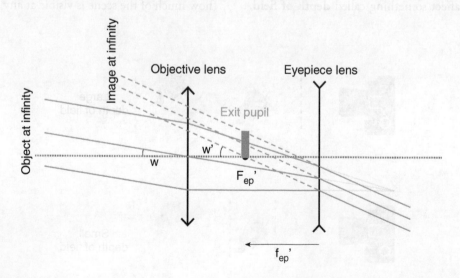

• **Fig. 13.5** Diagram of how rays from an object far away (infinity) are focused by a Galilean telescope. The exit pupil is shown in green, at the focal point of the eyepiece lens (F_{ep}'). The angle of the image relative to the optical axis (w') is larger than the angle of the object relative to the optical axis, highlighting that magnification has occurred.

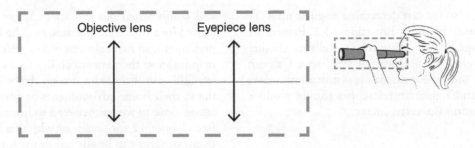

• **Fig. 13.6** Keplerian telescopes have two positively powered lenses.

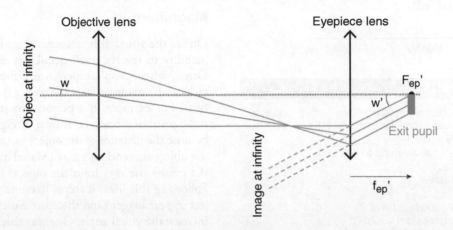

• **Fig. 13.7** Diagram of how rays from an object far away (infinity) are focused by a Keplerian telescope. The exit pupil is shown in green, at the focal point of the eyepiece lens (F_{ep}'). The angle of the image relative to the optical axis (w') is larger than the angle of the object relative to the optical axis, highlighting that magnification has occurred.

(see chapters 8 and 16 for more detail on aberrations), so to get around this, they usually only possess narrow apertures, which limit the light that can enter the instrument. This means that objects that are emitting low levels of light (e.g. a star in the sky) will be difficult to see. However, the good news is that we can get around this problem by using a mirror instead of lenses and installing a **reflecting telescope** (Fig. 13.8). These telescopes use a large concave mirror (positively powered) to collect light across a wide aperture and form a nice, magnified image. The mirror is usually chosen to be paraboloidal (aspherical) because the wide aperture would make spherical mirrors susceptible to those pesky spherical aberrations we talked about in chapter 6. Another advantage of a reflecting telescope is that they don't suffer from chromatic aberration (see chapter 8) because chromatic aberration can only occur if light is refracted, not reflected. So all round, this type of telescope is excellent.

Magnification

As we stated at the beginning of the telescope section, telescopes are designed to produce magnified images of objects, and we could see in Figs 13.5 and 13.7 that the magnification is dependent on the angular difference between the object relative to the optical axis (w) and the image relative to the optical axis (w'). This means that telescopic magnification is defined as **angular magnification (m)**. However, these angles are determined by the ratio between the powers of the **eyepiece lens (F_{ep})** and

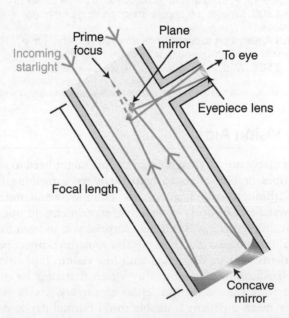

• **Fig. 13.8** Diagram of a reflecting telescope showing how light from a star (blue) is focused by the concave mirror with the wide aperture.

objective lens (F_o), so we can determine angular magnification relatively easily by using Equation 13.2. Remember as well, that the sign of the magnification tells us whether the image is upright ($+$) or inverted ($-$), so a Galilean telescope should produce positive magnification values (upright image), and Keplerian telescopes should produce negative magnification (inverted image).

Equation 13.2 $\quad m = -\dfrac{F_{ep}}{F_o}$

Equation 13.2 (explained)

$$mag. = -\frac{power\ of\ eyepiece\ lens}{power\ of\ objective\ lens}$$

DEMO QUESTION 13.1

A Galilean telescope has an eyepiece lens with a power of $-9.50D$, and it produces a magnification of $+2.5X$. What is the power of the objective lens?

    Step 1: Determine what we need to calculate
power of objective lens, F_o
    Step 2: Define variables
$F_{ep} = -9.50$
$m = +2.5$ *(the sign is important here)*
    Step 3: Determine necessary equation
$m = -(F_{ep} / F_o)$ *(Equation 13.2)*
    Step 4: Calculate
$m = -(F_{ep} / F_o)$
$2.5 = -(-9.5 / F_o)$
$F_o = -(-9.5 / 2.5)$
$F_o = +3.80D$
    (don't forget the $\pm$ sign!)

Practice Questions:

13.1.1 A Galilean telescope has an eyepiece lens with a power of $-5.00D$, and it produces a magnification of $+4X$. What is the power of the objective lens?

13.1.2 A Keplerian telescope has an eyepiece lens with a power of $+7.00D$ and an objective lens with a power of $+4.50D$. What is the angular magnification of the telescope?

13.1.3 A Keplerian telescope has an eyepiece lens with a power of $+6.25D$, and it produces a magnification of $-8.50X$. What is the power of the objective lens?

Low Vision Aids

It's relatively easy to imagine that people might need to use telescopes or binoculars to help them see something far away (through magnification), for example, astronomers, bird watchers, students completing experiments in optics labs at university. . . . But it may surprise you to learn that optical instruments like these are also sometimes prescribed to patients who are diagnosed with **low vision**. Low vision is a classification of poor-quality vision that can't be corrected with glasses, contact lenses or surgery, and it will usually mean a patient is unable to do normal day-to-day tasks like read, drive, watch TV or recognise their friends

and family when out and about.[2] Low vision itself can be caused by a myriad of diseases, but the key factor is that it's permanent, so management of low vision involves trying to help improve the patient's ability to use the sight they have left. This can include improving the brightness of the lighting in their home environments or advising patients to put lamps close to where they read to improve the illumination (see chapter 12 for details of why this is helpful). Alternatively, patients can be advised to use low vision aids such as magnifiers.

Magnifiers

One of the visual difficulties associated with low vision is an inability to resolve small detail, for example, written text. Often, when people experience difficulty in this way, the task can be made easier if the object is made bigger (magnified). For example, if a person was struggling to read the small print of a book (as shown in Fig. 13.9A), it might be because the distance of the object from the observer leads to the object subtending a small **visual angle** (angle formed at the eye by the rays from the object) (distant object (θ_d)). Following this idea, it seems like one way to make the object appear bigger (and therefore easier to see) would be to increase the visual angle. One way this can be achieved is by bringing the object closer to the observer (as shown in Fig. 13.9B). This would increase the visual angle (close object (θ_c)), which will make the object much larger on the retina; however, as I'm sure many of you can appreciate, it can be difficult to focus at very short distances away from the eye, especially as we advance in age, which might mean the object becomes blurry before it can be large enough to be clearly visible. An alternative solution, then, is to use a lens (between the observer and the object) that is able to produce a magnified image of the object, farther away from the observer (as shown in Fig. 13.9C). This works because the image is distant (so the observer can focus on it) but the visual angle is large, mimicking the scenario when the object was much closer. Overall, this means the desired outcome of the magnifier is to produce a virtual (upright) image that is larger than without the magnifier.

In general, **magnifiers** describe high-powered lenses that are designed to make the image of objects bigger through magnification. Magnifiers themselves can comprise a single-lens system (this is typical of **hand-held and flatform magnifiers**) or they might comprise a multiple lens system such as a **telescopic monocular.**[3] Remember though, not all telescope systems are created equally, so if a telescopic device is required, it should be one that produces an upright (virtual) image, otherwise they won't be much use to the individual at all! Overall, each type of magnification device will be useful for different types of tasks (summarised in Table 13.1); for example, a handheld magnifier can be useful for near-work, such as reading or watching videos on your mobile device (especially if it has a light so that it can illuminate the object), but you wouldn't be able to use one to look at something far away, like a train timetable screen or a specials

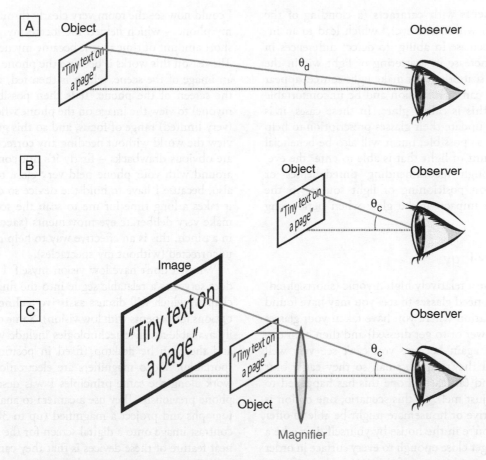

• **Fig. 13.9** Simplistic illustration showing link between visual angle (θ) and distance. When the object is far away from the observer (A), the visual angle is very small (θ_d, distant). If the object is brought closer to the observer (B), then the visual angle becomes much larger (θ_c, close), but the observer might find it difficult to focus on the object. The ideal solution in this scenario, then, is to use a magnifying lens (C) to make a small object produce a magnified, virtual image.

TABLE 13.1	Magnification Devices and Their Relative Features	
Magnification Device	**Useful For**
Hand-held magnifiers	Near-work (e.g. reading)
Spectacle magnifiers	Near-work (e.g. reading)
Stand magnifier	Near-work (e.g. reading)
Telescopic monoculars	Near-distance

board in a restaurant. In these cases a telescopic monocular would be far more useful.

Magnifiers and monoculars are therefore very useful for anyone who has issues with their vision, but unfortunately (a little like glasses and contact lenses) they aren't perfect. For example, magnifying lenses can induce aberrations (imperfections) in the image (see chapter 16 for more information on this), which is especially true if we attempt to utilise sections of the lens that are away from the optical centre, and it has a more detrimental effect in high-powered lenses (typical of those used in magnifiers). This means that very high-powered magnifiers will usually need to have a smaller

lens (to prevent aberrations), so if you need something magnified to quite a high degree, it will often have a smaller **field of view**. This can then lead to other issues, such as difficulty using the lens with both eyes (binocular viewing), which means that sometimes patients will have to occlude one eye in order to make effective use of the magnifier. Similarly, many of the spectacle magnifiers can have quite a limited **depth of field**, meaning that unless the object is positioned within the narrow range of appropriate distances, it will appear blurry. Overall, though, despite these limitations, low vision aids provide a great solution to the everyday difficulties that low vision patients can experience.

In addition to magnifiers and monoculars, there are a number of alternative low vision aids available, so if you're interested in this then I'd encourage you to do some research to find out more.

Adapted Lenses

Now we know that magnifiers can be useful for helping patients with low vision, but not all vision-related issues are to do with image size – sometimes patients can experience difficulty with glare[4] that affects their ability to see. This is often true for patients with **cataracts** (a clouding of the ocular media (lens) within the eye),[4] which lead to an increase in blur, a decrease in ability to detect differences in contrast, and an increase in scattering of light within the eye. Crucially, this scattering can make light sources appear very bright, which can affect vision and be uncomfortable for the patient – this is called **glare**. In these cases, it is beneficial to try to update their glasses prescription to help them see as clearly as possible, but it will also be beneficial to reduce the amount of light that is able to enter the eye, for example, through recommending tinted lenses or through advising on positioning of light sources in the home to limit the impact of the glare when performing tasks.

Assistive Technology

If, like me, you have a relatively high myopic (shortsighted) refractive error and need glasses to see, you may have found yourself in the situation where you have taken your glasses off (possibly to shower or to get dressed) and then been unable to find them again because you can't see very well without them, and they're quite small so they easily blur into the background (at least I hope this has happened to people other than just me!). In this scenario, one option is to hope that a relative or housemate might be able to offer assistance, but if you're in the house by yourself, it can be a bit of a struggle to get close enough to every surface in order to get it into focus (within your far point) and see if your glasses are sitting there, mocking you. However, a few years ago when this happened to me for the 1,000th time, I realised that I don't need to get close to all the surfaces, because I have a phone with a camera on it, and I can easily focus on the phone screen when it is held close to my face. So I grabbed my phone (which is large enough to find) and turned on the camera and was very pleased to discover that

I could now see the room very clearly through the screen on my phone – which helped me locate my glasses in such a short amount of time that it became my new personal best. The reason this works is because the phone camera captures an image of the scene, which is then fed, in a live view, to the screen of the phone. It is then possible for me (as a myope) to view the image on the phone when it's within my (very limited) range of focus, and so this gives me a way to view the world without needing any correction. Now, there are obvious drawbacks – firstly it's not convenient to walk around with your phone held very close to your face, but also, because I have to hold the device so close to my face, it takes a long time for me to scan the scene as I have to make very deliberate eye movements (**saccades**). However, in a pinch, this is an effective way to help me see when I'm uncorrected (without my spectacles).

Whilst I don't have low vision myself, I think this anecdote serves as a relatable segue into the final section of this chapter, which will discuss **assistive technology** (electronic options for patients with low vision). Some of the more readily available assistive technologies include video magnifiers, and they can be desktop (fixed in position) or handheld (portable). Video magnifiers are electronic magnifiers that work along the same principles I was describing with my phone previously. They use a camera to analyse text or photographs and project a magnified (up to 30×),[5] increased-contrast image onto a digital screen for the patient to see. A neat feature of these devices is that they can take snapshots, so patients can move around the screen at their preference. Also, because they utilise digital software, it is possible to buy video magnifiers that will read the text aloud, which can help hugely with understanding what is written if patients have low vision. Finally, these video magnifiers are not susceptible to the same small field of view and aberrations that handheld lens magnifiers are, but these advantages come at a cost as these video magnifiers are often far more expensive.

Test Your Knowledge

Try the questions below to see if you need to review any sections again. All answers are available in the back of the book.

TYK.13.1 What is an 'optical instrument'?

TYK.13.2 Could the human eye be classed as an optical instrument? Explain your answer.

TYK.13.3 If we wanted to focus our camera on something very far away, would we choose a 24 mm or 300 mm lens? Explain your answer.

TYK.13.4 Would you expect a Galilean telescope to have a positive or negative magnification? Explain your answer.

References

1. Dupré S. Inside the camera obscura: Kepler's experiment and theory of optical imagery. *Early Sci Med.* 2008;13(3):219-244.
2. Leat SJ, Legge GE, Bullimore MA. What is low vision. *Optom Vis Sci.* 1999;76:198-211.
3. NHS. *Low Visual Aids.* https://www.hey.nhs.uk/wp/wp-content/uploads/2020/07/Low-Visual-Aids.pdf. Accessed December 20, 2021.
4. Lasa MS, Podgor MJ, Datiles MB, Caruso RC, Magno BV. Glare sensitivity in early cataracts. *Br J Ophthalmol.* 1993;77(8):489-491.
5. RNIB. *Assistive Technology.* https://www.rnib.org.uk/sight-loss-advice/equality-rights-andemployment/staying-work/assistive-technology. Accessed February. Accessed February 7, 2022.

14
Polarisation

CHAPTER OUTLINE

OBJECTIVES

After working through this chapter, you should be able to:

Explain the difference between polarised and unpolarised light

Explain the process of polarisation by transmission

Explain the process of polarisation by refraction

Explain the process of polarisation by reflection

Explain the process of polarisation by scattering

Introduction

We've already discussed a lot about light and how it can be emitted from a source in all directions (e.g. like the sun), and more specifically we've talked about how light can be expressed as **waves**, travelling outwards from the source. This chapter will focus on how we can alter the orientation of those waves, through a process called **polarisation**.

Some Light Revision

(Pun intended.) When light is emitted from a light source, it can be described in terms of its wavefronts, light rays or light waves. To understand polarisation, we need to focus on light as a **wave**.

Imagine a single light wave is being emitted from a light source (in this case, possibly a laser), as shown in Fig. 14.1A. In this example, the light is oscillating vertically, which means its **electric field** (or **electric vector**) is also vertically oriented. We learned in chapter 1 that visible light is part of the electromagnetic spectrum, but we never specifically discussed that it is technically an **oscillating electric and magnetic field** (both of which are oriented perpendicular to one another). The oscillating electric field that forms the light has the potential to be able to affect electrons in other materials by causing them to start oscillating too. This oscillation

in other electrons forms part of the basic explanation of how polarisation works, but we don't need to get too bogged down in this right now.

If we now go back to thinking about our single light source, I think we can agree that it's relatively easy to imagine light as a single waveform with a vertically oriented electric field (and much easier to draw that way too); however, most light sources (the sun, LED bulbs) produce light that contains vibrations in all possible meridians (otherwise known as orientations/planes), as shown in Fig. 14.1B (which unfortunately is much harder to draw and visualise). In this case, the light is formed of many orientations of light, so the **electric field** changes orientation randomly over time.

When light vibrates in all directions like this (see Fig. 14.1B), it's considered to be **unpolarised**, because it has more than one orientation of vibration (and a slightly unpredictable electric field). However, it is possible to take unpolarised light and reduce it to a beam of light comprising vibrations that occur (mostly) within a single meridian, which we would then describe as **polarised** light. This process of transforming the unpolarised light into a polarised state is called **polarisation**, and polarisation can occur through a number of different methods, including: (1) **transmission**, (2) **reflection**, (3) **refraction** and (4) **scattering**. First, however, let's discuss types of polarisation.

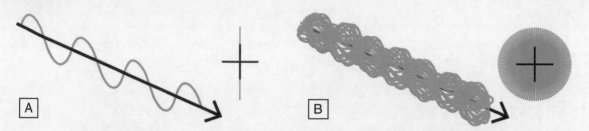

• **Fig. 14.1** Diagram showing how we usually think of light (a wave vibrating or oscillating in one orientation, in this case vertical (A)), and how natural light truly behaves (vibrating in all directions (B)).

Types of Polarisation

For light to become polarised, we need to limit the orientations (or confine the direction of the electric field vector). This can be done linearly, circularly or elliptically.

Linear polarisation occurs if the electric field of the light (orientation of the wave) is restricted to a single plane/orientation (Fig. 14.2A). This type of polarisation will be discussed most often within this chapter as it's the 'easiest' to understand. In contrast to this, **circular polarisation** comprises two linearly polarised (perpendicular) waves that possess a phase difference of 90° whilst possessing the same amplitude (Fig. 14.2B). In this case, the electric field produced by these waves will rotate as the waves move forward, in a circular shape. This can be clockwise or anticlockwise and is usually referred to as right-hand or left-hand circular polarisation, depending on which of the waves is 'ahead' (in terms of phase) of the other. If two linearly polarised (perpendicular) waves possess different amplitudes or a phase difference that varies from 90°, then this produces **elliptical polarisation** (Fig. 14.2C).

Now polarised light can also be classified as either **p-polarised** or **s-polarised** depending on how it is polarised relative to what's referred to as the **plane of incidence**. The plane of incidence can be thought of as a flat, completely imaginary surface on which the incident (and reflected) light exists – so, often, the plane of incidence is drawn perpendicular to the surface (Fig. 14.3). **P-polarised** light describes light that possesses an electric field that is **parallel** to the plane of incidence ('p' for parallel), whereas **s-polarised** light describes light with an electric field that is **perpendicular** to the plane of incidence ('s' for s'not parallel at all . . . or, technically, s for 'senkrecht', which is German for perpendicular). So in Fig. 14.3 if the reflected light was parallel to the plane of incidence (vertical) then it would be p-polarised, and if it was perpendicular to the plane of incidence (horizontal), it would be s-polarised.

Polarisation by Transmission

One of the most common man-made methods of polarising light is to use a material as a **polariser** (a system that can turn unpolarised light into a polarised state). These materials are specially designed to only transmit waves vibrating in a single direction (much like in the example in Fig. 14.4). Now, because this method of polarisation will transmit

vibrations of light parallel to the **transmission axis (or polarisation axis)** of the polariser, this method is often called **polarisation by transmission**. In Fig. 14.4, the polarising filter shown has a vertical transmission axis, so only vibrations oriented vertically will be transmitted through. All other vibration directions will be stopped by the filter, particularly those oriented perpendicularly to the transmission axis. An easy way to remember this is to liken it to the 'picket

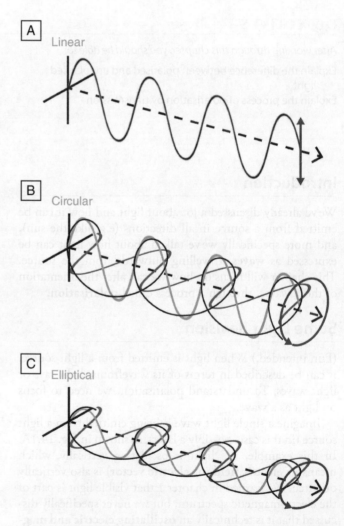

• **Fig. 14.2** Diagram showing linear polarised light (A), circular polarised light (B), and elliptical polarised light (C). Here the light is propagating from left to right as indicated by the black dashed line. Light waves are shown in blue, the electric field is shown in solid black and the type of polarisation is indicated in a bright pink.

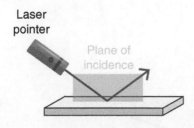

Laser
pointer

Plane of
incidence

• **Fig. 14.3** Diagram showing plane of incidence (light blue) as existing along the line of the incident and reflecting light (red). In this case it's perpendicular to the surface (grey).

fence' analogy.[1] This analogy assumes that a dog (for example) with a stick in its mouth will only be able to pass through a gap in a picket fence if the stick is vertical (meaning the dog will need to turn its head). Holding the stick horizontally will not work – just like with this example of polarisation!

This also means that if you put two perpendicularly aligned polarisers one after another, the light would become polarised as it transmits through the first polariser, but it would then get stopped by the second polariser. These are called **crossed polarisers** (Fig. 14.5).

Importantly, as these polarisers are technically stopping quite a good amount of light from passing through to the other side, there is a reduction in brightness (~50%) of the light after transmission. This helps form part of the

explanation as to why polarising filters make great lenses for sunglasses (but it isn't the whole story). The benefit of having polarised lenses is discussed towards the end of this chapter.

Polarisation by Reflection

Another method of polarising light can be to reflect it off a surface; in proper scientific terms this is due to the relationship between the **electric field** of the light relative to the **plane of incidence** upon the surface. Essentially, if the electric vector is perpendicular to the plane of incidence, then the light will be polarised in the same orientation as the electric vector. In a simple example, if we have incident light upon a horizontal surface (e.g. a lake), then the plane of incidence will be vertical (as shown in Fig. 14.6). This means that the light will ultimately end up being polarised to be parallel to the surface of the road (also horizontal), which will be *perpendicular* to the plane of incidence, making it s-polarised.

In simpler, more general terms, this all means that given the right conditions, the reflected light will be polarised parallel to the surface from which it was reflected, so for the majority of examples (snow, roads, lakes) the reflected light will be polarised in the horizontal plane, but in some cases (e.g. light reflecting off a window on a house) it will be polarised in the vertical plane.

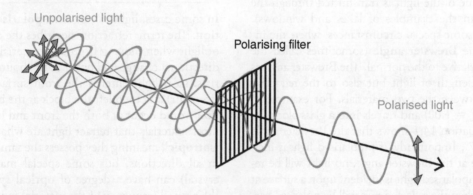

Unpolarised light

Polarising filter

Polarised light

• **Fig. 14.4** Polarisation by transmission shown with a filter that possesses a vertical transmission axis.

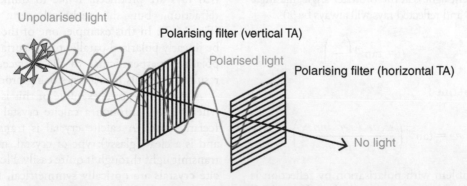

Unpolarised light

Polarising filter (vertical TA)

Polarised light

Polarising filter (horizontal TA)

No light

• **Fig. 14.5** Crossed polarisers (angled at 90° to each other) prevent light from transmitting through the system, because after passing through the first polariser with a vertical transmission axis (TA), the light is inappropriately oriented for transmitting through the second polariser with a horizontal TA.

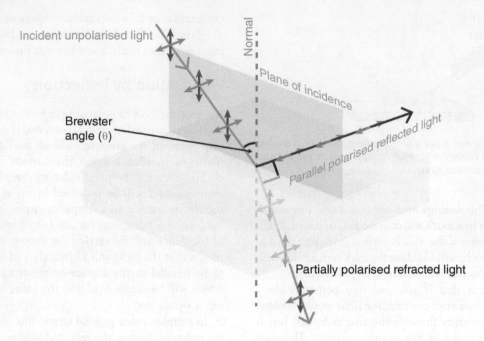

Incident unpolarised light

Normal

Plane of incidence

Brewster angle (θ)

Parallel polarised reflected light

Partially polarised refracted light

• **Fig. 14.6** Diagram showing Brewster angle (θ) with the example of unpolarised light incident upon a glass block. The angle between the refracted and reflected rays is 90°, and the reflected light is polarised parallel to the surface of the glass block.

An interesting feature of polarisation by reflection is that it can occur when some of the light is transmitted through the material too (like in the examples of lakes and windows). However, there are some special circumstances, where the incident light is at the **Brewster angle** (sometimes called the **polarising angle**) relative to the normal. The Brewster angle is related to the wavelength of light but also to the refractive index difference between the two materials. For example, if light starts in air ($n_1 = 1.00$) and travels into a glass block ($n_2 = 1.523$), then Equation 14.1 shows that the Brewster angle will be roughly 56.7°. Importantly, if p-polarised light is incident upon a surface at the Brewster angle, no light will be reflected, whereas if unpolarised light is incident upon a surface at the Brewster angle, then the reflected rays will be polarised parallel to the plane of the surface – in which case the remaining refracted light will be partially polarised (see Fig. 14.6). In all cases, when the incident light is at the Brewster angle, the angle between the refracted and reflected rays will always be 90°.

Equation 14.1

$$\theta = \tan^{-1}\left(\frac{n_2}{n_1}\right)$$

Equation 14.1 (explained)

$$Brewster\ angle = \tan^{-1}\left(\frac{second\ ref.\ index}{first\ ref.\ index}\right)$$

However, the problem with polarisation by reflection is that in the real world it can cause a great deal of **glare**, which is something we'll pick up on in the section 'Applications of Polarisation'.

Polarisation by Refraction

In some cases, light can become **polarised through refraction**. The term 'refraction' describes the change in direction of light when moving from one material into another. This directional change will occur at the boundaries of the materials, so if light entered the front surface of a glass block (from air) and then left the block at the back surface, refraction would occur at both the front and back surfaces. Now, most materials that refract light are what we call 'optically isotropic', meaning they possess the same optical properties in all directions, but some special materials (e.g. calcite crystal) can have a degree of **optical symmetry**, meaning the natural frequency of the material (and its propensity for transmitting light) will be different depending on the axis. When light enters this type of material, two linearly polarised rays are produced! I like to think of this as double refraction, but the technical term is **birefringence** (Fig. 14.7). In this example, one of the polarised rays will be linearly polarised parallel to the surface, and one will be polarised perpendicular to the surface, which ultimately results in two distinct images being produced.

A nice, real-world example of this is the image formed when viewed through a calcite crystal (sometimes called Iceland spar). A calcite crystal is transparent-translucent and is a clear (glassy) type of crystal, meaning that it can transmit light through it quite easily. However, because calcite crystals are optically symmetrical, they produce birefringence which produces two images of any object when viewed through the crystal. We can see a nice example of this in Fig. 14.8.

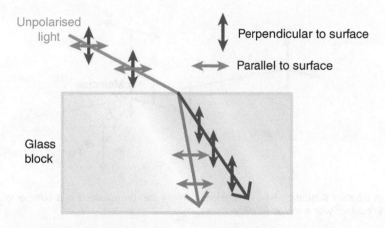

• **Fig. 14.7** Illustration showing incident light (blue ray) upon a glass block. At the front surface of the block, the light is split into two perpendicularly, linearly polarised rays, which will produce two images.

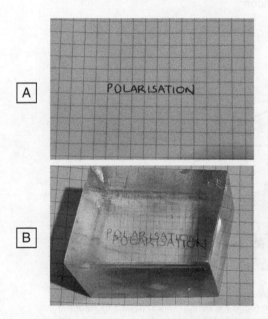

• **Fig. 14.8** An example of birefringence in a calcite crystal (also known as Iceland spar). You can see that without the crystal, the writing is neat(ish) and very clear (A), whereas when the crystal is placed on top of the writing, it produces two images of the writing and the square lines on the page (B). These two images will be produced by perpendicularly polarised light.

In clinical applications, the retinal nerve fibre layer (RNFL) in the eye is a birefringent material (meaning it splits light into two rays). If light is sent into the eye (let's say from a camera), and it passes through the RNFL, then the difference between the subsequent two rays will reveal a lot about the thickness of the RNFL, so this feature is used in some optical imaging for monitoring the health of the back of the eye.

Polarisation by Scattering

The final method of polarisation we're going to discuss in this chapter is **polarisation by scattering**. This method (just like it says on the tin) describes polarisation that occurs as

light is scattered as it travels through a medium. For example, when unpolarised white light from the sun travels through the Earth's atmosphere, it will come into contact with the various atoms that make up the atmosphere. This will set the electrons in the atoms into vibration, which causes them to produce their own electromagnetic wave that radiates out in all directions (Fig. 14.9). This newly generated wave then strikes neighbouring atoms, which causes a knock-on effect of the same vibration and production of electromagnetic waves, which are once again radiated out in all directions. This absorption and reemission of light waves is what causes the light to be 'scattered' within the medium.

For a real-world example, let's consider that the sun looks yellow at noon and red at sunset, and why the sky looks blue. When this absorption and reemission process happens with unpolarised sunlight, shorter (more blue) wavelengths within the sunlight are more easily polarised/scattered than the longer wavelengths. At noon, the light from the sun only has a relatively small amount of atmosphere to travel through, which limits the amount of polarisation that can happen (Fig. 14.10). However, the scattering of the blue wavelengths into the atmosphere makes the sky look blue, and as a consequence of them being removed from the white light of the sun, the sun appears shifted towards the longer side of the spectrum – making it appear yellow instead of white. Similarly, at sunrise and sunset, the light from the sun has much more atmosphere to travel through, which causes some of the slightly longer (more yellow) wavelengths to be scattered as well (see Fig. 14.10). This means that by the time the light from the sun reaches us at this time of day, the blue and yellow light will be scattered into the atmosphere (making the sky appear orange), and the appearance of the sun will be shifted further towards the long wavelength side of the spectrum, making it appear red.

Applications of Polarisation

Polarisation and polarising filters can be utilised effectively for a number of applications, including photography, glare-reducing sunglasses, and 3-dimensional (3D) films.

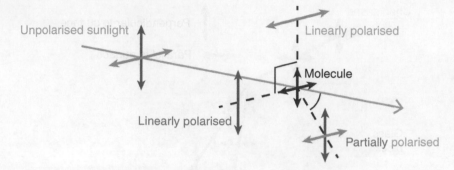

• **Fig. 14.9** A diagram illustrating how unpolarised sunlight can be polarised in a number of directions when making contact with a molecule in the atmosphere.

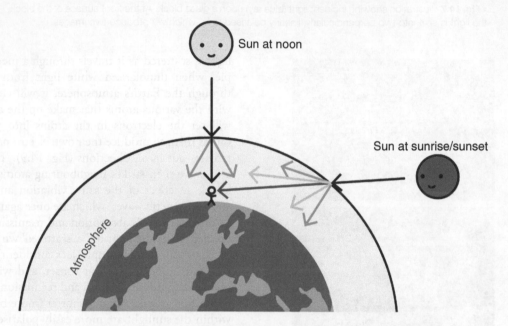

• **Fig. 14.10** An illustration of a person on Earth (not to scale) viewing the sun at noon and at sunrise/sunset. At sunrise/sunset the sunlight has farther to travel to reach the person, which means more of the light is scattered. This makes the sun appear redder as it gets nearer the horizon.

Photography

When taking photographs, polarised light (particularly that caused by reflection) can create a lot of glare and can affect the colour of certain objects within the image. Photographers then, can use a polarising filter on the front of their camera lens, which will reduce glare, darken the colour of the sky, and manage unwanted light reflections. Modern polarising filters are typically circular polarisers to make them maximally effective, as linear polarisers can affect the auto-focus capabilities of some cameras.

Sunglasses

Polarised sunglasses are often seen as a way for people selling sunglasses to charge you extra for the lenses, but they really do serve a purpose! These lenses are typically designed to remove the glare and reflections from polarised light reflected off water, roads, snow, etc. This means that most of the light they are trying to block out will be polarised parallel to the surface it's reflected from, which should (in most cases) be horizontal relative to the observer. This means that polarised lenses in sunglasses can be linearly polarised to only permit vertical light through (to remove all horizontal glare light from the scene). As discussed earlier in the chapter, this will also reduce the brightness of the scene, which highlights that they're effective for use as sunglasses. The advantage of polarised lenses is that the removal of the reflected light allows people to see into the water (so great for fishermen and sailors), and they can improve contrast of the scene (so also great for sportspeople like golfers). However, these lenses can also remove the light information from certain digital displays that emit polarised light, so if you've ever noticed that a digital sign appears to vanish at certain angles through your polarised lenses, it's because the light emitted is also polarised!

3D Films

Modern 3D films that require the cool, black-tinted specs (as opposed to the slightly less cool red and green specs) utilise principles of polarisation to make their scenes 'pop out' of the screen. They do this by using two 3D cameras to film two side-by-side, simultaneous shots of every scene which identifies the disparity (relative difference in position) between objects. If an object is closer to the cameras, it will appear to have larger disparity than an object far away. These scenes are then superimposed on top of one another using two projectors (which makes them look a little blurry – particularly for objects close to the camera – if viewing without the appropriate specs on). For linearly polarised films, these projectors will be set to emit light that is polarised in a particular orientation, but crucially, they need to be set differently to one another. For example, one projector might emit light linearly polarised vertically, and one might emit light linearly polarised horizontally. Your special glasses will have two different lenses – one set to allow through each type of polarised light; so for example, perhaps only vertically polarised light (from the first projector) can reach the left eye, and the opposite for the right eye. Our brains can then interpret and merge the two disparate images to achieve that sense of depth. However, an issue arises if we tilt our heads whilst in the cinema (or snuggle up to a loved one), because it changes the orientation of the polarising filter in the lenses and can prevent the light getting through properly, which is less than ideal. To fix this, projectors can utilise circular polarisation, which means head-tilting is OK again.

Test Your Knowledge

Try the questions below to see if you need to review any sections again. All answers are available in the back of the book.

TYK.14.1 Define 'unpolarised light'.
TYK.14.2 Explain the difference between circular and elliptical polarisation.
TYK.14.3 What type of light would be emitted through two identically oriented polarising filters?
TYK.14.4 Is light reflected off a lake more likely to be polarised in the horizontal or vertical plane?
TYK.14.5 Explain why the sun appears red at sunset.

Reference

1. Physics Classroom. Polarisation. n.d. https://www.physicsclassroom.com/class/light/Lesson-1/Polarization#:~:text=A%20picket%2Dfence%20analogy%20is,vibrates%20in%20a%20single%20plane. Accessed December 20, 2021.

15

Imaging the Eye and Measuring Refractive Error

CHAPTER OUTLINE

OBJECTIVES

After working through this chapter, you should be able to:

Explain why it is difficult to see the back of the eye and the anterior angle without the help of special devices

Explain how direct and indirect ophthalmoscopy works

Explain how direct and indirect gonioscopy works

Explain retinoscopy and how it works

Explain how applanation tonometry works

Introduction

In this chapter, we're going to use some of the knowledge we gained in previous chapters in order to start to understand some of the basic principles behind imaging the inside of the eye (which as you might imagine, requires special optical systems), before moving on to discuss how we can use optical physics to determine a person's refractive error and how applanation tonometry works.

Please note that this book is not designed to be a guide for how to perform these techniques safely in clinical practice; instead consider this an interesting summary of the underlying principles to help you understand the techniques.

Imaging the Eye

To start with, let's think about imaging the inside of the eye. Now, when I say 'imaging' here, I'm referring to the ability to produce an optical image of the inside of the eye. The reason for needing to do this would be to assess the health of a patient's eye, so it is an essential part of an optometrist's daily practice. However, if you've ever met another human being before you'll know that we can't just look directly into a person's eye, because in normal circumstances the pupil (the aperture in the iris leading to the back of the eye) appears black.

Why Can't We See Inside the Eye Anyway?

Let's begin by considering the reduced human eye that we learned about in chapter 5 (Fig. 15.1 for a refresher). This reduced eye assumes that the overall power of the eye will be +60.00D, and the retina (the sensory tissue at the back of the inside of the eye) will exist at the secondary focal point of the eye (+22.22 mm). This means that we can assume that light reflecting from the retina (forming an image of the retina) will possess a vergence of −60.00D when it reaches the front surface of the cornea, and that therefore the light leaving the patients' eye will have parallel vergence. Following this, we can start to understand that an in-focus image of the retina will be 'at infinity' (we can confirm this using vergence equations from chapter 2). This means that in fact, we absolutely should be able to see the retina from outside the eye, providing we can line ourselves up with the exit pupil of the eye (see chapter 13 for a reminder of this idea). However, there are two issues:

1. The inside of the eye is very dark, and we can only see illuminated objects (see chapter 1 for a review of this).
2. The human pupil is usually very small (4.3 mm[1]), which will severely restrict our **field of view**.

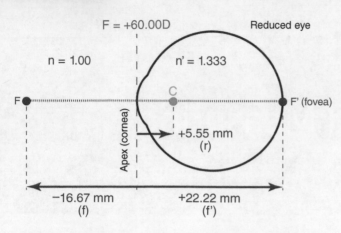

• **Fig. 15.1** Reduced model eye with power, distances, and refractive indices labelled appropriately.

Logically, then, if we could illuminate the inside of the eye somehow, and overcome the issue of the field of view, then it should be possible to see inside the eye.

Ophthalmoscopy

One method for viewing the back of the eye is called **ophthalmoscopy** (*ophthalmo-, eye; -scopy, view*), and there are two main types: **direct ophthalmoscopy** and **indirect ophthalmoscopy**.

Direct Ophthalmoscopy

Direct ophthalmoscopy requires the use of a hand-held device called an ophthalmoscope. This device sends parallel (zero vergence) light into the eye, which will then focus on

the retina, thanks to the focusing power of the cornea and lens. The light then travels along the same path back out of the eye, which means it leaves the eye as parallel light again. This parallel light can then approach the clinician's eye, which will form a lovely, focused image of the patient's retina on the clinician's retina and allow them to see exactly what's going on inside the patient's eye (Fig. 15.2).

The nice thing about direct ophthalmoscopy is that it produces a virtual (upright) image, so if the top of the image looks a bit suspect, then it means the top of the retina looks a bit suspect, and it's easy to relate the two (unlike with indirect ophthalmoscopy which produces a real, inverted image – see section 'Indirect Ophthalmoscopy' for more details).

Assuming that the clinician has corrected vision, and the patient is emmetropic (no refractive error), then the clinician will not need a lens of any power in order to see the patient's retina. Instead, the clinician will just need to get very close to the patient – we're talking 1 to 2 cm away – in order to be able to see through the patient's pupil. However, due to the size of the pupil, the clinician will still only be able to see a small amount of the retina at any one time (small field of view), which means they will need to change their viewing angle to see other parts of the retina (a bit like viewing through a keyhole – Fig. 15.3). This is why, if you've ever had this done, clinicians will wiggle around and do the ophthalmoscopy dance in front of you – they're attempting to see all the parts of your retina. The clinician will also usually ask the patient to move their gaze (upwards, up and to the right, rightwards, down and to the right, etc.) to help them view as much of the back of the eye as possible.

However, this method only allows the clinician to use one eye at a time (due to how close the clinician needs to be to the patient), which can be an issue if the clinician has

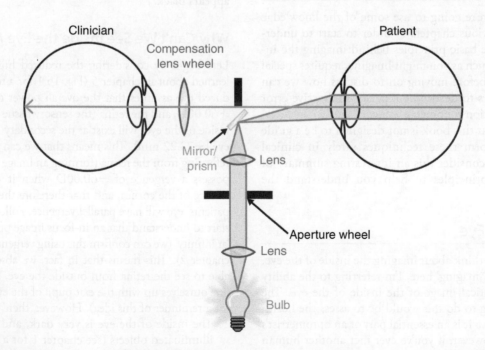

• **Fig. 15.2** Breakdown of how direct ophthalmoscopy images the patient's retina (right) to allow the clinician to see what it looks like (left).

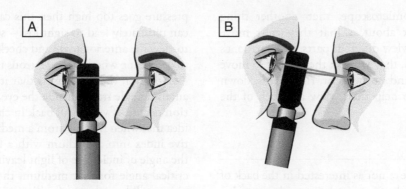

• **Fig. 15.3** Figure showing clinician using a direct ophthalmoscope to look at the patient's fovea (A) and then adjusting their position to look at the inferior (bottom) part of the patient's retina (B).

amblyopia or any other condition affecting the vision of a single eye.

The other, slightly complicated factor to think about is that if the patient (or clinician) has a refractive error, then the light from the ophthalmoscope will be focused incorrectly (either behind or in front) of the patient or clinician's retina, and so the ophthalmoscope will need to be adjusted to account for that.

Indirect Ophthalmoscopy

In contrast to direct ophthalmoscopy, **indirect ophthalmoscopy** allows the clinician to use two eyes (**stereoscopic viewing**) and utilises a high-power plus lens (e.g. +20.00D, +90.00D) called a **condensing lens**.[2] Light is shone through the condensing lens and focused on the patient's

retina, and, just like before, the light will reflect back out of the eye following along the same path and passing back through the condensing lens (Fig. 15.4). This lens then forms an image of the retina which is magnified but inverted (upside down and flipped left to right), which is passed to the clinician's retina in order for them to see the image. The field of view will be determined by the power of the condensing lens – so clinicians will usually have a preferred type of lens.

The advantages of the indirect ophthalmoscopy technique (compared to direct) are that the clinician can view the patient's retina using both eyes, and thanks to the power of the condensing lens, the field of view will be much greater. This method can be utilised using either a **head-mounted binocular indirect ophthalmoscope** (abbreviated as BIO) or with a **slit-lamp biomicroscope** (abbreviated as SL).

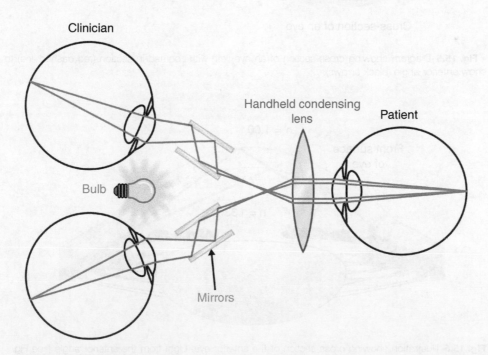

• **Fig. 15.4** Breakdown of how indirect ophthalmoscopy images the patient's retina (right) to allow the clinician to see what it looks like (left).

If using a slit-lamp biomicroscope, then another thing clinicians need to think about is that they can't move themselves very easily to view different parts of the patient's retina. To get around this, they will ask the patient to move their gaze (upwards, up and to the right, rightwards, down and to the right, etc.) to help them view as much of the fundus as possible.

Gonioscopy

Now, let's imagine that we're not as interested in the back of the eye, but instead we'd be interested to see the **anterior angle**. We haven't discussed much anatomy and physiology in this book, so you'll just have to trust me when I say that the anterior angle (the point where the inside surface of the cornea becomes the limbus and connects to the iris – shown by an arrow in Fig. 15.5) is an important site for **aqueous drainage**. Aqueous humour is the name for the fluid that exists in the front part of our eye, and it helps to nourish certain structures and also helps to maintain a certain **intraocular pressure (IOP)**. IOP is important because if the

pressure goes too high then this can lead to damage which can ultimately lead to sight loss – so it's useful for clinicians to view the anterior angle and check that it's healthy in order to determine whether the aqueous is able to drain effectively.

However, the problem is that it's not possible to see the anterior angle from outside the eye, as **total internal reflection** occurs. If you recall back in chapter 9 we discussed the idea that when moving from a medium with a higher refractive index into a medium with a lower refractive index, if the angle of incidence of light leaving the object exceeds the critical angle for that medium, then all the light from the object will be reflected *back* into the higher refractive index medium (which is appropriately called total internal reflection). This is what happens with the anterior angle in the eye (as seen in Fig. 15.6), where due to the refractive index difference between the aqueous and cornea (1.336 and 1.376), relative to the air (1.00), the light from the anterior angle meets the corneal surface at an angle that exceeds the critical angle (i_c). This causes it to reflect back into the anterior chamber – making it seemingly invisible to anyone outside of the eye.

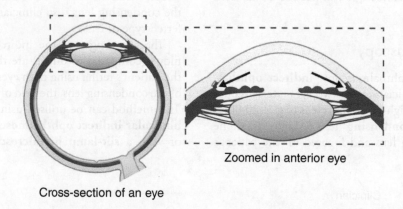

Cross-section of an eye   Zoomed in anterior eye

• **Fig. 15.5** Diagram showing cross-section of an eye (left) with zoomed-in section (red dashed line) to show anterior angle (black arrows).

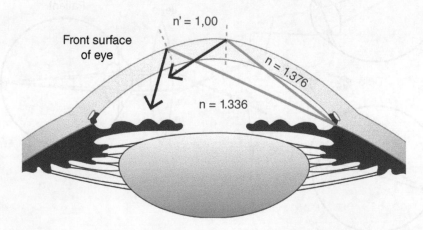

• **Fig. 15.6** Illustration showing cross-section of the anterior eye. Light from the anterior angle (see Fig. 15.5) suffers from total internal reflection due to the refractive index difference between the inside of the eye (relative to the outside).

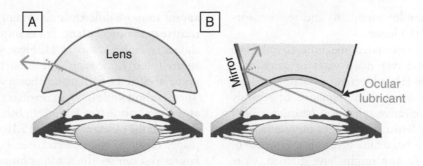

• **Fig. 15.7** Diagram illustrating how direct gonioscopy (A) and indirect gonioscopy (B) work.

In order to get around this, clinicians need to utilise a **goniolens** – a special lens for viewing the anterior angle. In general terms, these lenses come in two forms to allow clinicians to perform: direct gonioscopy (Fig. 15.7A) and indirect gonioscopy (Fig. 15.7B). Both techniques require a lens to be placed directly onto the front surface of the eye (so you'll be relieved to know that the eye will be anaesthetised first).

Direct Gonioscopy

Direct gonioscopy involves placing a special lens onto the front surface of the eye. This lens will be manufactured at a refractive index more similar to the eye than air, which means light from the anterior angle can pass into the lens itself. Then, the special (very steep) curve of the outer surface of the lens allows the light to leave the lens as it no longer exceeds the critical angle and therefore isn't susceptible to total internal reflection. This is a useful technique because it provides a 'direct' view of the angle, from all possible angles of viewing. However, the problem with direct gonioscopy is that it needs to be placed on the patient's eye whilst they are lying down, so a traditional optometric practice wouldn't be able to perform this technique.

Indirect Gonioscopy

Indirect gonioscopy relies on similar principles to the direct gonioscopy technique, but this time, the clinician will use powered mirrors instead of a lens. Indirect gonioscopy can involve either a **three-mirror goniolens** or a **four-mirror goniolens**, depending on what the clinician is looking for, and (to some extent) personal preference. As shown in Fig. 15.8A, three-mirror lenses can view the posterior pole of the eye by looking straight through (blue), or they can help the clinician view the equatorial section (yellow) using the trapezoid mirror (73°), or they can allow the clinician to view the ora serrata (green) using the rectangular mirror (67°). Finally, the clinician can use the **D-shape mirror** (59°) to view the anterior angle (pink). In contrast to this, a four-mirror goniolens (Fig. 15.8B) can only view the posterior pole (blue) and the anterior angle (pink) as it has four D-shape mirrors (59°) placed around the inside of the lens. As these lenses utilise a mirror reflection, they

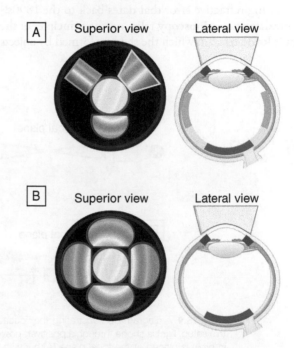

• **Fig. 15.8** Colour-coded illustration view of three-mirror goniolens (A) and four-mirror goniolens (B) from the superior view and the lateral view. Each mirror is outlined in a colour which is projected onto the cross-section view of the eye to show the area it makes visible.

produce an indirect view of the angle and require repositioning of the lens depending on which part of the angle the clinician wants to view.

Measuring Refractive Error

At this point in the chapter, we're going to slightly deviate away from health-related imaging and instead start to consider the refractive power (and associated refractive *error*) of the eye. We learned in chapter 5 that the human eye can possess spherical or cylindrical refractive errors (or both), with spherical refractive errors being defined as either too much power in all planes (myopia), requiring negative spherical lenses, or too little power across all planes (hyperopia), requiring positive spherical lenses. Cylindrical error, on the other hand, is defined as a difference in refractive power along a single plane (or meridian) and requires specialised cylindrical (or toric) lenses.

Apart from using an automated machine to calculate refractive errors, there are two main ways of assessing a patient's refractive error: (1) subjective refraction (asking patients what they can see with a sequence of sensibly chosen lenses) and (2) objective refraction (shining a light into the patient's eye and letting the laws of physics tell you what the error is likely to be, whilst utilising a sequence of sensibly chosen lenses). As you might have guessed, we're going to focus on objective refraction in this book, and in particular we're going to focus on a method called **retinoscopy** (or sometimes skiascopy), which is a technique for measuring refractive error that dates back to the 1800s![3]

Neutralisation retinoscopy relies on the principles of the **Foucault knife test,**[4] in which the shadow formed by objects appear to move differently depending on where the object is relative to the **focal plane**. For example, look at the diagrams shown in Figs. 15.9 to 15.11. Here, you can see that a light source (bulb) is focusing light through a condensing lens at a point labelled the focal plane (shown with dashed black lines). There is also a knife (grey, sharp object) which is either located at the focal plane (see Fig. 15.9); behind the focal plane, farther from the observer (see Fig. 15.10); or in front of the focal plane, closer to the observer (see Fig. 15.11). In all these figures you can see the shadows formed by the knife in each example. When the knife is at the focal plane but not obstructing the light rays (see Fig. 15.9A), no shadow is produced; however, if the knife is moved slightly upwards, it will quickly block the light (see Fig. 15.9B). This means that if the shadow quickly alternates between nonexistent and 'full coverage' when the knife is moved (as shown in Fig. 15.9), we

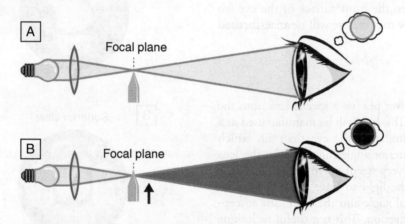

• **Fig. 15.9** A diagram demonstrating the Foucault knife test[4] with the knife placed at the focal plane. In this setup, light is shone through a positively powered lens to form a focus (focal plane). If the knife (shown in grey) is placed at the focal plane (A) but without obscuring the light, then it will allow all light to pass (not obstructing). If, however, it is moved slightly upwards (B), it will quickly block all the light completely, meaning the shadow is either 'full' or absent.

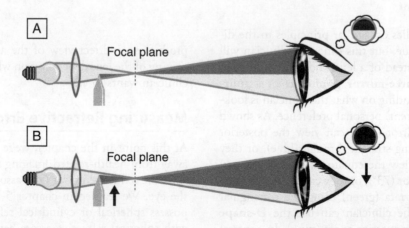

• **Fig. 15.10** A diagram demonstrating the Foucault knife test[4] with the knife placed farther from the observer than the focal plane. In this setup, light is shone through a positively powered lens to form a focus (focal plane). If the knife (shown in grey) is placed farther from the observer than the focal plane (A), then it will slightly obscure the light and produce an inverted shadow (after the light crosses following convergence). If the knife is then moved slightly upwards (B), it will move the shadow (and the remaining light) downwards in the opposite direction to the movement of the knife (against movement).

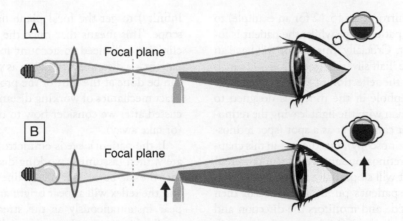

• **Fig. 15.11** A diagram demonstrating the Foucault knife test[4] with the knife placed closer to the observer than the focal plane. In this setup, light is shone through a positively powered lens to form a focus (focal plane). If the knife (shown in grey) is placed closer to the observer than the focal plane (A), then it will slightly obscure the light and produce an upright shadow (as the light continues in a straight line). If the knife is then moved slightly upwards (B) it will move the shadow (and the remaining light) upwards, in the same direction to the movement of the knife (with movement).

can assume the object is at the focal plane. Alternatively, when the knife is behind the focal plane, farther from the observer (see Fig. 15.10A), it produces an inverted shadow because the light converges at the focal plane and crosses to the opposite side. If this knife is then moved upwards (further into the light), then we can see from Fig. 15.10B that the shadow will move in the opposite direction. This is called an **against movement** because the shadow is moving in the opposite direction to the object, which suggests the object is farther from the observer than the focal plane. Finally, when the knife is in front of the focal plane, closer to the observer (see Fig. 15.11A), it produces a shadow that falls on the same

side as the knife. If this knife is then moved upwards (farther into the light), then Fig. 15.11B shows us that the corresponding shadow will move in the same direction as the object. This is called a **with movement** because the shadow is moving in the same direction as the object, which suggests the object is closer to the observer than the focal plane. This is informative to us because we can estimate the position of the knife relative to the focal plane (and vice versa) using the direction and appearance of the shadows.

Now, you may be thinking this is all well and good, but how does this relate to retinoscopy? Well, with retinoscopy a clinician uses a device called a (self-illuminated) **retinoscope**

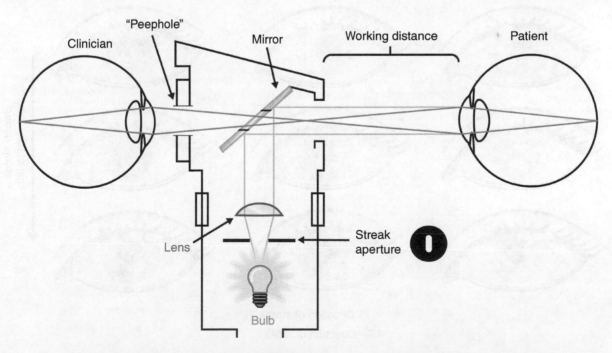

• **Fig. 15.12** Simplified illustration of how a self-illuminating retinoscope works, with light from the bulb passing through a positive lens before being reflected to the patient by a mirror. The mirror contains a 'peephole' so that the clinician can see the patient through the device.

which utilises an angled mirror (Fig. 15.12 for an example) to shine a bright light at the patient's eye whilst the patient is focusing on a 'distant' target. Crucially, this mirror will have an aperture ('peephole') or be 'half silvered' (see-through), which allows the clinician to see the reflection of the light (from the patient's retina). This peephole in the mirror is designed to align the view of the clinician with the light leaving the retinoscope, and the bright light can appear as a spot (spot retinoscopy) or a streak (streak retinoscopy), but the text in this chapter will focus on the streak retinoscope and a plane (unpowered) mirror. This streak of light will sit partially across the iris, and some of it will enter the patient's pupil. The clinician then moves the streak side-to-side and monitors the direction and shape of the light (and the shadow) visible through the pupil, which is shining off the back of the eye (this image of the light is called the **reflex**). The goal of retinoscopy is to line up the focal plane (far point; see chapter 5 for a reminder of this) of the eye with the 'entrance pupil' of the retinoscope – which, because the clinician will be 50 or 67 cm away from the patient, assumes that light from the patient's eye will need to converge to find the retinoscope's entrance pupil appropriately. However, remember that the patient will be focusing on a distant target (parallel vergence) because the clinician is trying to determine their distance refractive error, which means clinicians need to be very careful to make a note of exactly how far they are away from the patient. As we learned in chapter 2, vergence is related to distance, and as the patient is focusing on the distant target (infinity), the clinician will need to account for their relative 'closeness', as they will find that they need to add too much positive power (relative to

infinity) to get the focal plane lined up with their retinoscope. This means that once the reflex is 'neutralised', the clinician will need to account for their distance from the patient – a distance referred to as **working distance** – which can be done at the start of the procedure, or at the end. The exact mechanics of working distance calculations will be discussed after we consider how to decide which lenses to add (or take away).

If the patient's eye is emmetropic or corrected appropriately, then (assuming working distance has been accounted for) the far point will nicely line up with the retinoscope, and the reflex will appear bright and fill the pupil and disappear instantaneously as the streak moves away from the pupil; this is considered 'neutrality' – that is, the light is focusing appropriately on the retina (Fig. 15.13, *right*). However, if the reflex has a visible movement, or is dull (less bright), or if the reflex moves at a different speed to the streak, then a refractive error is present – that is, the light is not focusing appropriately on the retina and is instead focusing too far in front (**myopia**) or too far behind (**hyperopia**). The goal of retinoscopy is to place corrective lenses in front of the patient's eye until the reflex shows a 'reversal' (neutrality). The way to determine whether a positive lens or a negative lens is needed to correct the error is to look at the movement of the light (and shadow, like with the knife edge). If the reflex has a *with* movement, then it means the far point of the eye is virtual (or behind the clinician) – which indicates hyperopia – so a positive corrective lens is needed (Fig. 15.13, *left*). Alternatively, if the reflex has an *against* movement, then it means the far point of the eye is

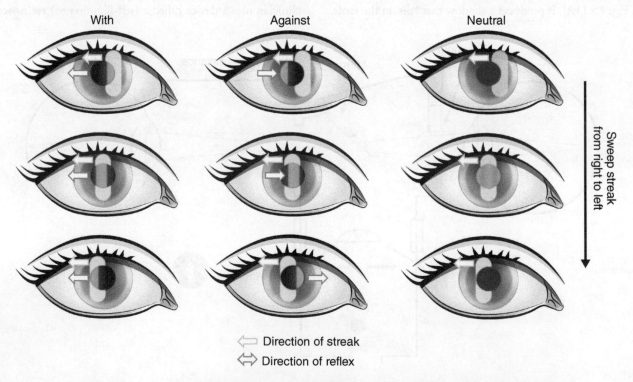

⇦ Direction of streak

⟺ Direction of reflex

• **Fig. 15.13** Illustration showing retinoscopy and associated reflex as the streak moves from right to left. Diagrams show what reflex looks like when: positive lenses need to be added (left), when negative lenses need to be added (middle), and when no lenses need to be added (right).

between the patient and the clinician – which indicates myopia – and so a negative corrective lens is needed (Fig. 15.13, *middle*). If the reflex moves at an angle that differs to that of the streak, this would indicate the presence of **astigmatism** (cylindrical error; see chapter 5).

The amount of refractive error present is determined by adding lenses (appropriately) until neutrality is reached; however, as we indicated a moment ago, this is influenced by the clinician's working distance. This means that to find the true refractive error, clinicians need to calculate the relative vergence assumed by their distance from the patient; for example, if they are sitting 67 cm away from the patient then they will be adding approximately +1.50D of vergence to the light leaving the patients' eye (L = n/l =1/+0.67 = +1.49) in order to focus it at their own eye. This means that at some point in the refraction process, the clinician will need to subtract this vergence from the estimate before determining the final prescription.[5] For example, if an experienced clinician was performing retinoscopy on me with my −6.75DS eyes, and they were sitting 67 cm away – they should find that they need to initially add −5.25DS of power to reach neutrality, but then subtract their working distance vergence (−5.25DS − (+1.50DS)) to determine that my true prescription is −6.75DS.

Applanation Tonometry

In this final section, we will briefly discuss how split-image prisms can be used to measure IOP. As we mentioned in the section on gonioscopy, it's important to monitor a patient's IOP because IOP that is too low or too high can lead to eye problems and vision loss.

Measurement of pressure is called tonometry, and the technique which we will discuss here is called **applanation tonometry** (or **contact tonometry**), which kind of means 'measure pressure by flattening'. In this case, an applanation tonometer can measure IOP by flattening the cornea over a set area. This relies on the **Imbert-Fick principle**,[6] which states that the pressure inside a sphere is related to the force required to flatten the surface of the sphere over a particular area (Equation 15.1).

Equation 15.1 $P = \dfrac{F}{A}$

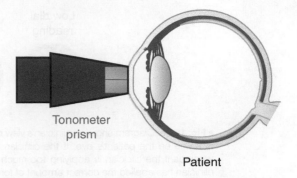

Tonometer prism

Patient

• **Fig. 15.14** Diagram showing applanation tonometry. The tonometer (with prisms inside) is in contact with the patient's eye, which is stained with fluorescein (yellow dye) to help show the meniscus of the tear film.

Equation 15.1 (explained) $Pressure = \dfrac{force}{area}$

In applanation tonometry, the tonometer will flatten an area of the cornea that corresponds to 3.06 mm in diameter,[6] and the IOP (mmHg) can be determined by the amount of force (grams) needed to flatten the cornea at this area, multiplied by 10 (Fig. 15.14). This means that the tonometer not only needs to be in contact with the front of the eye (but don't worry, the eye will have anaesthetic so it won't feel anything), but it also needs to apply a small amount of force. So, how does the clinician know when the cornea is truly and appropriately flattened?

In order to correctly flatten the cornea, the clinician will need to stain the front surface of the eye using a yellow dye called fluorescein.[5] This dye is useful because it highlights the tear film, so when the tonometer is positioned on the eye (in contact with the eye and tear film), the tear film produces a meniscus (curve in the surface) around the edge of the tonometer. This meniscus will be viewed through a split-image prism (two cylindrical lenses cut at opposite, diagonal angles to one another – Fig. 15.15) which (as its name suggests) splits the image of the spherical meniscus into two semi-circle halves called **mires**. The way the split-prisms are constructed means that the clinician can see how the mires align with one another (Fig. 15.16) to decide whether to add more force or less force until the balance is appropriate to record the IOP.

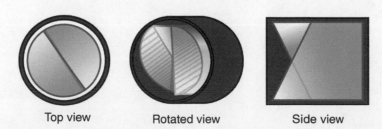

Top view   Rotated view   Side view

• **Fig. 15.15** Illustration showing how the tonometer works from three cross-sectional viewpoints. Inside, there is a split-image prism (two cylindrical lenses which have been cut to be oppositely angled).

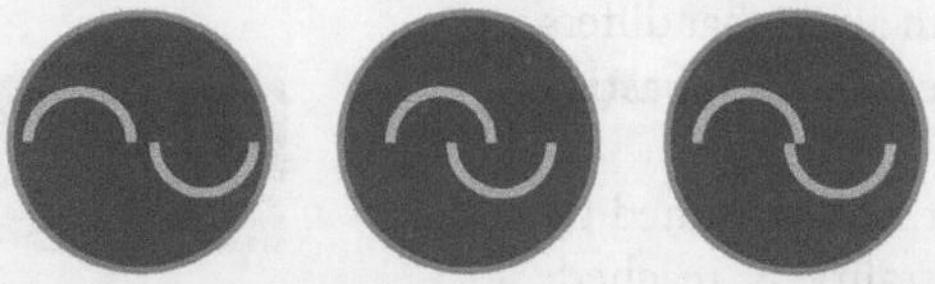

| Low dial reading | High dial reading | Correct alignment |

• **Fig. 15.16** Diagram showing clinician's view of the mires (yellow lines) which are apparent when pressure is made on the patient's eye. If the clinician is applying too little force, the mires will be too far apart, whereas if the clinician is applying too much force, the mires will be overlapping too much. When the clinician has applied the correct amount of force, the mires will be aligned as shown on the right with the inner edges in contact.

Test Your Knowledge

Try the questions below to see if you need to review any sections again. All answers are available in the back of the book.

TYK.15.1 Why is it not possible to see the back of a patient's eye without the help of a special device?

TYK.15.2 Is a slit-lamp biomicroscope a form of direct or indirect ophthalmoscopy?

TYK.15.3 Why is it advantageous to the clinician to ask the patient to move their gaze when performing ophthalmoscopy?

TYK.15.4 Explain why the anterior angle of the eye is not visible without the help of a special lens.

TYK.15.5 On a three-mirror goniolens, which mirror would allow the clinician to view the anterior angle?

TYK.15.6 Explain what an against movement would look like during retinoscopy.

TYK.15.7 If a clinician performed retinoscopy on a patient at a working distance of 50 cm, what spherical power would they need to account for in the final refractive error?

TYK.15.8 What equation does applanation tonometry rely on for calculating intraocular pressure (IOP)?

References

1. Aminihajibashi S, Hagen T, Foldal MD, Laeng B, Espeseth T. Individual differences in resting-state pupil size: evidence for association between working memory capacity and pupil size variability. *Int J Psychophysiol*. 2019;140:1-7.
2. Sherman S E The history of the ophthalmoscope. In: Henkes H, Zrenner C, eds. History of Ophthalmology (Sub auspiciis Academiae Ophthalmologicae Internationalis). Dordrecht: Springer; 1989:221-228.
3. Corboy JM. *The Retinoscopy Book: An Introductory Manual for Eye Care Professionals*. 5th ed. USA: SLACK Incorporated; 2003.
4. Hallak J. Reflections on retinoscopy. *Am J Optom Physiol Opt*. 1976;53(2):224-228.
5. Elliott DB. *Clinical Procedures in Primary Eye Care*. 5th ed. Amsterdam: Elsevier Health Sciences; 2020.
6. Rhee D. *Color Atlas & Synopsis of Clinical Ophthalmology: Glaucoma*. 3rd ed. The Netherlands: Wolters Kluwer; 2019.

16

Wavefront Aberrations and Adaptive Optics

OBJECTIVES

After working through this chapter, you should be able to:

Define a wavefront aberration

Explain how aberrations can affect the resultant image

Explain a Zernike polynomial

Understand how aberrometers can quantify aberrations

Explain how adaptive optics systems can improve image resolution

Introduction

We've already discussed **aberrations** (imperfections in the image) in previous chapters when we've considered spherical aberrations and chromatic aberrations. This chapter will focus on aberrations more generally before explaining why they're such a nuisance, and how to get rid of them.

Wavefront Aberrations

In a perfect **optical system** that produces an image, all the light rays from the object would be perfectly focused to form a complete, comprehensive and accurate representation of the object (e.g. Fig. 16.1A). For example, if we think of our eyes as optical systems, the goal of the eye is to focus a clear image of the world onto the back of our eyes so that we can see in perfect clarity. However, as you'll be familiar with your own eyes, you know that this isn't the case. If we need glasses, then we'll see blurry images without our correction, and even if we don't need glasses, we might struggle to focus on things too close or too far away. These are examples of imperfections in the image which are called **wavefront aberrations** (because these aberrations exist in the wavefront). In its most basic form, the term 'aberration' describes a failure of light rays to converge sensibly at a point of focus. This means that the rays will, in some way,

be **blurring** (less focused; Fig. 16.1B) or **distorting** (warped in shape somehow; Fig. 16.1C) the image.

And, slightly frustratingly, these aberrations exist in almost all optical systems (lenses, imaging systems, eyeballs). This can lead to issues such as: blurry vision for people in the real world, or blurry images being taken of the back of a patient's eye. We will go into more detail on these aberrations and their effects throughout this chapter.

Types of Aberrations

Before we go into detail of how aberrations can cause problems, let's start by discussing the type of aberrations that can be induced. In the previous section we started to distinguish between blurring relative to distorting, but in actuality, we can break it down a lot more by not only classifying the type of aberration but also classifying how impactful the aberration is. One way to do this is to use **Zernike polynomials**,[1] which turn the induced aberrations into a mathematical construct so we can tell how disruptive one aberration might be relative to another. In this case, each aberration can be assigned a value that is either positive or negative, and these values will predict alterations in the shape and quality of the image. Zernike polynomials are expressed in the form Z_n^m, where the subscript n defines the **order** of the aberration, and the superscript m defines

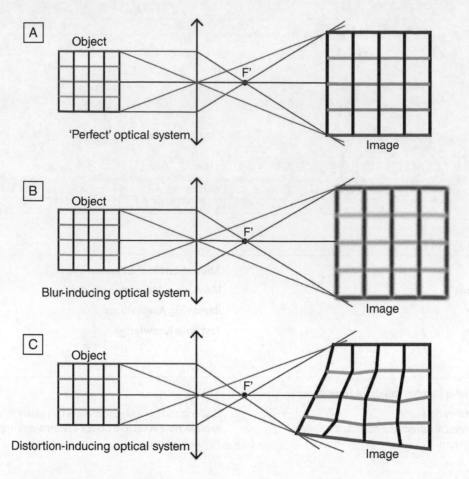

A - Object - 'Perfect' optical system - F' - Image

B - Object - Blur-inducing optical system - F' - Image

C - Object - Distortion-inducing optical system - F' - Image

• **Fig. 16.1** Diagram showing examples of how optical systems should focus light to form a clear image (A), and how they can induce blur (B) and distortion (C).

the **angular frequency** (how many times the wavefront pattern repeats itself every 2π radians). Fig. 16.2 shows a view of the polynomials labelled and described.

In optometric practice, the angular frequency aligns with the number of planes of the cornea that the aberration affects – for example, you can imagine that a 'tilt' aberration would only affect one plane (horizontal or vertical), so its angular frequency is 1 (−1 or +1 depending on the direction). Also, typically, aberrations with a *negative* angular frequency are aligned in the vertical plane, whereas aberrations with a *positive* angular frequency are aligned in the horizontal plane. To provide a clinically relevant example, in chapter 5 we discussed that people can have **astigmatism** (a refractive error along a particular plane within the eye). In Fig. 16.2 we can see that astigmatism is a second-order wavefront aberration with either a +2 or −2 angular frequency.

Aberrations in Lenses

Lenses are used in optical instruments (and glasses) in order to focus light in a set way. This means that you could be forgiven for thinking that all light is refracted through the lens equally, but in reality this isn't the case. The **optical centre** of the lens will possess the clearest image, but as light moves away from the optical centre, more and more aberrations (imperfections)

will be induced (Fig. 16.3). This is particularly true for high-powered lenses where the lenses need to be thicker in order to produce the power required.

If we wear glasses, we can demo this ourselves, otherwise we can use Fig. 16.4 to help think about it. Lenses need to have curved surfaces in order to focus light correctly, but with two curved surfaces, the shape of the lens will vary from the centre relative to the edges. In Fig. 16.4 you can see that the edges of the convex and concave lenses begin to resemble prisms, which is a clear indicator that they will start to introduce **prismatic effects**. As light moves away from the optical centre of a glasses lens, the light will undergo prismatic changes, which will affect the quality of the image seen by the wearer. If you have a pair of glasses, try looking through the edges of the lens – it should be less clear than when you wear them normally, because it's introducing these pesky aberrations.

Aberrations in the Human Eye

If we now take a moment to think of some common-sense biology, we know that the goal of the eye is to refract light in such a way that incoming light focuses on the back of the eye, and we also know that if a person has a particular refractive error, then there may be some blurring (e.g. defocus).

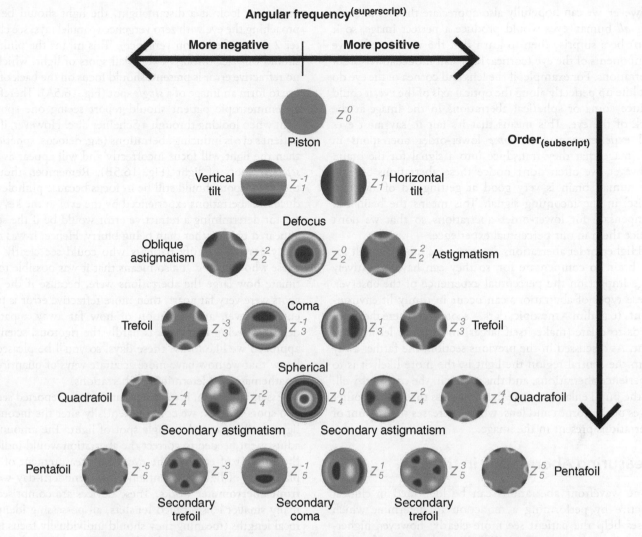

• **Fig. 16.2** Illustration of the first five orders of Zernike polynomial aberrations. Black text describes the type of aberration (e.g. 'defocus') whilst green text identifies the polynomial. Order increases linearly in a downward direction (e.g. 'Piston' at the top has an order of 0, whereas 'Pentafoil' at the bottom has an order of 5). Angular frequency increases outwards from the middle, with the left side being negative and the right side being positive.

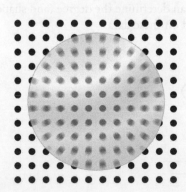

• **Fig. 16.3** Diagram showing a lens on top of a grid of black circles. When the circles are refracting through the edges of the lens, they experience greater amounts of distortion compared to the central region.

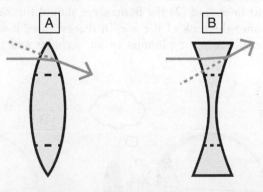

• **Fig. 16.4** Diagram showing light (blue) refracting through the edges of a convex (A) and concave (B) lens. Black dashed lines illustrate that the edges of a lens become prism shaped, whereas blue dashed lines indicate that the image will be displaced upwards (convex, A) or downwards (concave, B) due to the prismatic effects at the lens edges.

However, we can hopefully also appreciate that it's unlikely that *all* human eyes would produce a perfect image, so it won't be a surprise then to learn that the various refractive components of the eye (cornea, lens) can induce lower-order aberrations. For example, if the lens and cornea of the eye do not line up perfectly along the optical axis of the eye, it could induce coma or spherical aberrations in the image at the back of the eye. This means that it's fair to say most eyes will experience at least *some* lower-order aberrations in the image that they transduce into a signal for the brain. However, we often don't notice these aberrations because the human brain is very good at getting rid of low-level 'noise' in the incoming signal. This means the brain can compensate for lower-order aberrations so that we don't notice them in our perceptual experience.

Higher-order aberrations, however, are more difficult for the brain to compensate for, so they can have a relatively large impact on the perceptual experience of the observer. These types of aberrations can occur in dimly lit environments (e.g. dim – mesopic; dark – scotopic) where the pupil needs to dilate (make itself larger) in order to let in more light. As discussed in the previous section, the farther away from the central region the light is, the more likely it is to experience aberrations, and this is true in the cornea as well. As the pupil enlarges, more light can pass through the outer edges of the cornea and lens, which increases the amount of aberrations present in the image.

Measuring Aberrations in the Eye

Some wavefront aberrations can be identified in clinical practice by performing a refraction to determine which lenses help the patient see more clearly; however, higher-order aberrations are more difficult to identify, so for these we need to utilise a device called an **aberrometer** (*aberr-*, aberration; *-ometer*, measurement).

Historically, one of the first aberrometers was devised by Christoph Scheiner in 1619,[2] when he realised that a two-pinhole occluder could identify if a person was able to see clearly or not. This device is called a **Scheiner disc** and works under the principles that (1) light can only travel in straight lines, and (2) the human eye should focus distant light onto the back of the eye. In theory, then, if you put two small, adjacent pinholes in an occluder and ask the patient to look at a distant light, the light should be approaching the eye with zero vergence (parallel rays; see chapter 2 for a refresher on vergence). This means the pinholes should only let through two small spots of light, which, if no refractive error is present, should focus on the back of the eye to form an image of a *single* spot (Fig. 16.5A). Therefore, an emmetropic patient should report seeing one spot of light when looking through a Scheiner disc. However, if the patient's eye is inducing aberrations (e.g. defocus, spherical), then the light will focus incorrectly and will appear as two *separate* spots of light (Fig. 16.5B). Remember, though, these two spots should still be in focus because pinholes reduce the aberrations experienced by the eye, so the key factor for determining a refractive error would be if the spots appeared twice rather than being blurry. Hence, it was relatively easy to identify patients who could see clearly and those who couldn't. It also means that it was possible to estimate how large the aberrations were, because if the two spots were very far apart, then more refractive error is present. However, an estimation of how far away a patient describes seeing two spots is hardly the rigorous, scientific approach we like to use these days, so you'll be pleased to know that we now have more accurate ways of quantifying (mathematically determining) aberrations.

Essentially, then, if we had a patient who reported seeing two spots of light, we could potentially alter the incoming light until it formed a single spot of light. The amount of adjustment needed to correct the aberration would indicate the amount of error in the eye. This measurement of displacement of light is essentially how a modern-day **wavefront aberrometer** works. These devices are comprised of many smaller lenses called **lenslets**, all possessing identical focal lengths (meaning they should individually focus light in the same way). These lenslets are designed to focus incoming light onto a sensor that can measure how much light deviates from what would be expected if the incoming light was an aberration-free wavefront. In Fig. 16.6 you can see that a perfect wavefront would cause the lenslets to focus light on all the intersections of the sensor – meaning they are all evenly distributed and have undergone no aberrations. However, if aberrations are present (Fig. 16.7), then the light will be focused inappropriately on the sensor, and the sensor can determine the degree (and shape) of the aberration based on these data.

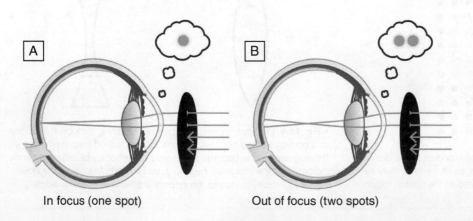

In focus (one spot)   Out of focus (two spots)

• **Fig. 16.5** Diagram showing how a Scheiner disc would work in an eye with no refractive error (A) which would experience a single spot of light, relative to an eye with refractive error (B) which would experience two spots of light.

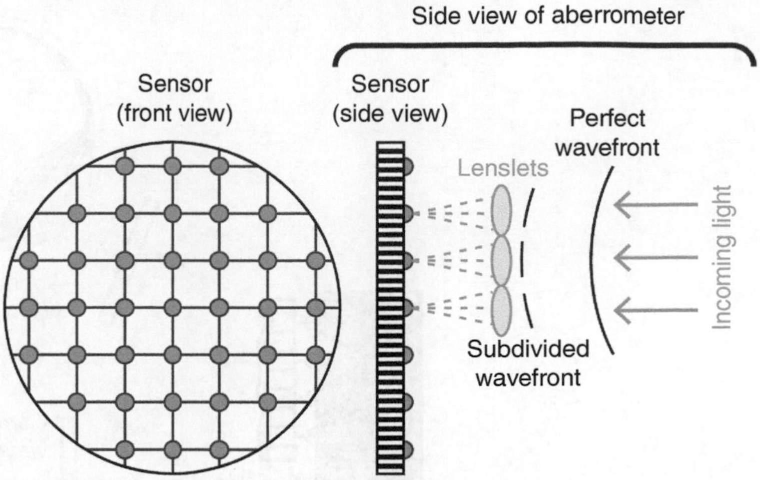

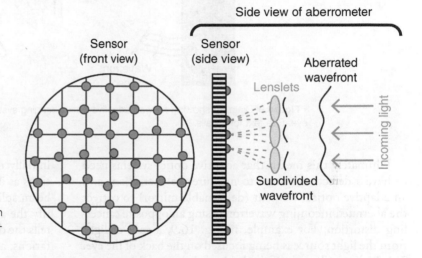

• **Fig. 16.6** Diagram of aberrometer focusing light through the lenslets onto the sensor. Incoming light is free of aberrations, so the resulting image is free of distortions and blur.

• **Fig. 16.7** Diagram of aberrometer focusing light through the lenslets onto the sensor. Incoming light contains aberrations, so the resulting image is distorted.

Removing Aberrations

Up to this point in the chapter, we've considered what an aberration is and what impact it can have on vision, and we've discussed how to quantify the degree of aberration present in an image. However, the most useful reason for measuring aberrations is to remove them from the image. This can be achieved with refractive errors in the eye through prescribing corrective lenses or contact lenses, but what about aberrations present in medical images?

In clinical terms, the problem with aberrations in the eye is that they distort images that we can take of the back of eye itself. You can imagine that if light focuses on the retina with some lower-order aberrations present and we wanted to take a photo of the back of the eye, the resulting image would also contain these lower-order aberrations because the light from our camera (or microscope) will experience the aberrations of the eye as it passes into the eye and as it reflects back out again. This is troubling because it limits the resolution (clarity) of the images we can take of the back of the eye, which means clinicians might miss small changes in health. It is therefore in our interest to be able to (1) detect the aberrations in the first place, (2) quantify the aberrations, (3) localise the aberrations and (4) be able to rapidly adjust/adapt the optical system to compensate for any aberrations

in the image. Thankfully imaging systems can achieve this very successfully through the principles of **adaptive optics**.

The term 'adaptive optics' refers to any optical system (or imaging system) that can adapt to compensate for any aberrations introduced between the object (e.g. the back of the eye) and the image. The goal is to remove the aberrations to improve the overall quality and resolution of the final image. When imaging the human eye, adaptive optics systems compensate for the eye's aberrations by utilising a rapidly **deformable mirror** (>100 Hz) which is constantly adjusted by monitoring the incoming light and changing (deforming) the shape of the mirror in order to undo the aberrations (Fig. 16.8).

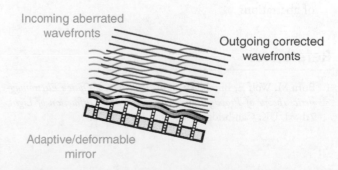

• **Fig. 16.8** Diagram showing how a deformable mirror could change its shape to correct (and remove) aberrations in an image.

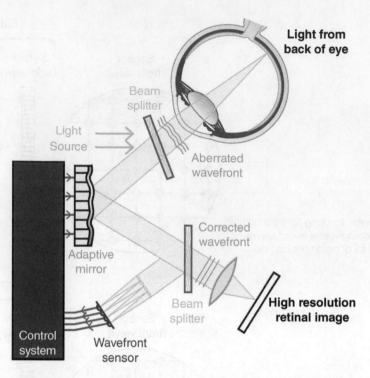

• **Fig. 16.9** Diagram showing how an adaptive optics imaging system could photograph the back of the eye. See text for details.

Ultimately this means that adaptive optics systems need to have a detection system to measure the aberrations and an adaptive optical element (deformable mirror) to correct the aberrated incoming wavefront using an opposite cancelling distortion. For example, in Fig. 16.9, a spot of light from the light source is being focused on the back of the eye. This is then reflected off the back of the eye and leaves out of the front of the eye to pass through the beam splitter, but at this point it now contains aberrations from the eye. The light is then reflected off the deformable mirror (though

initially the mirror won't be able to cancel out the aberrations as it doesn't yet know what to do) and reflected off a beam splitter towards a wavefront sensor which will quantify the aberrations in the image. The control system then tells the deformable mirror how to compensate for the aberrations, and the deformable mirror works its magic to produce a corrected wavefront and a high-resolution final image. The trick is that this system is constantly updating and adapting so it can even account for small eye movements and changes in accommodation in the eye itself.

Test Your Knowledge

Try the questions below to see if you need to review any sections again. All answers are available in the back of the book.

TYK.16.1 What is an aberration?

TYK.16.2 Which part of a lens induces the greatest amount of aberration?

TYK.16.3 In terms of Zernike polynomials, what 'order' of aberration is **defocus**?

TYK.16.4 Explain how a Scheiner disc can identify the presence of a refractive error.

TYK.16.5 Explain how adaptive optics systems can take high-resolution images.

References

1. Born M, Wolf E, Bhatia AB, et al. *Principles of Optics: Electromagnetic Theory of Propagation, Interference and Diffraction of Light.* 7th ed. UK: Cambridge University Press; 1999.

2. Morris BCW. The Scheiner optometer. *Clin Exp Optom.* 1966;49(11):321–329.

17

Optical Coherence Tomography

OBJECTIVES

After working through this chapter, you should be able to:

Explain what interference is and how it can be used to measure distances

Explain what OCT stands for

Explain (in simple terms) how time-domain OCT works

Explain (in simple terms) how Fourier-domain OCT works

Explain (in simple terms) how swept-source OCT works

Describe clinical applications of OCT

Introduction

This chapter will focus on the exciting world of **optical coherence tomography (OCT)** imaging, which is currently considered the 'gold standard' of imaging the eye. However, OCT relies on the wave theory of light, so we need to start with some light revision (as always, pun intended).

Some Light Revision

In chapter 10 we discussed that light can be thought of as a **wave**, and that multiple waves can superimpose on top of one another (by arriving at a point at the same time) and combine to produce a **resultant wave**. This resultant wave may have a smaller or larger amplitude (brightness or intensity) depending on how the waves interact. Remember, as well, that if the waves are **coherent** (meaning they possess the same wavelength and frequency), then they will produce either **constructive** or **destructive interference**. The type (and extent) of the interference will depend on whether the waves arrive **in-phase** (path difference a whole multiple of the wavelength) to produce constructive interference (an increase in amplitude) or if they arrive **out-of-phase** (path difference half a wavelength out) to produce

destructive interference (a decrease in amplitude). Fig. 17.1 shows a reminder of this.

In chapter 10 we also discussed that the path difference travelled by two beams of light can help us measure distances. This requires two identical waves (which can be from a single light source split into two) to travel separate distances before meeting again at a detector which can quantify the resultant amplitude and determine the relative path difference. This has been discussed before in the context of the **Michelson interferometer**, which we will review in the next section.

The Interferometer

The simplest interferometer to start with is the Michelson interferometer, which utilises light from a coherent light source and splits it into two (Fig. 17.2). One of the paths of light travels to a moveable mirror a known distance away, whilst the other path of light travels to something we want to measure the distance of. In the case of the Michelson interferometer, the second path of light travels to a fixed mirror.

As discussed in chapter 10, the idea of this setup is that by moving the moveable mirror set amounts, the interference pattern at the detector will cycle through constructive

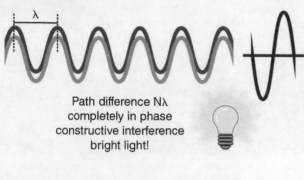

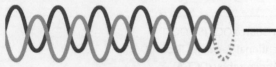

Path difference Nλ
completely in phase
constructive interference
bright light!

Path difference N+0.5λ
completely out of phase
destructive interference
no light

• **Fig. 17.1** Diagram showing difference between constructive interference (top) and destructive interference (bottom). The resultant amplitudes are shown in black on the right-hand side.

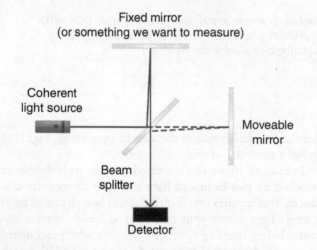

Fixed mirror
(or something we want to measure)

Coherent
light source

Moveable
mirror

Beam
splitter

Detector

• **Fig. 17.2** Diagram of a Michelson interferometer.

interference (increase in amplitude) and destructive interference (decrease in amplitude). For example, if we move the mirror by a distance that equates to 0.25 of the wavelength of the light, then the path difference will equate to 0.5 of the wavelength (as the light will experience +0.25 approaching the mirror and +0.25 after reflecting, totalling +0.5). This means that, providing we know the wavelength of the light, by measuring the interference at the detector we can determine the distance the light has travelled.

This is, in relatively simple terms, how OCT works.

What Is OCT?

OCT is a method of structurally imaging the individual layers of the eye. Typically this is used to image the retinal

layers at the back of the eye, but it can also be used to image the anterior eye as well. If we use the example of imaging the retinal layers, OCT utilises the principles of interferometry to measure how light reflects from each of the individual layers in order to determine the distance they are away from the detector (Fig. 17.3). This distance information can then be transformed into a black-and-white image of the layers, which can help to monitor health and disease.

Interferometry and OCT

As discussed, OCT systems utilise these principles of interferometry in order to image the layers of the eye, but there are several different types of OCT system.

Fibre-Based Time-Domain OCT (TD-OCT)

The first type of OCT is called **fibre-based time-domain OCT** (or **TD-OCT** for short). This method of OCT utilises a **moveable mirror** (just like in the Michelson interferometer) which means it measures the interference patterns over time as the mirror is moved (hence why it's called a time-domain). They usually use a **low-coherence, near-infrared light source** which is produced using a **superluminescent diode**. Fig. 17.4 shows roughly how the system works (you'll notice it's very similar to that of the Michelson interferometer), but with a lens system for helping to image side to side (laterally) across the back of the eye. One of the paths of light is incident upon the moveable mirror (**reference beam**), whilst the other is incident upon the eye (**measurement beam**), and the measurement beam is reflected, or backscattered, from the back of the eye with different delay times which are dependent on the optical properties of the tissue and the distance away from the light source. The software within the system can then interpret the interference fringe (or **reflectance**) profiles as they pass through the detector in order to determine the depth of the tissue

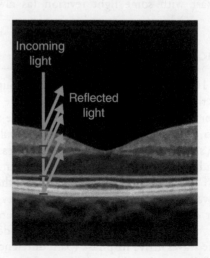

Incoming
light

Reflected
light

• **Fig. 17.3** Illustration of an optical coherence tomography (OCT) image of retinal layers (shown in shades of grey), with representative light reflecting off the layers back to the detector (shown in blue).

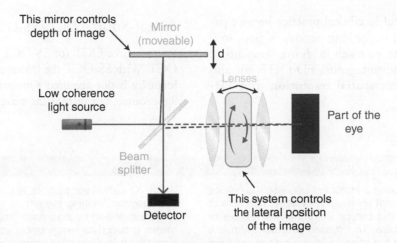

This mirror controls
depth of image

Mirror
(moveable)

d

Low coherence
light source

Lenses

Part of the
eye

Beam
splitter

This system controls
the lateral position
of the image

Detector

• **Fig. 17.4** Diagram of fibre-based time-domain optical coherence tomography (TD-OCT) system imaging part of the eye (shown in purple on the right). Notice that the system uses a moveable mirror to image in depth.

and produce the nice black-and-white image of conventional OCT (as shown in Fig. 17.4). Importantly, because these images reveal cross-sectional views of the retina, they are imaging the z-plane (as opposed to the x-y, transverse plane; Fig. 17.5). However, of all the types of OCT, this system is slow and of the lowest resolution (lowest-quality images).

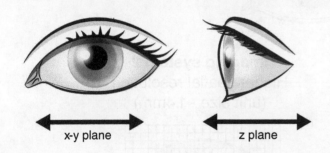

x-y plane

z plane

• **Fig. 17.5** Illustration showing the difference between imaging in the x-y (face-on) plane and the z (depth) plane.

Fibre-Based Fourier-Domain OCT (FD-OCT)

The second type of OCT is called **fibre-based Fourier-domain OCT** (or **FD-OCT** for short; also sometimes called **spectral domain or SD-OCT**). In this case, instead of recording interference (and intensity) at different locations of the reference mirror, the interference is recorded as a function of wavelengths (or frequencies) of light. This is achieved by using a broadband light source (containing multiple wavelengths centred on ~850 nm) and then inserting a diffraction grating or spectrometer in the system just before the detector. The detector then looks at the interference profiles of each of the wavelengths/frequencies (hence the name *Fourier*-domain) which is called **spectral interference** (Fig. 17.6). The advantage of this technique is that the depth information from the eye can be acquired simultaneously (without moving the mirror over time), which allows it to take images much faster than TD-OCT; therefore, we can describe it as having a faster **acquisition time**. Fast

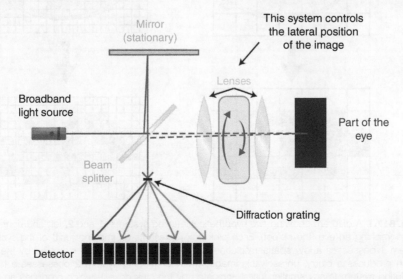

This system controls
the lateral position
of the image

Mirror
(stationary)

Lenses

Broadband
light source

Part of the
eye

Beam
splitter

Diffraction grating

Detector

• **Fig. 17.6** Diagram of a fibre-based Fourier-domain optical coherence tomography (FD-OCT) system imaging part of the eye (shown in purple on the right). Notice that the system uses a diffraction grating to measure spectral interference.

acquisition times are useful in clinical practice because patients usually don't like to sit for long periods of time, so if high-resolution images can be taken in shorter amounts of time, then this is very advantageous. FD-OCT can also acquire images at a higher **spatial resolution** than TD-OCT (Box 17.1).

Swept-Source OCT (SS-OCT)

Swept-source OCT (or SS-OCT for short) is a type of FD-OCT. With SS-OCT the frequency-(wavelength)-dependent intensity is not acquired simultaneously using a broadband light source, but instead the wavelength of the light source is

---

• Box 17.1   Spatial Resolution

The concept of spatial resolution is important because this defines the level of structural detail that an imaging system is capable of capturing. In simple terms, this can be likened to the number of megapixels in a digital camera. This means a system with low spatial resolution would blur the image a lot more than a system capable of producing a higher spatial resolution. Fig. B17.1 shows an object (the eye) which is going to be imaged by two systems. The one on the left has a lower spatial resolution (shown by the larger size of the imaging 'units'), which means the resultant image

will be almost unrecognizable, and a lot of details will be missing. However, the imaging system on the right has a higher spatial resolution (shown by the smaller size of the imaging 'units'), which means it becomes recognisable as an eye again, and you can even start to make out the shape and the position of the pupil. The potential clinical consequence of using a system with a low spatial resolution is that a clinician may be unable to detect small changes or subtle indications of pathology, so in general terms the higher the resolution (and smaller the imaging 'units'), the better.

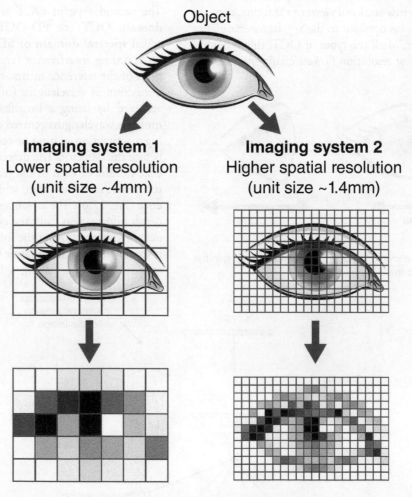

• **Fig. B17.1** A diagram showing two hypothetical imaging systems (1 and 2, left and right, respectively) photographing an eye (the object). Each pink box represents an imaging 'unit' of the system. Imaging system 1 possesses a low spatial-resolution system (fewer larger 'units', indicated by the pink boxes), which produces a blurry, unresolvable image, whereas imaging system 2 possesses a higher spatial-resolution system (many smaller 'units', indicated by the pink boxes), which produces an image that is beginning to resemble the original.

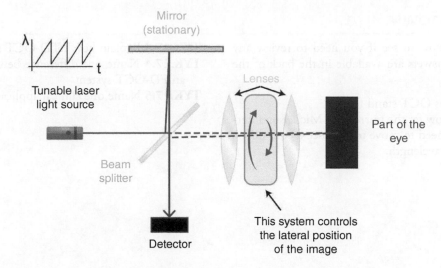

• **Fig. 17.7** Diagram of SS-OCT system imaging part of the eye (shown in purple on the right). Notice that the system uses a tunable laser as the light source.

tuned to sweep (hence swept . . .) through a narrow range of wavelengths sequentially, as shown in Fig. 17.7. Crucially, however, this range will be centred on approximately 1050 nm, indicating that SS-OCT utilises a longer wavelength of light relative to FD-OCT. The advantage of using longer wavelengths is that the tissue penetration is greater, meaning it is possible to image deeper into the eye (even down to the level of the choroid – the vascular layer behind the retina), but the pitfalls of using a longer wavelength light source is that the spatial resolution can be reduced. The good news, however, is that it is possible to slightly improve the spatial resolution through enhancements built into the imaging system's software. Ultimately, the advantages of SS-OCT relative to TD-OCT and FD-OCT are that it maintains a high resolution whilst also possessing the fastest acquisition time, and it allows imaging of deeper tissue structures.

Conventional Versus En Face

Conventional OCT scans will typically image tissue structures in depth, meaning that data from these scans will show cross-sectional views of the part of the eye being imaged, which is very useful in a clinical environment, as optometrists and ophthalmologists can scroll through sections of the retina to assess health and monitor changes over time. However, it is also now possible to use OCT systems to produce **en face** (face-up) scans (also called **C-scans**). These scans can build on the OCT system's ability to image in depth by adding confocal analysis of the data. This produces a high-resolution image of the retina in the x-y (transverse) plane, meaning they can reveal flat, face-on images of the eye at any specified depth, for example, at the outer retinal level or the choroidal level. Overall, these additional data can provide further information of subtle, very small-scale changes in retinal tissue, which is helping researchers learn more about the anatomical changes associated with disease.

OCT Angiography (OCT-A)

One final type of OCT imaging that we will consider here is **OCT angiography (OCT-A),** which utilises en face scanning methods. The word angiography means 'vessel' (angio-) measurement (-graphy), highlighting that this type of OCT serves as a noninvasive method of imaging blood vessels in the eye. More specifically, it works by comparing the reflectance of the light from red blood cells that are moving within the retinal and choroidal vessels; therefore, it is imaging changes in the reflectance profile in the same location over time. In very simple terms, this works because moving red blood cells will induce more of a change in the reflectance profile than stationary layers of tissue, and it's possible for the software to analyse this difference between moving and static tissue to estimate where the blood vessels are and how fast the blood is moving through them.

Clinical Applications

OCT is a system that allows us to see high-resolution images of individual layers in structures of the eye – which is advantageous to standard fundus photography because it has higher resolution and has the ability to image in depth. Therefore, it's incredibly useful as a technique for imaging the health of the eye because clinicians can clearly see if any pathology is present in deep layers of the tissue and because it's so high resolution it can also give an incredibly accurate representation of any anatomical changes associated with pathology over time, at the level of a few micrometres.

It also allows precise measurements of distance (e.g. how thick the retinal nerve fibre layer is, or how long the axial depth of the eyeball is), and it can help to measure the shape of the cornea (e.g. in keratoconus or to see how well a contact lens is sitting on the front surface of the eye).

Test Your Knowledge

Try the questions below to see if you need to review any sections again. All answers are available in the back of the book.

TYK.17.1 What does OCT stand for?

TYK.17.2 Explain how far the mirror in a Michelson interferometer would need to move to produce a path difference of a whole wavelength.

TYK.17.3 Explain how a TD-OCT system works.

TYK.17.4 Name one difference between a TD-OCT and an FD-OCT system.

TYK.17.5 Name one clinical application of OCT.

Experiments to Do at Home

18

Create Your Own Camera Obscura

OBJECTIVES

After working through this chapter, you should be able to:

Explain how a pinhole produces an image

Create your own camera obscura

Introduction

As we discussed very briefly in chapter 13, a 'camera obscura' is an imaging device that utilises the theory behind pinhole photography. When light emanating from an object shines through a pinhole, it produces an upside-down image. This is because light rays from the tip of the object (e.g. the top of the mug in Fig. 18.1) travel in a straight line through the pinhole and end up near the floor, whilst light rays from the base of the object travel in a straight line through the pinhole and end up near the ceiling. When these rays form a focus, it necessarily produces an inverted image.

The Experiment

In order to see how this works, it's best to make our own. To do this, we'll need a pinhole aperture and something to project the image onto (Fig. 18.2).

Equipment Required

- A pencil
- A drawing pin/needle/something with which to make a very small hole
- Two pieces of A4-sized black card (if you don't have black card, a cereal box might do)
- Tape of some kind
- Scissors
- Tracing paper or equivalently **translucent** material that, when held up to a lamp, is diffusely illuminated but does

not show a clear image of the lamp through the material (e.g. a translucent sandwich bag or the bag from inside a cereal box – if these are too transparent, you can double up the layers)

Method

1. Cut an 8 cm strip off the first piece of black card as shown in Fig. 18.3. Set the 8 cm strip to one side for now.
2. Take the remaining part of the first piece of black card and roll it up to make a tube (tube 1 in Fig. 18.4). Tape to secure. The diameter of the tube should be roughly 6 cm, so overlapping is allowed.
3. Roll up the second (uncut) piece of black card to fit inside the first tube. This needs to fit very snugly, so I recommend rolling it up small, placing it inside the first tube, and then letting it expand inside. Carefully remove this narrower tube and secure with tape (tube 2 in Fig. 18.4). You should now have two tubes of slightly different length and diameter (with the wider tube being shorter in length).
4. Now secure the translucent element (e.g. tracing paper) over the edge of tube 2 as shown in Fig. 18.5. This is the screen on which the image will appear, so make sure it's tight and flat.
5. Collect the remining 8 cm strip of black card and tube 1 (the shorter tube). Draw around the tube to create a circular template on the card, then draw a slightly bigger circle and connect the two circles with radial lines (as shown in Fig. 18.6).

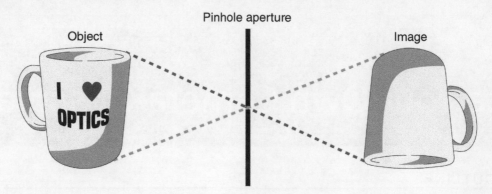

Object   Pinhole aperture   Image

• **Fig. 18.1** Diagram showing path of light rays from a mug, producing an upside-down image in a pinhole camera. The image is also flipped left to right, so in the image (on the right), the text will be facing the other way (which is why it's missing).

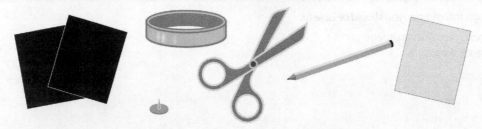

• **Fig. 18.2** Illustration of required materials.

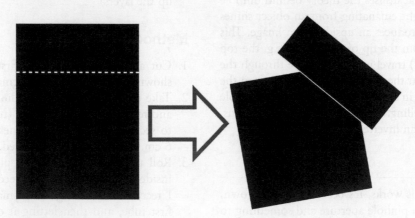

• **Fig. 18.3** Diagram of step 1 of method – cut an 8 cm strip off one of the pieces of card.

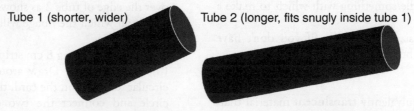

Tube 1 (shorter, wider)   Tube 2 (longer, fits snugly inside tube 1)

• **Fig. 18.4** There should be two tubes – a short, wide one (tube 1) and a narrow, long one (tube 2).

Tube 2

• **Fig. 18.5** The translucent material needs to be taped nice and tight on the end of the narrow, long tube (tube 2).

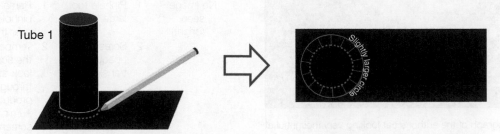

Tube 1

slightly larger circle

• **Fig. 18.6** Use the short, wide tube (tube 1) to draw a circle on the spare 8 cm strip of card (left). Then draw a larger circle around it and connect the two with radial lines (right).

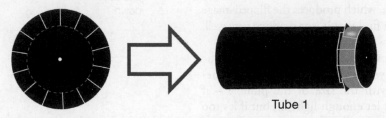

Tube 1

• **Fig. 18.7** When cut and pierced, the 'toothy circle' (left) should then be attached to one end of the short, wide tube (tube 1).

6. Cut the larger circle out of the card, and then cut the radial lines to make 'teeth' around the inside circle.

7. Use your drawing pin (or equivalent) to make a pinhole in the centre of the inner circle; you should now have something like that shown in Fig. 18.7.

8. Attach the toothy circle to tube 1 using tape (see Fig. 18.7).

9. Place the 'screen' end of tube 2 inside tube 1 (the screen needs to be inside the tube to make sure the image isn't affected by other light sources). You've now made your camera obscura (Fig. 18.8)!

10. Point the pinhole end towards something well lit (this works best outdoors on a sunny day) to see an upside-down image form on the screen. You can adjust the distance of the screen from the pinhole by pushing the inner tube closer and farther away. This should change the size of the image seen on the screen (which should be inside the tube).

Results

Hopefully your camera obscura was able to produce a clear, upside-down image of the world (e.g. Fig. 18.9). The reason

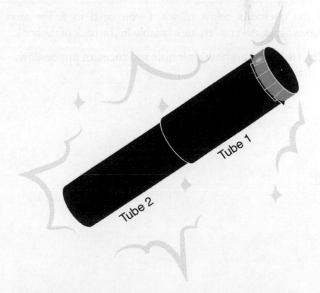

Tube 1

Tube 2

• **Fig. 18.8** The narrow, long tube (tube 2) goes screen-side first inside the short, wide tube (tube 1).

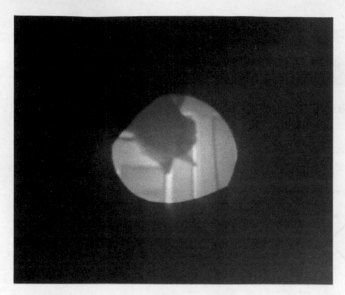

• **Fig. 18.9** A photograph of the author's cat looking very thoughtful at the window. The photograph was taken through the author's camera obscura.

this works is because the pinhole on the front affects how light can travel inside the camera, which produces the flipped image on the screen inside. If you find that it isn't working very well, you can troubleshoot the issue using Table 18.1 as a guide.

As a rough guide, however, make sure to point the camera at something very well lit (e.g. a tree in the sunshine) and maybe experiment with the size of the pinhole – if it's too small then it won't let enough light in, but if it's too big then the image will be very blurry.

As with all experiments, if it didn't work out (even after trouble-shooting) then you should think about what you could do to improve the method next time.

Test Your Knowledge

Try the questions below to see if you need to review any sections again. All answers are available in the back of the book.

TYK.18.1 Explain how a pinhole produces an upside-down image.

TYK.18.2 Explain why moving the screen away from the pinhole produces a larger image.

TABLE 18.1	**Trouble-Shooting the Camera Obscura**	
Reported Issue	**Potential Problem**	**Potential Solution**
No image seen (dark)	1. Pinhole too small 2. Object not bright enough	1. Make pinhole larger 2. Shine a torch on an object and try again
No image seen (bright)	1. Pinhole too large 2. Screen too opaque/translucent	1. Remake a smaller pinhole and stick over the original 2. Temporarily remove the screen tube and look at a light source through it – it should produce diffuse illumination of the screen without producing a visible image of the light
Image seen but not upside down	1. Pinhole too large 2. Looking through camera the wrong-way round	1. Remake a smaller pinhole and stick over the original 2. Make sure you're looking through the empty end of the screen tube, with the pinhole closest to the object

19

Create a Blue Sky at Home

OBJECTIVES

After working through this chapter, you should be able to:

Create a demonstration of polarisation by scattering

Explain how polarisation by scattering works

Introduction

As a brief recap, in chapter 14 we discussed how light can be made to only have one (or at least very few) orientations of electric field if it undergoes a process of **polarisation**. This is important because light from the sun is **unpolarised**, meaning that the light is vibrating in all orientations, and therefore the orientation of the electric field varies randomly over time. One way in which this natural sunlight can become polarised is through **polarisation by scattering** in which the light from the sun will be scattered (and polarised) when it comes into contact with molecules in the atmosphere. In particular, shorter wavelengths (within the sunlight) are scattered more easily than the longer wavelengths, which means that as light travels through the atmosphere, it scatters shorter (blue) wavelengths into the atmosphere (making the sky look blue), which subsequently makes the light from the sun appear to be shifted slightly towards the longer wavelengths (making the sun look more yellow).

In this experiment we are going to investigate this principle by making our very own atmosphere in a glass and using a torch as our 'sun'.

The Experiment

For this experiment we are going to attempt to prove that when light travels through a busy medium (like the atmosphere), it will scatter shorter wavelengths more than longer wavelengths. This will be achieved by creating an atmosphere (milky water in a glass) and seeing what the sun (a torch light) looks like as it passes through the atmosphere.

Before starting the experiment, please make sure you have all the equipment you need (and a mobile device to record your results!).

Equipment Required

- A clear glass (a reasonable size glass, no pattern if possible)
- A white-light torch (mobile phone lights work OK, but torches work better)
- Some cold tap water
- A small amount of milk
- Something to stir the mixture with
- Optional (but advised): a towel or kitchen roll to mop up water/milk spillages

Method

1. Fill the glass with cold water.
2. Shine the torch from behind the glass, directly towards yourself.
3. Make a note of the colour of the torch light – hopefully it looks quite white (unaffected by travelling through the water).
4. Make a note of the colour of the water – hopefully it looks quite clear.
5. Make a note of the colour of the milk (before we put it into the water) – hopefully it looks white.
6. Now add a very tiny amount of milk into the water (if you add too much then the experiment won't work, so it's better to add too little than too much!).

You may need to stir the mixture to make it work appropriately.

7. Shine the torch from behind the glass, directly towards yourself.
8. Make a note of the colour of the torch light – hopefully it looks more yellow.
9. Keep adding milk until the torch light begins to become convincingly yellow in appearance.
10. Make a note of the colour of the milky water – hopefully it looks to be bluer than without the light.
11. Now keep the torch still but view the milky water from above the glass; take notice of what's happened to the colour – does it look bluer with the torch than without?

Results

Hopefully you could see that the torch light magically (or scientifically and predictably) changed colour to become more yellow-orange when the milk was added to the water, and that the milky water became blue. The reason this works is because the milk in the water scatters the light from the torch through **polarisation by scattering** (Fig. 19.1). As we learned in chapter 14, shorter wavelength (blue) light scatters more easily than longer wavelength light, so as a result of this the blue light from the torch ends up diffusing through the milk, making it look bluer, and the light source will look more yellow (due to the missing blue). However, if you find that the experiment isn't working very well, you can troubleshoot the issue using Table 19.1 as a guide.

As with all experiments, if it didn't work out (even after troubleshooting), then you should think about what you could do to improve the method next time.

You can also watch me do a demonstration of the experiment on the associated Elsevier website (Fig. 19.2).

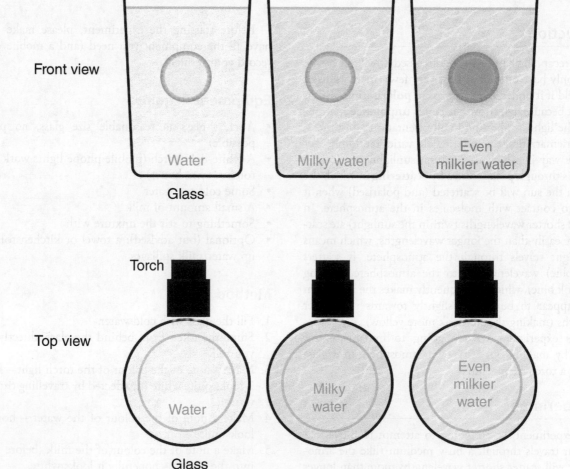

• **Fig. 19.1** Illustration of the effect viewed from the front of the glass (top) and the top of the glass (bottom). As the water becomes milkier (right), the light from the torch will experience polarisation by scattering, which will make the torch light seem more yellow (top) and the milky water look bluer (bottom).

TABLE 19.1	Troubleshooting the Polarisation Experiment	
Reported Issue	**Potential Problem**	**Potential Solution**
Light source does not turn orange (but milk turns blue)	1. Light source producing diffuse light 2. Not enough milk added	1. Angle the light source slightly downwards towards the table – this will mean the light that reaches you is less diffuse (alternatively, try a different light source) 2. Add more milk and try again
Light source disappears when milk is added	1. Too much milk added 2. Light source too low intensity	1. Replace the water and try again – this time add the milk a tiny drop at a time 2. Try to find a brighter light source

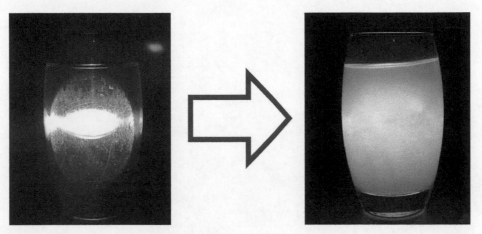

• **Fig. 19.2** Two stills taken from the associated video version of the experiment being completed by the author. The left image shows the bright white light being transmitted through the clear water in the glass. The right image shows the torchlight becoming more yellow/orange once the milk is introduced. It is also clear that the milk has taken on a blueish hue.

Test Your Knowledge

Try the questions below to see if you need to review any sections again. All answers are available in the back of the book.

TYK.19.1 Explain why the torch looks more yellow as we add more milk.

TYK.19.2 Explain why using a red light source wouldn't work.

20

Create a Prism

CHAPTER OUTLINE

OBJECTIVES

After working through this chapter, you should be able to:

Explain why light can disperse through water if a mirror is
   introduced

Explain dispersion

Introduction

Looking back over the book so far, in chapter 1 we learned that white light (e.g. sunlight) contains all wavelengths of visible light, and in chapter 8 we discussed that these wavelengths of light can be **dispersed** to be independently visible (e.g. in the case of a rainbow where white light disperses through a raindrop, or when light travels through a **prism**).

   Dispersion is something that we'll have experienced ourselves in real life if we've ever seen light pass through a crystal ornament in a window – it makes a rainbow pattern appear. This rainbow pattern is simply the white (incident) light from the sun dispersing (splitting out into its constituent wavelengths), which makes it appear to be lots of colours instead of just white. This phenomenon occurs because the wavelength of the light is directly related to how much refraction it undergoes as it travels from one material to another. There is an old adage '*blue bends best*' which is supposed to help us remember that shorter wavelength light (e.g. blue) will refract to a greater degree than longer wavelength light (e.g. red) when dispersion takes place.

   As any science teacher will probably tell you, the best way to understand this process is to get your hands on a prism and see the effect first-hand. Unfortunately, optical prisms aren't that common around the home, so instead I'd like to encourage you to build your own prism.

   For this experiment we are going to create our own prism at home in order to split white light into the colours of the rainbow – which will also allow us to see first-hand how

changing the apical angle will affect the deviation (and the amount of dispersion).

The Experiment

Our 'at-home' prism experiment works best (and is most impressive) when constructed outside on a sunny day, but it can also work very effectively if you have a torch that produces white light. The only thing to note is that the torch light might make a slightly less-convincing rainbow, depending on its particular spectrum, so please bear this in mind when completing the experiment outlined here.

   Before starting the experiment, please make sure you have all the equipment you need (and a mobile device to record your results!).

Equipment Required

- A tray or a bowl that can be filled with water
- A plane (flat) mirror that can be placed in the tray/bowl
- Something to see the dispersed light on (e.g. piece of paper or a wall)
- *Optional: something to secure the mirror in place, for example, a stone to rest it on or some tape (just in case it makes setting up the experiment easier)*

Method

1. **Fill the tray/bowl with water** – make sure there is enough water that the mirror would be at least partially

submerged if placed in the tray/bowl at an angle. I've found that this works best with at least 2 inches of water, so please bear this in mind when selecting your tray.

2. **Place the mirror into the tray/ bowl** – it must be at an oblique angle (e.g. 45°) and must be at least partially submerged. This is made easiest by taping the edge of the mirror to the edge of the tray or by resting it on something (or if you have someone helping you, one of you can hold the mirror in place).

3. **Place the tray/bowl in a location where the sun will shine directly onto the water,** or **angle the torch so that it is shining into the water, towards the mirror.**

4. **Hold the paper parallel to the tray/bowl above the water and look to see if you've produced dispersion** (see Figs. 20.1 and 20.2 for a demonstration of this).

5. Now change the angle of the mirror (or increase the amount of water) and note what happens to the rainbow – does it change, or does it stay the same?

Results

This works because as the light is refracted through the water, then reflected at the mirror, and then refracted as it leaves the water again, it behaves as raindrops do in the sky to produce a rainbow! All the wavelengths that make up white light will refract at different angles, so by refracting them twice, we are refracting them to such an extent that they become separated – this is **dispersion**.

However, if you find that it isn't working very well, you can troubleshoot the issue using Table 20.1 as a guide.

As with all experiments, if it didn't work out (even after troubleshooting), then you should think about what you could do to improve the method next time.

You can also watch me do a demonstration of the experiment on the associated Elsevier website.

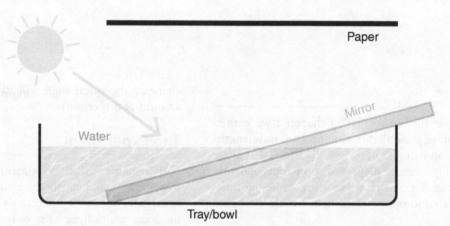

Paper

Mirror

Water

Tray/bowl

• **Fig. 20.1** An illustration of the setup for this experiment. Please note that the sun can be replaced with a torch if necessary.

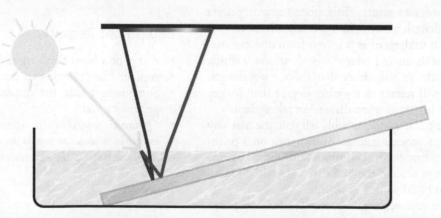

• **Fig. 20.2** As the white light from the sun (or torch) refracts through the water and reflects back out again, the wavelengths that make up white light are dispersed to form a rainbow.

TABLE 20.1	Troubleshooting the Homemade Prism	
Reported Issue	Potential Problem	Potential Solution
No rainbow visible	1. Mirror not angled properly 2. Light source not angled properly 3. Water not deep enough	1. Try altering the angle of the mirror as shown in the video demo on the Elsevier website 2. Try altering the angle of the light source as shown in the video demo on the Elsevier website 3. Add more water (you may need a deeper bowl)

Test Your Knowledge

Try the questions below to see if you need to review any sections again. All answers are available in the back of the book.

TYK.20.1 Explain why the white light produces a rainbow when it passes through the setup described in this chapter.

TYK.20.2 Explain what you think would happen if you changed the angle of the light approaching our homemade prisms.

21

Measure the Speed of Light

CHAPTER OUTLINE

OBJECTIVES

After working through this chapter, you should be able to:

Explain how microwaves heat food using interference
Explain how we can use chocolate to measure the speed of light

Introduction

In chapter 1 we briefly mentioned different types of electro-magnetic radiation, one of which involved a type of energy you can find in most kitchens – **microwaves**. As a quick recap, microwaves are a form of electromagnetic energy comprising wavelengths that fall between infrared and radio waves, meaning that in general terms their wavelengths are relatively long, and they exert relatively low energy compared to other types of energy (e.g. UV) (Fig. 21.1).

Now, it's probably no surprise to hear that one of the most easy-to-understand practical uses of microwave radiation is for the generation of heat (thermal energy) in a microwave oven. This means that every time you convert an item of food from a chilled substance into its molten lava counterpart in the microwave, you're technically doing a scientific experiment that utilises **interference** properties of electromagnetic radiation (see chapter 10). This is possible because the microwave energy is absorbed by fats, sugars, proteins and water, causing them to heat up. The microwaves also interfere with each other causing the formation of hot spots in the food in locations where **constructive interference** takes place. This can be likened to the 'bright maxima' we discussed in chapter 10, but instead of bright light, it produces hot spots. If your microwave contains a turntable, then the turntable serves to dissipate these hot spots, enabling food to be cooked more evenly, and if your microwave doesn't contain a turntable, then instead it will contain a built-in, rotating motor which serves the same purpose.

The hot spots generated by the constructive interference are related to the **wavelength** of the microwaves, as anywhere two peaks or two troughs align, there will be maximum heat produced (Fig. 21.2). This means that the distance between the hot spots will equate to **half** of the wavelength.

The Experiment

In order to find the wavelength of the microwaves in our microwave ovens, we purposely want to create hot spots within the oven – thereby cooking something incredibly unevenly. . . . This means we will need to remove the turntable from the microwave before we begin.

Please note: if your microwave does not contain a turntable (or if the turntable can't be removed), then unfortunately you won't be able to do this experiment unless you borrow someone else's microwave.

Notes of Caution

- Microwaves produce heat. Be careful not to burn yourself, particularly as the turntable used to distribute the heat is not being used.
- Do not place metal objects in the microwave oven. Microwaves reflect off metal and will damage the internal workings of the microwave oven.
- Do not use the microwave without food inside; if there is nowhere for the microwaves to go, they will damage the microwave oven.

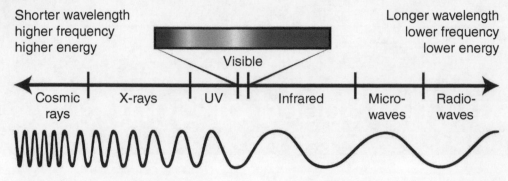

Shorter wavelength
higher frequency
higher energy

Longer wavelength
lower frequency
lower energy

Visible

Cosmic rays · X-rays · UV · Infrared · Micro-waves · Radio-waves

• **Fig. 21.1** Diagram of the electromagnetic spectrum (EMS) showing the relationship between wavelength, frequency and energy.

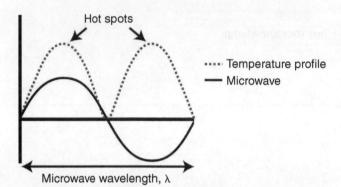

Hot spots

···· Temperature profile
— Microwave

Microwave wavelength, λ

• **Fig. 21.2** Diagram showing the amplitude profile and wavelength of a microwave (black line). As the amplitude increases, the energy also increases, meaning that both the peak and the trough of the microwave profile will produce the highest amount of intensity (heat). This means that the microwave will produce two hot spots (shown in red dashed lines) whose distance will equate to half a wavelength (distance between peak to trough).

Equipment Required

• Microwave oven that utilises a removable turntable
• A 10 cm+ bar of chocolate (select one that's tasty and then you can eat it afterwards)
• A timer
• A ruler

Method

1. **Prepare the chocolate to be as flat as possible** (e.g. grating the bumps off the chocolate).
2. Read the frequency (v) of the microwave off the label on the back of the microwave oven or by consulting the manual, and **make a note of it somewhere**. It is usually given in megahertz (MHz), which must be converted to hertz (Hz). Convert from MHz to Hz by multiplying by 10^6 (e.g. 2,450 MHz = 2,450,000,000 Hz).
3. **Remove the turntable** from the microwave oven.
4. **Place the prepared chocolate onto a microwave-proof tray and then place in the microwave**.
5. **Microwave the chocolate in short, 5-second bursts** and examine the food after each burst. You are looking for the point at which the chocolate *just* begins to melt. Two (or more) areas of melting will occur.

6. **Once visible, measure the distance between the two hot spots with a ruler**. Convert this measurement into metres and multiply by 2 to get the wavelength (λ).
7. Calculate the speed of light using the equation below:

$$\text{speed of light} = \text{wavelength} \times \text{frequency}$$

This is often written as:

$$c = \lambda v$$

Results

The actual speed of light is **299,792,458 m s^{-1}**. How do your results compare?

If you find that the results don't match up with the real speed of light, or if you're struggling to locate the hot spots, you can troubleshoot the issue using Table 21.1 as a guide.

TABLE 21.1 Troubleshooting the Speed of Light Experiment

Reported Issue	Potential Problem	Potential Solution
Chocolate melts	1. Left in microwave too long	1. Try shorter bursts (e.g. 3 seconds)
Hot spots are really large	1. Left in microwave too long	1. Try shorter bursts (e.g. 3 seconds)
	2. Chocolate was moved during process	2. Make sure not to disturb the chocolate whilst doing the experiment – can you check for hot spots without removing it from the microwave?
Distance between hot spots is too small/too large	1. Chocolate was moved during process	1. Make sure not to disturb the chocolate whilst doing the experiment – can you check for hot spots without removing it from the microwave?
	2. Distance was not measured from equivalent points	2. Make sure to measure from one edge to the equivalent edge (e.g. left of one hot spot to left of other hot spot) for maximum accuracy

As with all experiments, if it didn't work out then you should think about what you could do to improve the method next time.

You can also watch me do a demonstration of the experiment on the associated Elsevier website.

Test Your Knowledge

Try the questions below to see if you need to review any sections again. All answers are available in the back of the book.

TYK.21.1 Explain why the distance between the hot spots is equal to half the wavelength of a microwave.

TYK.21.2 Explain why we needed to take the turntable out of the microwave for it to work.

22
Create a 'Cornea'

OBJECTIVES

After working through this chapter, you should be able to:

Explain how the human eye focuses distant light on the retina

Explain the different contributions of refractive index and curvature on an image

Introduction

In this book we've learned a lot about light and how it interacts with both flat (plane) and curved surfaces. We've also learned that when light moves from a material of one refractive index to another, it will undergo **refraction** (a change in direction). We've also touched on the idea that the human eye (see chapter 5 for revision on this) is able to focus light on the back of the eye through two key characteristics:

1. The **cornea** (front of the eye) is a **different refractive index** to that of air (cornea 1.376; air 1.00), which allows refraction to take place. Importantly the fluid inside the eye that sits behind the cornea (the **aqueous**) is a similar refractive index to the cornea.
2. The **cornea** is a **convex, curved shape**, which means it has **dioptric power**. This allows the cornea to add convergence to the incoming light (Fig. 22.1).

This is important because it shows us that the basic focusing of distant light onto the back of the eye has nothing to do with any muscles (which is a common misconception) and can therefore not be 'trained'. Instead, if a **refractive error** is present and light focuses too early (myopia) or too late (hyperopia), it can only be corrected by altering the **vergence** of the light before it enters the eye (glasses or contact lenses), or by changing the shape of the cornea (refractive surgery). To prove this, this chapter will explain how we can make a mock (relatively huge) cornea at home using common household items.

The Experiment

The goal of this experiment is to show that the refractive index change alone would not be enough for the eye to focus light over such a short distance (corresponding to the length of the eyeball); instead we're going to prove that it's the curvature of the cornea that adds all the power. To that end we need to produce a convex surface that's a different refractive index to air and see how the image compares to a flat surface that's a different refractive index to air. Please note, however, that there will be quite a size difference between our homemade 'cornea' and a real cornea, so the radius of curvature is not equivalent and so our homemade cornea will not have a power equivalent to a real cornea. Instead, it will serve to demonstrate the basic principles.

Before starting the experiment, please make sure you have all the equipment you need (and a mobile device to record your results!).

Equipment Required

- An empty, *clear* plastic 2 L fizzy drink bottle – note the shape of the bottle is quite important so try to find one that looks like the one in Fig. 22.2.
- A pair of scissors
- A felt-tip pen or marker of some kind
- An empty, clear plastic *flat* tub; this could be a food storage container or an empty packet of sliced cheese – anything that's flat, plastic and completely clear.

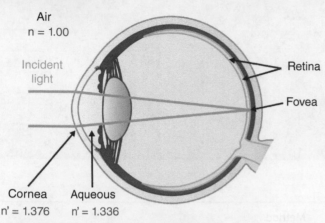

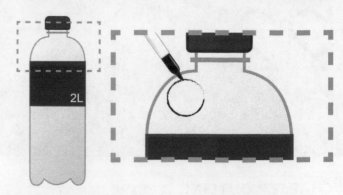

• **Fig. 22.1** An illustration of a cross-section of a human eye with light (blue lines) entering through the cornea (labelled) and being focused onto the fovea in the retina (labelled). The refractive index of air (n = 1.00) and the refractive index of the cornea (n′ = 1.376) and aqueous (n′ = 1.336) are labelled for information.

• **Fig. 22.3** A diagram showing how to produce the disc from the 2 L bottle, which will act as the front surface of our 'cornea'.

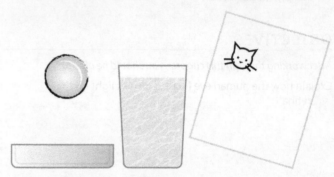

• **Fig. 22.4** After cutting out the disc, this is the equipment we will be using for the experiment itself.

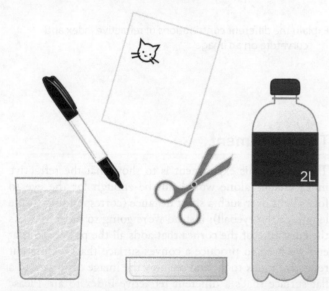

• **Fig. 22.2** A diagram of all the equipment needed for this experiment, including: a pen, scissors, water, a clear flat plastic tub, a 2 L empty plastic bottle and a doodle or some writing on a piece of paper. Please note that the 2 L bottle needs to be clear plastic and needs to be this shape (round 'shoulders' near the top).

- Water
- An object that can be laid flat on the table, which we will look at through our homemade cornea; this could be a drawing on a piece of paper (like in Fig. 22.2) or possibly something written down, but please don't use anything electrical, valuable or important, because there is a small risk of spilling the water onto the object.
- *Optional (but advised): a towel or kitchen roll to mop up water spillages*

Method

1. **Using the pen, draw a circle shape on the top 'shoulder' area of the 2 L bottle** (like shown in Fig. 22.3). Make

sure the circle is a reasonable size (at least 5 cm in diameter). It does not have to be perfectly spherical.

2. **Using the scissors, cut out the plastic disc from the top of the 2 L bottle** – you should now have the disc, the flat plastic tub, the water and the object remaining (Fig. 22.4).

3. **Create (or source) the object** – for me, I like to do a little doodle on a piece of paper (see Fig. 22.4), but you can just write a single word if you feel more comfortable doing that (please see the associated video content on Elsevier's website for a demonstration of this experiment).

4. **Place the object flat onto the table.**

5. **Look at the object through the empty, flat plastic tub.** It shouldn't change.

6. **Now look at the object through the empty, curved plastic disc.** It still shouldn't change.

7. **Pour some of the water (at least 0.5 cm deep) into the clear, flat plastic tub and hold it ~1 cm above the object.**

8. **Look through the water (like shown in Fig. 22.5) to see what the object looks like.** You should be able to see that, as you move the flat tub (filled with water) over the object, the image of the object looks the same (though possibly slightly wobbly due to the water). It should not be magnified, or upside down. It will just be a virtual (upright), same-size image.

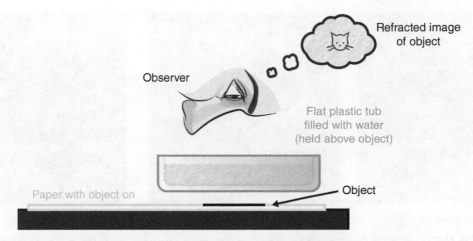

• **Fig. 22.5** The first part of the experiment involves looking at the image of the object through the 'flat lens' (water inside the flat plastic tub). This diagram is a side view of how the experiment should be done and illustrates the best setup for optimal viewing.

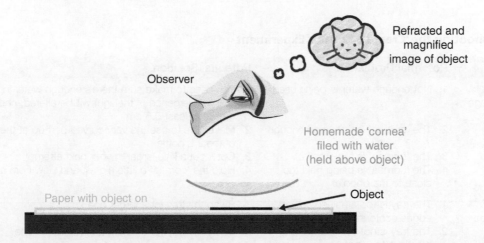

• **Fig. 22.6** The second part of the experiment involves looking at the image of the object through the 'cornea' (water inside the convex disc). This diagram is a side view of how the experiment should be done and illustrates the best setup for optimal viewing.

9. **Now put the tub to one side and pour some water into the plastic disc we cut out of the 2 L bottle –** this is our fake cornea.
10. **Carefully hold the disc ~1 cm above the object** (this is where most water spillage happens). The disc should be convex, with its apex pointing towards the table.
11. **Look through the water in the disc (like shown in Fig. 22.6) to see what the object looks like.** You should be able to see that, as you move the disc (filled with water) over the object, the image of the object looks different (though still probably slightly wobbly due to the water). This time the image should be magnified and virtual (upright).
12. Try changing the distance from the object to the 'cornea' – what does it do to the image?

Results

Fig. 22.7 shows some screenshots from my own attempt at this experiment (the full version can be viewed on Elsevier's website), and hopefully your experiment found the same thing. Ideally, when you looked at the object through the 'flat lens' (the water in the flat plastic tub), there should have been no real difference in the image of the object and the object itself. This is because when light travels through a flat-surface material that has a different refractive index to the material in which the object exists (in our case, this is air), it might change the position of the image, but it wouldn't change the image characteristics. However, when we hold our convex 'cornea' over the image, the combination of the curved surface and the refractive index difference means that our 'cornea' is positively powered. This is evidence of the fact that the image appears to be magnified (something that is impossible with a negatively powered lens – see chapters 3 and 7 for review on image formation).

This shows that it is simply the combination of the **curvature of the cornea** and the **refractive index difference** (of the cornea relative to the air) that enables our eyes to focus light over such a short distance.

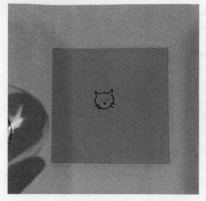
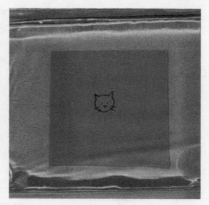
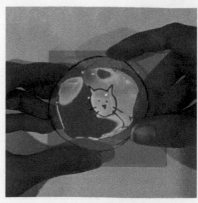

No 'lens'   Flat 'lens'   'Cornea'

• **Fig. 22.7** Screenshots from the video version of me completing the experiment at home. The left image shows my 'object' (drawing of a cat) without any involvement from my watery lenses. The middle image shows the image of the object as seen through the 'flat lens' (water in the flat plastic tub). The image on the right shows the image of the object as seen through the convex 'cornea', and it is clearly magnified.

TABLE 22.1	Troubleshooting the 'Create a Cornea' Experiment	
Reported Issue	**Potential Problem**	**Potential Solution**
'Cornea' does not magnify the image	1. Not enough water is being used	1. You need to make sure there's enough water in the 'cornea' that the vergence of the light will be altered; check to see if there's at least 0.5 cm
	2. The 'cornea' isn't curved enough	2. Make sure to use the very curved part up at the top 'shoulder' of the 2 L bottle
	3. The 'cornea' is too small	3. Cut it out a little larger in your next attempt
	4. The 'cornea' is being held too close to the doodle	4. Hold the 'cornea' a little higher, and view from above
The flat tray also affects the image	1. The tray is too small so curved edges confound the results	1. Swap the tray for a larger one
	2. The tray is not truly flat, or the plastic is too thick	2. Swap the tray for a flatter, thinner plastic one

Bonus – did you happen to notice that the image was sometimes a little distorted near the edges of the 'cornea'? Can you use the information from chapter 16 to explain what's happening here?

Also, as ever, if you find that the experiment isn't working very well, you can troubleshoot the issue using Table 22.1 as a guide.

Test Your Knowledge

Try the questions below to see if you need to review any sections again. All answers are available in the back of the book.

TYK.22.1 Explain how the human eye can focus distant light onto the back of the eye.

TYK.22.2 Why did we use water for the refractive index difference?

As with all experiments, if it didn't work out (even after troubleshooting), then you should think about what you could do to improve the method next time.

You can also watch me do a demonstration of the experiment on the associated Elsevier website.

TYK.22.3 Explain why the image is sometimes a little distorted near the edges of the 'cornea' in our demonstration (see Fig. 22.7 for an example of this distortion).

TYK.22.4 If we had filled our lenses with glycerine (a viscous, clear liquid of refractive index 1.47), do you think the results would have been the same? Discuss your thoughts.

23

Kitchen Thin Film Interference

OBJECTIVES

After working through this chapter, you should be able to:

Explain 'thin film interference'

Explain why the interference pattern is colourful

Produce a thin film demonstration of your own

Introduction

Before we delve deep into the wonderful world of **thin film interference**, let's take a moment to remind ourselves what **interference** is in the first place (you can also review chapter 10 for additional revision on this). Interference (in optics) describes the variation in wave amplitude that occurs when multiple waves (e.g. of light) interact with one another. The type of interference (and amplitude of the resultant, combined wave) is determined by the relative phase difference or path difference of the individual waves. Fig. 23.1A shows an example of light interfering constructively, with two in-phase blue waves shown (phase difference 0°) and a path difference that equates to a whole wavelength ($n\lambda$). This leads to an increase in amplitude in the resultant wave (shown in orange). Contrarily, Fig. 23.1B shows an example of light interfering destructively, with the two out-of-phase blue waves (phase difference 180°) and a path difference that equates to half a wavelength ($n + 0.5\lambda$). This leads to a decrease in amplitude in the resultant wave (shown in orange; the example in Fig. 23.1B is complete destructive interference, meaning the resultant amplitude is zero). The important part of this is that the difference in path length of the waves will determine the interference.

A great example of interference in the real world is **thin film interference**, where light will partially reflect off the front and back surfaces of a very thin film – which essentially reflects two versions of the light back towards you. This allows the light to produce interference which will either produce a reflection (constructive) or not (destructive). Interestingly, if white light (comprising lots of wavelengths) is incident upon one of these films, the individual wavelengths of light will interfere differently with one another, which produces a nice rainbow pattern of interference. Again, the key factor determining this is the path difference, so the angle of the approaching light plays a role, but crucially the thickness of the film does too (see Fig. 23.2).

This chapter aims to allow you to see this for yourself whilst also demonstrating that the thickness of the film plays a key role in the observed interference pattern. This means we're going to make our own thin films!

The Experiment

The goal of this experiment is to show that the path differences in light can be introduced when it reflects off the front and back surfaces of a thin film and to show that the thickness determines the shape of the pattern. To that end we need to make our own thin film that varies in thickness, and we need to shine some white light through it.

Before starting the experiment, please make sure you have all the equipment you need (and a mobile device to record your results!).

Equipment Required

- Some cold water in a dish or tub of some kind
- Some liquid soap for washing dishes (or bubble-blowing mixture, if you have it)

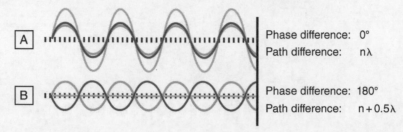

• **Fig. 23.1** Illustration showing blue waves producing constructive (A) and destructive (B) interference. Orange waves show approximate resultant waves.

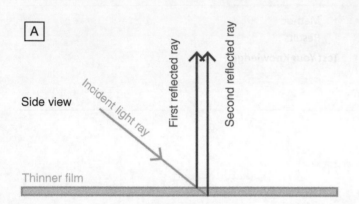

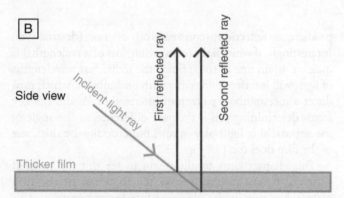

• **Fig. 23.2** Diagram showing that thickness of the film will alter the path difference between the two reflected rays of light. If the film is thinner (A), the waves have less of a path difference than if the film is thicker (B).

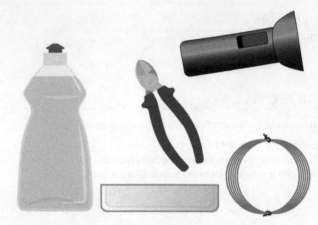

• **Fig. 23.3** An illustration of the materials required for this experiment.

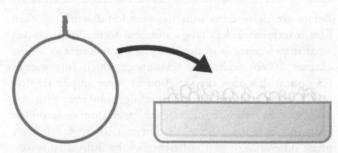

• **Fig. 23.4** Illustration showing the required shape of the wire (left) that needs to be placed in the soap mixture (right) to produce the film.

- A light source (torch or mobile phone light)
- Something with an aperture (e.g. a metal bangle that you wouldn't mind getting soapy and wet) or some craft wire (the thinner the wire the better) and wire cutters (as shown in Fig. 23.3)
- *Optional (but advised): a towel or kitchen roll to mop up water spillages*

Method

1. If you have an object with an aperture then skip this step; otherwise, cut approximately 10 to 15 cm of wire with the wire cutters and shape to form a circle (it doesn't have to be a perfect circle). Twist the wire ends together to keep it nice (and give you something to hold on to) like shown in Fig. 23.4.

2. **Add one part liquid soap with five parts water and mix together enthusiastically** (to make bubbles and have a fun time). If using bubble-blowing mixture, simply pour the bubble mixture into the bowl. Also, look at the bubbles in the mixture – are they rainbow coloured? If so, this is thin film interference!

3. **Dip the wire ring (or object with aperture) into the soapy liquid and carefully remove it so that it retains a thin film of the soap mixture** (like a bubble-blower wand; see Fig. 23.4). If the film disappears at any point whilst completing the experiment, simply repeat this step.

4. **Hold the ring (or object with aperture) vertically and shine the torch on it from whichever angle gives you the best view of the interference pattern.**

5. **Make a note of what you can see** (you may need to adjust the torch to get the best view, and sometimes the pattern takes a few seconds to materialise) – **there should be rainbow stripes present in the film.**

6. **Make a note of how the stripes vary as you go down the film – do they change at all?**

Results

Fig. 23.5 shows a photograph I took when I attempted this experiment, and although it turned out to be extremely difficult to photograph, I'm hopeful that you can see the interference patterns coming through nicely in the picture (particularly near the top of the ring). There is also a patch of destructive interference visible at the very top of the film, which is where the film is so thin that all visible wavelengths destructively interfere with one another. There is also evidence that the interference stripes change in thickness as they get nearer the bottom of the film, though this is likely more visible in your own version which you can see live at home.

Let's explore why this change in stripe thickness happens with the help of a diagram (Fig. 23.6). In Fig. 23.6 you can see a front view and a side (cross-sectional) view of the film. Remember in the introduction of the chapter we said that the angle of the incident light and the thickness of the film would impact the interference pattern? Well, what you might not have realised is how relatively small changes in thickness can have a relatively large impact on the interference pattern. In our experiment, we held the film vertically, which meant that the thickness was uneven across the film because gravity is applying its forces to the film, making it thicker towards the bottom of the film itself. This means that when light reflects from the top part of the film, it will

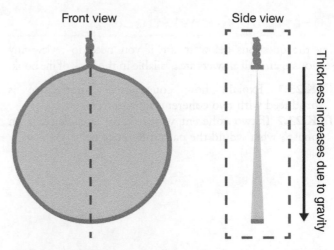

• **Fig. 23.6** A diagram of a cross section of the film (right) showing how the thickness varies vertically.

experience a different pattern of path differences to the light at the bottom of the film. You should try this experiment again, but this time hold the film horizontally. What would you expect to see?

Also, as ever, if you find that the experiment isn't working very well, you can troubleshoot the issue using Table 23.1 as a guide.

As with all experiments, if it didn't work out (even after troubleshooting), then you should think about what you could do to improve the method next time.

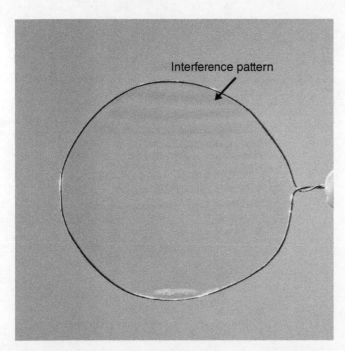

• **Fig. 23.5** A photograph of the interference pattern I made when I tried this experiment at home.

TABLE 23.1	Troubleshooting the Thin Film Interference Experiment		
Reported Issue	**Potential Problem**		**Potential Solution**
Soap film pops before interference can be viewed	1. Mixture is too watery		1. Add more washing-up liquid, or leave to stand (covered) overnight – this makes it bubblier
	2. The ring is too large, so the weight of the soap is too great		2. Try using a smaller ring
Interference is not visible	1. Lighting is not maximally effective		1. Remember that interference can only occur if light is present; I found this worked best in well-lit rooms, against a dark background, with a torch lighting the ring from the side
	2. Film is too thick		2. This can happen if the mixture is too soapy or if the ring is too large – try a smaller ring and a more watery mixture

Test Your Knowledge

Try the questions below to see if you need to review any sections again. All answers are available in the back of the book.

TYK.23.1 Explain how constructive interference is produced with two coherent light sources.

TYK.23.2 If two coherent waves arrive at a detector 'in phase', what would the path difference be?

TYK.23.3 Explain why the interference pattern varies vertically in our experiment.

TYK.23.4 Why do you think there's no visible interference pattern towards the very top of the film (see Fig. 23.5)?

SECTION 5

Question Answers

Answers to Practice Questions

Below are some representative answers to the 'practice questions' that appear within any chapters where we need to learn to apply some maths. They're designed to help you focus your learning, so make sure you have a go at answering them yourself before you take a peek at the answers!

Chapter 2

2.1.1 If an object is placed 12 cm in front of a surface, what is the object's vergence at the point where light from the object meets the surface?

$l = -0.12$
$n = 1.00$
$L = n/l$
$L = 1.00/ -0.12$
$L = -8.33D$

2.1.2 If an object is placed 7 cm in front of a surface, what is the object's vergence at the point where light from the object meets the surface?

$l = -0.07$
$n = 1.00$
$L = n/l$
$L = 1.00 / -0.07$
$L = -14.29D$

2.2.1 If a light ray is incident on a glass block (refractive index 1.523) at an angle of 35°, what is the angle of refraction?

$i = 35°$
$n = 1.00$
$n' = 1.523$
$n (\sin i) = n' (\sin i')$
$1.00 (\sin 35) = 1.523 (\sin i')$
$0.5735../ 1.523 = (\sin i')$
$0.3766.. = (\sin i')$
$\sin^{-1} (0.3766..) = i'$
$i' = 22.12°$

2.2.2 If a light ray is incident on a piece of plastic (refractive index 1.498) at an angle of 25°, what is the angle of refraction?

$i = 25°$
$n = 1.00$
$n' = 1.498$
$n (\sin i) = n' (\sin i')$
$1.00 (\sin 25) = 1.498 (\sin i')$
$0.4226.. / 1.498 = (\sin i')$
$0.2821.. = (\sin i')$
$\sin^{-1} (0.2821..) = i'$
$i' = 16.39°$

2.2.3 If a light ray refracts out of a glass block (refractive index 1.523) at an angle of 20°, what was the angle of incidence at the back surface?

$i' = 20°$
$n = 1.523$ (because the light is leaving the glass block)
$n' = 1.00$ (because the light is moving into air)
$n (\sin i) = n' (\sin i')$
$1.523 (\sin i) = 1.00 (\sin 20)$
$1.523 (\sin i) = 0.3420..$
$(\sin i) = 0.3420.. / 1.523$
$(\sin i) = 0.2246..$
$i = \sin^{-1} (0.2246..)$
$i = 12.98°$

2.3.1 Calculate the lateral displacement of a light ray that enters a 3-cm-wide glass block (refractive index 1.523) at an angle of 31°.

$i_1 = 31°$
$n = 1.00$
$n' = 1.523$
$d = 0.03$
$n (\sin i) = n' (\sin i')$
$1.00 (\sin 31) = 1.523 (\sin i')$
$0.5150../ 1.523 = (\sin i')$
$0.3381.. = (\sin i')$
$\sin^{-1} (0.3381..) = i'$
$i' = 19.77..°$
$s = (d (\sin (i_1 - i_1'))) / (\cos (i_1'))$
$s = (0.03 (\sin(31 - 19.77..))) / (\cos (19.77..))$
$s = 0.006211 m$
$s = 0.62 cm$

2.3.2 Calculate the lateral displacement of a light ray that enters a 11-cm-wide glass block (refractive index 1.523) at an angle of 29°.

$i_1 = 29°$
$n = 1.00$
$n' = 1.523$
$d = 0.11$
$n (\sin i) = n' (\sin i')$
$1.00 (\sin 29) = 1.523 (\sin i')$
$0.4848.. / 1.523 = (\sin i')$
$0.3183.. = (\sin i')$
$\sin^{-1} (0.3183..) = i'$
$i' = 18.56..°$
$s = (d (\sin (i_1 - i_1'))) / (\cos (i_1'))$
$s = (0.11 (\sin(29 - 18.56..))) / (\cos (18.56..))$
$s = 0.02102 m$
$s = 2.10 cm$

2.4.1 Determine the power of a convex spherical glass surface (refractive index 1.523) with a radius of curvature of 18 cm.

r = +0.18 m
n = 1.00
n' = 1.523
F = (n' − n) / r
F = (1.523 − 1.00) / 0.18
F = +2.91D

2.4.2 Determine the power of a concave spherical glass surface (refractive index 1.523) with a radius of curvature of 10 cm.

r = −0.1 m
n = 1.00
n' = 1.523
F = (n' − n) / r
F = (1.523 − 1.00) / −0.1
F = −5.23D

2.4.3 Determine the power of a convex spherical glass surface (refractive index 1.523) with a radius of curvature of 50 cm.

r = +0.5 m
n = 1.00
n' = 1.523
F = (n' − n) / r
F = (1.523 − 1.00) / 0.5
F = +1.05D

2.5.1 An object is placed 10 cm in front of a convex spherical glass surface (refractive index 1.523) with a radius of curvature of 8 cm. Where does the image form?

l = −0.1 m
r = +0.08 m
n = 1.00
n' = 1.523
F = (n' − n) / r
F = (1.523 − 1.00) / 0.08
F = +6.54..D
L = n / l
L = 1.00 / −0.1
L = −10
L' = L + F
L' = −10 + 6.54..
L' = −3.46..
l' = n' / L'
l' = 1.523 / −3.46..
l' = −0.4399 m
l' = −43.99 cm

2.5.2 An object is placed 30 cm in front of a concave spherical glass surface (refractive index 1.523) with a radius of curvature of 15 cm. Where does the image form?

l = −0.3 m
r = −0.15 m
n = 1.00
n' = 1.523

F = (n' − n) / r
F = (1.523 − 1.00) / −0.15
F = −3.49..D
L = n / l
L = 1.00 / −0.3
L = −3.33..
L' = L + F
L' = −3.49.. + −3.33..
L' = −6.82
l' = n' / L'
l' = 1.523 / −6.82
l' = −0.2233 m
l' = −22.33 cm

Chapter 3

3.1.1 A biconcave thin lens has a front surface power of −4.00D and a back surface power of −8.00D. What is the overall power of this lens?

F_1 = −4.00D
F_2 = −8.00D
F = F_1 + F_2
F = −4.00 + −8.00
F = −12.00D

3.1.2 A plus meniscus thin lens has a front surface power of +6.50D and a back surface power of −2.00D. What is the overall power of this lens?

F_1 = +6.50D
F_2 = −2.00D
F = F_1 + F_2
F = 6.50 + −2.00
F = +4.50D

3.2.1 A biconvex thin lens has a focal length of 30 cm. What is its power?

n' = 1.00
f' = +0.30
F = n' / f'
F = 1.00 / +0.3
F = +3.33D

3.2.2 A biconcave thin lens has a focal length of 11 cm. What is its power?

n' = 1.00
f' = −0.11
F = n' / f'
F = 1.00 / −0.11
F = −9.09D

3.2.3 A biconvex thin lens has a focal length of 25 cm. What is its power in water (refractive index 1.333)?

n' = 1.333
f' = +0.25
F = n' / f'
F = 1.333 / +0.25
F = +5.32D

3.2.4 A biconcave thin lens has a power of −4.00D. What is its focal length?

$n' = 1.00$
$F = -4.00D$
$f' = n' / F$
$f' = 1.00 / -4.00$
$f' = -0.25$ m or -25.00 cm

3.3.1 An object is placed 50 cm in front of a biconvex thin lens with a power of +10.00D. Where does the image form?

$l = -0.50$ m
$F = +10.00D$
$n = 1.00$
$n' = 1.00$
$L = n / l$
$L = 1.00 / -0.50$
$L = -2.00$
$L' = L + F$
$L' = -2.00 + +10.00$
$L' = +8.00$
$l' = n' / L'$
$l' = 1.00 / +8.00$
$l' = +0.125$ m or $+12.50$ cm (right of lens)

3.3.2 An object is placed 35 cm in front of a biconcave thin lens with a power of −12.00D. What is the magnification of the image?

$l = -0.35$ m
$F = -12.00D$
$n = 1.00$
$n' = 1.00$
$L = n / l$
$L = 1.00 / -0.35$
$L = -2.86..$
$L' = L + F$
$L' = -2.86.. + -12.00$
$L' = -14.86..$
$m = L / L'$
$m = -2.86.. / -14.86..$
$m = +0.19X$

3.3.3 An object is placed 15 cm in front of a biconcave thin lens with a focal length of 20 cm. Where does the image form?

$l = -0.15$ m
$f' = -0.20$ m
$n = 1.00$
$n' = 1.00$
$F = n' / f'$
$F = 1.00 / -0.20$
$F = -5.00D$
$L = n / l$
$L = 1.00 / -0.15$
$L = -6.67..$
$L' = L + F$
$L' = -6.67.. + -5.00$
$L' = -11.67..$

$l' = n' / L'$
$l' = 1.00 / -11.67$
$l' = -0.0857$ m or -8.57 cm (left of lens)

3.4.1 Two thin lenses of powers +1.00D and +5.50D are in contact with each other. If an object is placed 10 cm in front of the first lens, where does the image form?

$l = -0.10$ m
$F_1 = +1.00D$
$F_2 = +5.50D$
$n = 1.00$
$n' = 1.00$
$F_e = F_1 + F_2$
$F_e = +1.00 + +5.50$
$F_e = +6.50D$
$L = n / l$
$L = 1.00 / -0.10$
$L = -10.00$
$L' = L + F_e$
$L' = -10 + 6.50$
$L' = -3.50$
$l' = n' / L'$
$l' = 1.00 / -3.50$
$l' = -0.2857$ m or -28.57 cm (left of lenses)

3.4.2 Two thin lenses of powers +6.50D and −4.25D are in contact with each other. If an object is placed 40 cm in front of the first lens, what is the linear magnification?

$l = -0.40$ m
$F_1 = +6.50D$
$F_2 = -4.25D$
$n = 1.00$
$n' = 1.00$
$F_e = F_1 + F_2$
$F_e = +6.50 + -4.25$
$F_e = +2.25D$
$L = n / l$
$L = 1.00 / -0.40$
$L = -2.50$
$L' = L + F_e$
$L' = -2.50 + 2.25$
$L' = -0.25$
$m = L / L'$
$m = -2.50 / -0.25$
$m = +10.00X$

3.4.3 Three thin lenses of powers +1.00D, −3.50D and +6.75D are in contact with each other. If an object is placed 25 cm in front of the first lens, where does the image form?

$l = -0.25$ m
$F_1 = +1.00D$
$F_2 = -3.50D$
$F_3 = +6.75D$
$n = 1.00$
$n' = 1.00$
$F_e = F_1 + F_2 + F_3$
$F_e = +1.00 + -3.50 + +6.75$

$F_e = +4.25D$

$L = n / l$

$L = 1.00 / -0.25$

$L = -4.00$

$L' = L + F_e$

$L' = -4 + 4.25$

$L' = +0.25$

$l' = n' / L'$

$l' = 1.00 / +0.25$

$l' = +4.00$ m or $+400.00$ cm (right of lenses)

3.5.1 Two thin lenses of powers +4.50D and −1.00D are separated by a distance of 5 cm. What is the back vertex power of the system?

$F_1 = +4.50D$

$F_2 = -1.00D$

$d = 0.05$ m

$F_v' = (F_1 + F_2 - dF_1F_2) / (1 - dF_1)$

$F_v' = (+4.50 + -1.00 - (0.05)(+4.50)(-1.00)) / (1 - (0.05)(+4.50))$

$F_v' = +4.81D$

3.5.2 Two thin lenses of powers +8.50D and −9.00D are separated by a distance of 11 cm. What is the front vertex power of the system?

$F_1 = +8.50D$

$F_2 = -9.00D$

$d = 0.11$ m

$F_v = (F_1 + F_2 - dF_1F_2) / (1 - dF_2)$

$F_v = (+8.50 + -9.00 - (0.11)(+8.50)(-9.00)) / (1 - (0.11)(-9.00))$

$F_v = +3.98D$

3.6.1 Two thin lenses of powers +5.75D and −3.00D are separated by a distance of 8 cm. What is the back vertex focal length of the system?

$F_1 = +5.75D$

$F_2 = -3.00D$

$d = 0.08$ m

$F_v' = (F_1 + F_2 - dF_1F_2) / (1 - dF_1)$

$F_v' = (+5.75 + -3.00 - (0.08)(+5.75)(-3.00)) / (1 - (0.08)(+5.75))$

$F_v' = +7.65..D$

$f_v' = n / F_v'$

$f_v' = 1 / +7.65..$

$f_v' = +0.1308$ m or $+13.08$ cm

3.6.2 Two thin lenses of powers −6.50D and −2.00D are separated by a distance of 11 cm. What is the front vertex focal length of the system?

$F_1 = -6.50D$

$F_2 = -2.00D$

$d = 0.11$ m

$F_v = (F_1 + F_2 - dF_1F_2) / (1 - dF_2)$

$F_v = (-6.50 + -2.00 - (0.11)(-6.50)(-2.00)) / (1 - (0.11)(-2.00))$

$F_v = -8.14..$

$f_v = -(n / F_v)$

$f_v = -(1 / -8.14...)$

$f_v = -0.1229$ m or -12.29 cm

3.7.1 Two thin lenses of powers +5.00D and +1.00D are separated by a distance of 15 cm. If an object is placed 25 cm in front of the first lens, where will the image form?

$F_1 = +5.00D$

$F_2 = +1.00D$

$d = 0.15$ m

$l_1 = -0.25$ m

$n = 1.00$

$n' = 1.00$

$L_1 = n / l_1$

$L_1 = 1.00 / -0.25$

$L_1 = -4.00$

$L_1' = L_1 + F_1$

$L_1' = -4.00 + +5.00$

$L_1' = +1.00$

$L_2 = L_1' / (1 - dL_1')$

$L_2 = +1.00 / (1 - (0.15 \times 1.00))$

$L_2 = +1.176...$

$L_2' = L_2 + F_2$

$L_2' = +1.176... + 1.00$

$L_2' = +2.176...$

$l_2' = n' / L_2'$

$l_2' = 1.00 / +2.176...$

$l_2' = +0.4595$ m or $+45.95$ cm

3.7.2 Two thin lenses of powers −2.50D and +8.25D are separated by a distance of 8 cm. If an object is placed 10 cm in front of the first lens, where will the image form?

$F_1 = -2.50D$

$F_2 = +8.25D$

$d = 0.08$ m

$l_1 = -0.1$ m

$n = 1.00$

$n' = 1.00$

$L_1 = n / l_1$

$L_1 = 1.00 / -0.1$

$L_1 = -10.00$

$L_1' = L_1 + F_1$

$L_1' = -10.00 + -2.50$

$L_1' = -12.50$

$L_2 = L_1' / (1 - dL_1')$

$L_2 = -12.50 / (1 - (0.08 \times -12.50))$

$L_2 = -6.25$

$L_2' = L_2 + F_2$

$L_2' = -6.25 + 8.25$

$L_2' = +2.00$

$l_2' = n' / L_2'$

$l_2' = 1.00 / +2.00$

$l_2' = +0.50$ m or $+50.00$ cm

3.8.1 Two thin lenses of powers $+6.00D$ and $+1.75D$ are separated by a distance of 10 cm. What is the equivalent power?

$F_1 = +6.00D$
$F_2 = +1.75D$
$d = 0.1$ m
$F_e = F_1 + F_2 - (dF_1F_2)$
$F_e = (+6.00) + (+1.75) - (0.1 \times (+6.00) \times (+1.75))$
$F_e = +6.70D$

3.8.2 Two thin lenses of powers $-2.25D$ and $+8.00D$ are separated by a distance of 11.5 cm. What is the equivalent power?

$F_1 = -2.25D$
$F_2 = +8.00D$
$d = 0.115$ m
$F_e = F_1 + F_2 - (dF_1F_2)$
$F_e = (-2.25) + (+8.00) - (0.115 \times (-2.25) \times (+8.00))$
$F_e = +7.82D$

3.9.1 Two thin lenses of powers $-3.50D$ and $+6.75D$ are separated by a distance of 10 cm. What is the secondary equivalent focal length of the system?

$F_1 = -3.50D$
$F_2 = +6.75D$
$d = 0.1$ m
$n = 1.00$
$F_e = F_1 + F_2 - (dF_1F_2)$
$F_e = (-3.50) + (+6.75) - (0.1 \times (-3.50) \times (+6.75))$
$F_e = +5.61..$
$f_e' = n / F_e$
$f_e' = 1 / +5.61..$
$f_e' = +0.1782$ m or $+17.82$ cm

3.9.2 Two thin lenses of powers $-2.25D$ and $+10.00D$ are separated by a distance of 50 cm. What is the primary equivalent focal length of the system?

$F_1 = -2.25D$
$F_2 = +10.00D$
$d = 0.5$ m
$n = 1.00$
$F_e = F_1 + F_2 - (dF_1F_2)$
$F_e = (-2.25) + (+10.00) - (0.5 \times (-2.25) \times (+10))$
$F_e = +19.00$
$f_e = -(n / F_e)$
$f_e = -(1 / 19..)$
$f_e = -0.0526$ m or -5.26 cm

3.9.3 A multiple lens system has a secondary equivalent focal length of $+25$ cm. What is the primary equivalent focal length of the system?

$f_e' = +0.25$ m
$f_e = - f_e'$
$f_e = -0.25$ m or -25.00 cm

3.10.1 Two thin lenses of powers $-4.00D$ and $+10.00D$ are separated by a distance of 5 cm. If an object is placed 25 cm in front of the primary focal point of the system, where will the image form?

$F_1 = -4.00D$
$F_2 = +10.00D$
$d = 0.05$ m
$x = -0.25$ m
$n = 1.00$
$n' = 1.00$
$F_e = F_1 + F_2 - (dF_1F_2)$
$F_e = (-4.00) + (+10.00) - (0.05 \times (-4.00) \times (+10.00))$
$F_e = +8$
$f_e' = n / F_e$
$f_e' = 1 / +8$
$f_e' = +0.125$ m
$(f_e')^2 = -xx'$
$(0.125)^2 = - (-0.25) x'$
$0.0156.. / -0.25 = -x'$
$-0.0625 = -x'$
$x' = +0.0625$ m or $+6.25$ cm

3.10.2 Two thin lenses of powers $+3.25D$ and $+2.00D$ are separated by a distance of 14 cm. If an object is placed 16 cm in front of the primary focal point of the system, where will the image form?

$F_1 = +3.25D$
$F_2 = +2.00D$
$d = 0.14$ m
$x = -0.16$ m
$n = 1.00$
$n' = 1.00$
$F_e = F_1 + F_2 - (dF_1F_2)$
$F_e = (+3.25) + (+2.00) - (0.14 \times (+3.25) \times (+2.00))$
$F_e = +4.34$
$f_e' = n / F_e$
$f_e' = 1 / +4.34$
$f_e' = + 0.2304..$m
$(f_e')^2 = -xx'$
$(0.2304..)^2 = - (-0.16) x'$
$0.0531.. / -0.16 = -x'$
$-0.3318 = -x'$
$x' = +0.3318$ m or $+33.18$ cm

3.10.3 A multiple lens system has a secondary equivalent focal length of $+23.25$ cm. If an object is placed 10 cm in front of the primary focal point of the system, where will the image form?

$f_e = +0.2325$ m
$x = -0.1$ m
$n = 1.00$
$n' = 1.00$
$(f_e')^2 = -xx'$

$(0.2325)^2 = - (-0.1) x'$
$0.0541.. / -0.1 = -x'$
$-0.5406 = -x'$
$x' = +0.5406$ m or $+54.06$ cm

3.11.1 Two thin lenses of powers -2.50D and $+3.00$D are separated by a distance of 3 cm. If an object is placed 45 cm in front of the primary focal point of the system, what is the linear magnification of the image?
$F_1 = -2.50$D
$F_2 = +3.00$D
$d = 0.03$ m
$x = -0.45$ m
$n = 1.00$
$n' = 1.00$
$F_e = F_1 + F_2 - (dF_1F_2)$
$F_e = (-2.50) + (+3.00) - (0.030 \times (-2.50) \times (+3.00))$
$F_e = +0.725$
$f_e' = n / F_e$
$f_e' = 1 / +0.725$
$f_e' = +1.38..$m
$(f_e')^2 = -xx'$
$(1.38..)^2 = - (-0.45) x'$
$1.902.. / -0.45 = -x'$
$-4.23.. = -x'$
$x' = +4.23..$m
$m = -x'F_e$
$m = - (+4.23..)(+0.725)$
$m = -3.07$X

3.11.2 Two thin lenses of powers $+3.25$D and $+7.00$D are separated by a distance of 19 cm. If an object is placed 8 cm in front of the primary focal point of the system, what is the linear magnification of the image?
$F_1 = +3.25$D
$F_2 = +7.00$D
$d = 0.19$ m
$x = -0.08$ m
$n = 1.00$
$n' = 1.00$
$F_e = F_1 + F_2 - (dF_1F_2)$
$F_e = (+3.25) + (+7) - (0.19 \times (+3.25) \times (+7.00))$
$F_e = +5.93..$
$f_e' = n / F_e$
$f_e' = 1 / +5.93..$
$f_e' = +0.1687..$m
$(f_e')^2 = -xx'$
$(0.1687..)^2 = - (-0.08) x'$
$0.0284.. / -0.08 = -x'$
$-0.3558.. = -x'$
$x' = +0.3558..$m
$m = -x'F_e$
$m = - (+0.3558..)(+5.93..)$
$m = -2.11$x

Chapter 4

4.1.1 A 7-cm-wide planoconvex lens has a radius of curvature of 12 cm. What is the sag of the lens?
$y = 0.035$ m
$r = 0.12$
$s = r - \sqrt{(r^2 - y^2)}$
$s = 0.12 - \sqrt{(0.12^2 - 0.035^2)}$
$s = 0.005218$ m
$s = 0.52$ cm

4.1.2 A 4-cm-wide planoconvex lens has a radius of curvature of 50 cm. What is the sag of the lens?
$y = 0.02$ m
$r = 0.5$
$s = r - \sqrt{(r^2 - y^2)}$
$s = 0.5 - \sqrt{(0.5^2 - 0.02^2)}$
$s = 0.0004$ m
$s = 0.04$ cm

4.1.3 A 5-cm-wide planoconvex lens has a radius of curvature of 10 cm. What is the sag of the lens?
$y = 0.025$ m
$r = 0.1$
$s = r - \sqrt{(r^2 - y^2)}$
$s = 0.1 - \sqrt{(0.1^2 - 0.025^2)}$
$s = 0.00318$ m
$s = 0.32$ cm

4.2.1 A thick lens (refractive index 1.523) has a convex front surface with a radius of curvature of 25 cm. What is the power of the front surface?
$n_1' = 1.523$
$r_1 = +0.25$ m
$n_1 = 1.00$
$F_1 = (n_1' - n_1) / r_1$
$F_1 = (1.523 - 1.00) / 0.25$
$F_1 = +2.09$D

4.2.2 A thick lens (refractive index 1.523) has a concave back surface with a radius of curvature of 25 cm. What is the power of the back surface?
$n_2' = 1.000$
$r_2 = +0.25$ m
$n_2 = 1.523$
$F_1 = (n_2' - n_2) / r_2$
$F_1 = (1.00 - 1.523) / +0.25$
$F_1 = -2.09$D

4.2.3 A 5-cm-thick lens (refractive index 1.523) has a front surface power of -2.00D and a back surface power of $+4.00$D. What is the power of the lens?
$t = 0.05$ m
$n_g = 1.523$
$F_1 = -2.00$D

$F_2 = +4.00D$
$n = 1.00$
$\bar{t} = t / n_g$
$\bar{t} = 0.05 / 1.523$
$\bar{t} = 0.0328..$
$F_e = F_1 + F_2 - \bar{t}\, F_1 F_2$
$F_e = -2.00 + 4.00 - (0.0328... \times -2.00 \times 4.00)$
$F_e = +2.26D$

4.3.1 Imagine a 0.8 cm thick biconvex lens (surface powers +1.00D and +3.50D; refractive index 1.523). Where is the secondary principal plane, relative to the back surface of the lens?
$F_1 = +1.00D$
$F_2 = +3.50D$
$t = 0.008\ m$
$n = 1.00$
$n_g = 1.523$
$\bar{t} = t / n_g$
$\bar{t} = 0.008 / 1.523$
$\bar{t} = 0.0053..$
$F_v' = (F_1 + F_2 - \bar{t}\, F_1 F_2) / (1 - \bar{t}\, F_1)$
$F_v' = (1.00 + 3.5 - 0.0053..\times1.00\times3.5) / (1 - (0.0053..\times 1.00)$
$F_v' = +4.51..$
$f_v' = n / F_v'$
$f_v' = 1.00 / +4.51..$
$f_v' = +0.2220..$
$F_e = F_1 + F_2 - \bar{t}\, F_1 F_2$
$F_e = 1.00 + 3.5 - 0.0053..\times1.00\times3.5$
$F_e = +4.48..$
$f_e' = n / F_e$
$f_e' = 1.00 / +4.48..$
$f_e' = +0.2231..$
$A_2P' = e' = f_v' - f_e'$
$A_2P' = e' = +0.2220.. - +0.2231..$
$A_2P' = e' = -0.0012\ m$
Or 0.12 cm left of the back lens

4.3.2 Imagine a 1-cm-thick biconvex lens (surface powers +2.00D and +6.25D; refractive index 1.523). Where is the primary principal plane, relative to the back surface of the lens?
$F_1 = +2.00D$
$F_2 = +6.25D$
$t = 0.01\ m$
$n = 1.00$
$n_g = 1.523$
$\bar{t} = t / n_g$
$\bar{t} = 0.01 / 1.523$
$\bar{t} = 0.0066..$
$F_v = (F_1 + F_2 - \bar{t}\, F_1 F_2) / (1 - \bar{t}\, F_2)$
$F_v = (2.00 + 6.25 - 0.0066..\times2\times6.25) / (1 - (0.0066..\times6.25)$
$F_v = +8.52..$
$f_v = -(n / F_v)$
$f_v = -(1.00 / +8.52..)$
$f_v = -0.1174..$
$F_e = F_1 + F_2 - \bar{t}\, F_1 F_2$
$F_e = 2.00 + 6.25 - 0.0053..\times2.00\times6.25$

$F_e = +8.17..$
$f_e = -(n / F_e)$
$f_e = -(1.00 / +8.17..)$
$f_e = -0.1224..$
$A_1P = e = f_v - f_e$
$A_1P = e = -0.1174.. - -0.1224..$
$A_1P = e = +0.0050\ m$
Primary principal plane is +0.5 cm right of front surface and is therefore −0.5 cm left of the back surface of the lens.

4.4.1 An object is placed 10 cm in front of a 4-cm-thick biconvex lens (refractive index 1.523) with a front surface power of +4.00D and a back surface power of +5.00D. Where does the image form relative to the back surface of the lens?
$l_1 = -0.10\ m$
$F_1 = +4.00D$
$F_2 = +5.00D$
$t = 0.04\ m$
$n = 1.00$
$n' = 1.523$
$L_1 = n_1 / l_1$
$L_1 = 1.00 / -0.10$
$L_1 = -10.00$
$L_1' = L_1 + F_1$
$L_1' = -10.00 + 4.00$
$L_1' = -6.00$
$l_1' = n_1' / L_1'$
$l_1' = 1.523 / -6.00$
$l_1' = -0.2538..$
$l_2 = l_1' - t$
$l_2 = -0.2538... - 0.04$
$l_2 = -0.2938...$
$L_2 = n_2 / l_2$
$L_2 = 1.523 / -0.2938...$
$L_2 = -5.18...$
$L_2' = L_2 + F_2$
$L_2' = -5.18... + 5.00$
$L_2' = -0.1832...$
$l_2' = n_2' / L_2'$
$l_2' = 1.00 / -0.1832...$
$l_2' = -5.4582\ m\ or\ -545.82\ cm$

4.4.2 An object is placed 20 cm in front of a 1.5-cm-thick biconcave lens (refractive index 1.523) with a front surface power of −2.50D and a back surface power of −3.00D. Where does the image form relative to the back surface of the lens?
$l_1 = -0.20\ m$
$F_1 = -2.50D$
$F_2 = -3.00D$
$t = 0.015\ m$
$n = 1.00$
$n' = 1.523$
$L_1 = n_1 / l_1$
$L_1 = 1.00 / -0.20$
$L_1 = -5.00$
$L_1' = L_1 + F_1$

$L_1' = -5.00 + -2.50$
$L_1' = -7.50$
$l_1' = n_1' / L_1'$
$l_1' = 1.523 / -7.50$
$l_1' = -0.2031..$
$l_2 = l_1' - \tau$
$l_2 = -0.2031... - 0.015$
$l_2 = -0.2181...$
$L_2 = n_2 / l_2$
$L_2 = 1.523 / -0.2181...$
$L_2 = -6.98...$
$L_2' = L_2 + F_2$
$L_2' = -6.98... + -3.00$
$L_2' = -9.98...$
$l_2' = n_2' / L_2'$
$l_2' = 1.00 / -9.98...$
$l_2' = -0.1002$ m or -10.02 cm

4.5.1 An object is placed 11 cm in front of a 4-cm-thick biconvex lens (refractive index 1.523) with a front surface power of +2.00D and a back surface power of +5.00D. Where does the image form relative to the back surface of the lens?

$l_1 = -0.11$ m
$F_1 = +2.00D$
$F_2 = +5.00D$
$t = 0.04$ m
$n = 1.00$
$n' = 1.523$
$L_1 = n_1 / l_1$
$L_1 = 1.00 / -0.11$
$L_1 = -9.09..$
$L_1' = L_1 + F_1$
$L_1' = -9.09.. + 2$
$L_1' = -7.09..$
$\bar{t} = t / n_g$
$\bar{t} = 0.04 / 1.523$
$\bar{t} = 0.026..$
$L_2 = L_1' / (1 - \bar{t} L_1')$
$L_2 = -7.09../ (1 - (0.026.. \times -7.09..))$
$L_2 = -5.98..$
$L_2' = L_2 + F_2$
$L_2' = -5.98... + 5.00$
$L_2' = -0.98...$
$l_2' = n_2' / L_2'$
$l_2' = 1.00 / -0.98...$
$l_2' = -1.0229$ m or -102.29 cm

4.5.2 An object is placed 25 cm in front of a 3-cm-thick biconcave lens (refractive index 1.523) with a front surface power of −1.50D and a back surface power of −5.00D. Where does the image form relative to the back surface of the lens?

$l_1 = -0.25$ m
$F_1 = -1.50D$
$F_2 = -5.00D$
$t = 0.03$ m

$n = 1.00$
$n' = 1.523$
$L_1 = n_1 / l_1$
$L_1 = 1.00 / -0.25$
$L_1 = -4.00$
$L_1' = L_1 + F_1$
$L_1' = -4.00 + -1.50$
$L_1' = -5.50$
$\bar{t} = t / n_g$
$\bar{t} = 0.03 / 1.523$
$\bar{t} = 0.020..$
$L_2 = L_1' / (1 - \bar{t} L_1')$
$L_2 = -5.50/ (1 - (0.020..\times -5.50))$
$L_2 = -4.96..$
$L_2' = L_2 + F_2$
$L_2' = -4.96... + -5.00$
$L_2' = -9.96...$
$l_2' = n_2' / L_2'$
$l_2' = 1.00 / -9.96...$
$l_2' = -0.1004$ m or -10.04 cm

Chapter 6

6.1.1 Two plane mirrors are inclined at an angle of 35° towards one another. What will the angle of deviation be?

$a = 35°$
$d = 360 - 2a$
$d = 360 - 2(35)$
$d = 360 - 70$
$d = 290°$

6.1.2 Two plane mirrors are inclined at an angle of 41.5° towards one another. What will the angle of deviation be?

$a = 41.5°$
$d = 360 - 2a$
$d = 360 - 2(41.5)$
$d = 360 - 83$
$d = 277°$

6.2.1 A convex spherical mirror has a radius of curvature of 100 cm. What is its power?

$r = +1$ m
$n = 1.00$
$f = r / 2$
$f = 1/ 2$
$f = +0.5$ m
$F = - (n / f)$
$F = - (1.00 / +0.5)$
$F = -2.00D$

6.2.2 A concave spherical mirror has a focal length of 50 cm. What is its power?

$f = -0.5$ m
$n = 1.00$
$F = - (n / f)$
$F = - (1.00 / -0.5)$
$F = +2.00D$

6.3.1 An object is placed 10 cm in front of a convex spherical mirror with a radius of curvature of 20 cm. Where does the image form?

$l = -0.1$ m
$r = +0.20$ m
$n = 1.00$
$f = r / 2$
$f = +0.20 / 2$
$f = +0.10$
$F = - (n / f)$
$F = - (1.00 / +0.10)$
$F = -10.00D$
$L = n / l$
$L = 1.00 / -0.1$
$L = -10$
$L' = L + F$
$L' = -10 + -10$
$L' = -20$
$l' = - (n' / L')$
$l' = - (1.00 / -20)$
$l' = +0.05$ m or $+5.00$ cm

6.3.2 An object is placed 30 cm in front of a concave spherical mirror with a power of +5.00D. Where does the image form?

$l = -0.3$ m
$F = +5.00D$
$n = 1.00$
$L = n / l$
$L = 1.00 / -0.3$
$L = -3.33..$
$L' = L + F$
$L' = -3.33.. + -5$
$L' = +1.67..$
$l' = - (n' / L')$
$l' = - (1.00 / 1.67..)$
$l' = -0.60$ m or -60.00 cm

6.4.1 An object is placed 20 cm in front of a convex spherical mirror with a radius of curvature of 30 cm. Where does the image form?

$l = -0.20$ m
$r = +0.30$ m
$n = 1.00$
$(1 / l') + (1 / l) = (2 / r)$
$(1 / l') + (1 / -0.20) = (2 / 0.3)$
$(1 / l') = 11.67..$
$l' = 1 / 11.67..$
$l' = +0.0857$ m or $+8.57$ cm

6.4.2 An object is placed 25 cm in front of a concave spherical mirror with a power of +5.00D. Where does the image form?

$l = -0.25$ m
$F = +5.00D$
$n = 1.00$
$f = - (n / F)$
$f = - (1.00 / +5.00)$

$f = -0.20$
$(1 / l') + (1 / l) = (1 / f)$
$(1 / l') + (1 / -0.25) = (1 / -0.20)$
$(1 / l') = -1$
$l' = 1 / -1$
$l' = -1.00$ m or -100.00 cm

6.5.1 An object is placed 20 cm in front of a concave spherical mirror with a radius of curvature of 60 cm. What is the magnification of the image?

$l = -0.20$ m
$r = -0.60$ m
$n = 1.00$
$(1 / l') + (1 / l) = (2 / r)$
$(1 / l') + (1 / -0.20) = (2 / -0.60)$
$(1 / l') = 1.67..$
$l' = 1 / 1.67..$
$l' = +0.60$ m
$m = - (l' / l)$
$m = - (+0.6 / -0.2)$
$m = +3.00X$ (magnified, upright, virtual)

6.5.2 An object is placed 30 cm in front of a concave spherical mirror of power +10.00D. What is the magnification of the image?

$l = -0.30$ m
$F = +10.00D$
$n = 1.00$
$f = - (n / F)$
$f = - (1.00 / +10.00)$
$f = -0.10$
$(1 / l') + (1 / l) = (1 / f)$
$(1 / l') + (1 / -0.30) = (1 / -0.10)$
$(1 / l') = -6.67..$
$l' = 1 / -6.67..$
$l' = -0.15$ m
$m = - (l' / l)$
$m = - (-0.15 / -0.3)$
$m = -0.50X$ (minified, inverted, real)

Chapter 8

8.1.1 What is the chromatic aberration of a crown glass lens with a power of +20.00D?

$V = 60$
$F = +20.00D$
$CA = F / V$
$CA = 20.00 / 60$
$CA = 0.33$

8.1.2 What is the chromatic aberration of a flint glass lens with a power of +10.00D?

$V = 30$
$F = +10.00D$
$CA = F / V$
$CA = 10.00 / 30$
$CA = 0.33$

8.2.1 What power of flint glass would be required to remove chromatic aberration from a lens made partly of crown glass (+8.00D)?

$V_c = 60$

$V_f = 30$

$F_c = +8.00D$

$CA = 0$

$CA = (F_c / V_c) + (F_f / V_f)$

$0 = (8.00 / 60) + (F_f / 30)$

$-0.133.. = F_f / 30$

$-0.133.. \times 30 = F_f$

$-4.00D = F_f$

8.2.2 What power of crown glass would be required to remove chromatic aberration from a lens made partly of flint glass (+2.00D)?

$V_c = 60$

$V_f = 30$

$F_f = +2.00D$

$CA = 0$

$CA = (F_c / V_c) + (F_f / V_f)$

$0 = (F_c / 60) + (2.00 / 30)$

$-0.067.. = F_c / 60$

$-0.067.. \times 60 = F_c$

$-4.00D = F_f$

Chapter 9

9.1.1 A ray of light is incident upon a prism at an angle of 20° and leaves the prism at an angle of 40°. If the prism has an apical angle of 55°, what is the angle of deviation of the light?

$i_1 = 20°$

$i_2' = 40°$

$a = 55°$

$d = (i_1 + i_2') - a$

$d = (20 + 40) - 55$

$d = 5°$

9.1.2 A ray of light is incident upon a prism at an angle of 21.2° and leaves the prism at an angle of 58.5°. If the prism has an apical angle of 30°, what is the angle of deviation of the light?

$i_1 = 21.2°$

$i_2' = 58.5°$

$a = 30°$

$d = (i_1 + i_2') - a$

$d = (21.2 + 58.5) - 30$

$d = 49.7°$

9.2.1 Calculate the minimum angle of deviation of a prism constructed of refractive index 1.498 of apical angle 60°.

$n_p = 1.498$

$n_s = 1.00$

$a = 60$

$n_s (\sin 0.5(a + d_{min})) = n_p (\sin (0.5 \times a))$

$1.00 (\sin 0.5(60 + d_{min})) = 1.498 (\sin (0.5 \times 60))$

$\sin 0.5(60 + d_{min}) = 1.498 (\sin (0.5 \times 60))$

$\sin 0.5(60 + d_{min}) = 0.749$

$0.5(60 + d_{min}) = \sin^{-1}(0.749)$

$0.5(60 + d_{min}) = 48.50..$

$30 + 0.5(d_{min}) = 48.50..$

$0.5(d_{min}) = 48.50.. -30$

$0.5(d_{min}) = 18.50..$

$d_{min} = 18.50.. / 0.5$

$d_{min} = 37.01°$

9.2.2 Calculate the minimum angle of deviation of a prism constructed of refractive index 1.65 of apical angle 30°.

$n_p = 1.65$

$n_s = 1.00$

$a = 30$

$n_s (\sin 0.5(a + d_{min})) = n_p (\sin (0.5 \times a))$

$1.00 (\sin 0.5(30 + d_{min})) = 1.65 (\sin (0.5 \times 30))$

$\sin 0.5(30 + d_{min}) = 1.65 (\sin (0.5 \times 30))$

$\sin 0.5(30 + d_{min}) = 0.427..$

$0.5(30 + d_{min}) = \sin^{-1}(0.427..)$

$0.5(30 + d_{min}) = 25.28..$

$15 + 0.5(d_{min}) = 25.28..$

$0.5(d_{min}) = 25.28.. -15$

$0.5(d_{min}) = 10.28..$

$d_{min} = 10.28.. / 0.5$

$d_{min} = 20.56°$

9.3.1 Determine the smallest angle of incidence at the first face of an equilateral triangular prism of refractive index 1.498 for light to just pass through the second face. The apical angle of the prism is 50°.

$n_p = 1.498$

$n_s = 1.00$

$a = 50$

$\sin(i_c) = 1 / n_p$

$\sin(i_c) = 1 / 1.498$

$i_c = \sin^{-1} (1 / 1.498)$

$i_c = 41.88..°$

$i_2 = i_c$

$i_1' = a - i_2$

$i_1' = 50 - 41.88..$

$i_1' = 8.12..°$

$n_s (\sin i_1) = n_p (\sin i_1')$

$1.00 (\sin i_1) = 1.498 (\sin 8.12..)$

$\sin i_1 = 1.498 (\sin 8.12..) / 1$

$i_1 = \sin^{-1} (1.498 (\sin 8.12..))$

$i_1 = 12.22°$

9.3.2 Determine the smallest angle of incidence at the first face of an equilateral triangular prism of refractive index 1.523 for light to just pass through the second face. The apical angle of the prism is 55°.

$n_p = 1.523$

$n_s = 1.00$

$a = 55$

$\sin(i_c) = 1 / n_p$

$\sin(i_c) = 1 / 1.523$

$i_c = \sin^{-1}(1 / 1.523)$
$i_c = 41.04..°$
$i_2 = i_c$
$i_1' = a - i_2$
$i_1' = 55 - 41.048..$
$i_1' = 13.96..°$
$n_s(\sin i_1) = n_p(\sin i_1')$
$1.00(\sin i_1) = 1.523(\sin 13.96..)$
$\sin i_1 = 1.523(\sin 13.96..) / 1$
$i_1 = \sin^{-1}(1.523(\sin 13.96..))$
$i_1 = 21.55°$

9.3.3 Determine the smallest angle of incidence at the first face of an equilateral triangular prism of refractive index 1.65 for light to just pass through the second face. The apical angle of the prism is 45°.
$n_p = 1.65$
$n_s = 1.00$
$a = 45$
$\sin(i_c) = 1 / n_p$
$\sin(i_c) = 1 / 1.65$
$i_c = \sin^{-1}(1 / 1.65)$
$i_c = 37.31..°$
$i_2 = i_c$
$i_1' = a - i_2$
$i_1' = 45 - 37.31..$
$i_1' = 7.69..°$
$n_s(\sin i_1) = n_p(\sin i_1')$
$1.00(\sin i_1) = 1.65(\sin 7.69..)$
$\sin i_1 = 1.65(\sin 7.69..) / 1$
$i_1 = \sin^{-1}(1.65(\sin 7.69..))$
$i_1 = 12.76°$

9.4.1 A prism produces 5 m of displacement at 100 m. What is its power?
$x = 500$ cm
$y = 10,000$ cm
$P = (100)(x/y)$
$P = (100)(500 / 10,000)$
$P = 5^\Delta$

9.4.2 A prism produces 15 cm of displacement at 65 cm. What is its power?
$x = 15$ cm
$y = 65$ cm
$P = (100)(x/y)$
$P = (100)(15 / 65)$
$P = 23.08^\Delta$

9.5.1 How much prism power will be induced if a patient looks through their −2.50DS lens 2 mm left of the optical centre?
$F = -2.50$DS
$c = 0.2$ cm
$P = cF$

$P = 0.2 \times -2.50$
$P = -0.5^\Delta$

9.5.2 How much prism power will be induced if a patient looks through their +4.25DS lens 1 mm right of the optical centre?
$F = +4.25$DS
$c = 0.1$ cm
$P = cF$
$P = 0.1 \times 4.25$
$P = 0.43^\Delta$

Chapter 10

10.1.1 A single slit is placed 40 cm in front of a wall. If the first and second maxima are 8 cm apart from one another, what is the angle of diffraction?
$L = 0.4$ m
$y = 0.08$ m
$\sin \phi = y / \sqrt{(L^2 + y^2)}$
$\sin \phi = 0.08 / \sqrt{(0.4^2 + 0.08^2)}$
$\phi = \sin^{-1}(0.1961..)$
$\phi = 11.31°$

10.1.2 A single slit is placed 55 cm in front of a wall. If the first and second maxima are 18 cm apart from one another, what is the angle of diffraction?
$L = 0.55$ m
$y = 0.18$ m
$\sin \phi = y / \sqrt{(L^2 + y^2)}$
$\sin \phi = 0.18 / \sqrt{(0.55^2 + 0.18^2)}$
$\phi = \sin^{-1}(0.3110..)$
$\phi = 18.12°$

Chapter 12

12.1.1 Calculate the planar angle shown as '?' in the following image:

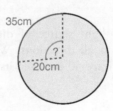

$c = 0.35$ m
$R = 0.2$ m
$\theta = c / R$
$\theta = 0.35 / 0.2$
$\theta = 1.75$
(π radians)
$\theta = 1.75 / \pi$
$\theta = 0.56 \pi$ rad
(degrees)

$\theta = 1.75 * (180 / \pi)$
$\theta = 100.27°$

12.1.2 Calculate the planar angle shown as '?' in the following image:

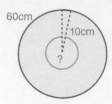

$c = 0.6$ m
$R = 0.1$ m
$\theta = c / R$
$\theta = 0.6 / 0.1$
$\theta = 6$
(π radians)
$\theta = 6 / \pi$
$\theta = 1.91 \ \pi$ rad
(degrees)
$\theta = 6 * (180 / \pi)$
$\theta = 343.77°$

12.2.1 A spherical light source of diameter 2 m emits 1500 lm uniformly in all directions. What is the average illuminance on a surface 2 m from its centre?
$\phi = 1500$
$R = 1$ m
$d = 2$ m
$\omega = 4\pi$
$I = \phi / \omega$
$I = 1500 / 4\pi$
$I = 119.37$ cd
$E = I / d^2$
$E = 119.37.. / 2^2$
$E = 159 / 9$
$E = 29.84$ lx

12.2.2 A spherical light source of diameter 2 m emits 300 lm uniformly in all directions. What is the average illuminance on a surface 50 cm from its centre?
$\phi = 300$
$R = 1$ m

$d = 0.5$ m
$\omega = 4\pi$
$I = \phi / \omega$
$I = 300 / 4\pi$
$I = 23.87..$cd
$E = I / d^2$
$E = 23.87.. / 0.5^2$
$E = 23.87.. / 0.25$
$E = 95.49$ lx

Chapter 13

13.1.1 A Galilean telescope has an eyepiece lens with a power of -5.00D, and it produces a magnification of $+4$X. What is the power of the objective lens?
$F_{ep} = -5.00$D
$m = +4$
$m = - (F_{ep} / F_o)$
$F_o = - (-5.00 / 4)$
$F_o = +1.25$D

13.1.2 A Keplerian telescope has an eyepiece lens with a power of $+7.00$D and an objective lens with a power of $+4.50$D. What is the angular magnification of the telescope?
$F_{ep} = +7.00$D
$F_o = +4.50$D
$m = - (F_{ep} / F_o)$
$m = - (7 / 4.5)$
$m = -1.56$X

13.1.3 A Keplerian telescope has an eyepiece lens with a power of $+6.25$D and it produces a magnification of -8.50X. What is the power of the objective lens?
$F_{ep} = 6.25$
$m = -8.5$
$m = - (F_{ep} / F_o)$
$F_o = - (6.25 / -8.5)$
$F_o = +0.74$D

Answers to Test Your Knowledge Questions

Below are some representative answers to the 'Test Your Knowledge' questions that appear at the end of every chapter. They're designed to help you focus your learning, so make sure you have a go at answering them before you take a peek at the answers!

Chapter 1

TYK.1.1 How do we measure 'wavelength'?
From two equal points on the wave, for example, from peak to peak or trough to trough.

TYK.1.2 Does ultraviolet light have higher or lower energy than visible light?
Ultraviolet light has higher energy than visible light (because it has a shorter wavelength and higher frequency).

TYK.1.3 Does ultraviolet light have a longer or shorter wavelength than visible light?
Ultraviolet light has a smaller wavelength than visible light.

TYK.1.4 Think about a regular table. Do you think light approaching the table is absorbed, reflected, transmitted or a combination of a few of these?
Light needs to be reflected for us to be able to see it, but it will be absorbing some of the light as well. This is particularly true for black or brown tables.

TYK.1.5 What colour would be produced if we combined green and red wavelengths?
Yellow.

TYK.1.6 What is a shadow?
A shadow is an absence of (at least some) light produced when an obstacle blocks the path of the light source.

Chapter 2

TYK.2.1 What is a collection of light rays called?
A pencil.

TYK.2.2 What does parallel vergence tell us about the origin of the light rays?
The rays have come from far away (infinity) because the wavefronts are flat relative to one another (zero vergence).

TYK.2.3 How do we decide whether an object distance will be negative or positive?
Object distance will always be negative because light starts at the object, and our convention states that light travels from left (where the object is) to right. We also always measure *from* the surface, so object distances will always be measured against the direction of light and therefore always be negative.

TYK.2.4 If a light ray moved from a medium with a refractive index of 1.00 into a medium with a refractive index of 1.523, would it bend towards or away from the normal?
It would bend towards the normal.

TYK.2.5 If you work out that following refraction an image will have a vergence of +4.00D, are the rays converging or diverging?
Converging (positive vergence suggests they are converging).

TYK.2.6 Would a concave spherical surface possess a negative or positive power? Why?
A concave spherical surface would possess a negative power because the centre of curvature will be on the left, meaning the radius of curvature (r) will be negative.

Chapter 3

TYK.3.1 What is the definition of a thin lens?
A lens in which the thickness is small enough (relative to the radius of curvature of each surface) that it's assumed that the refractive index of the lens material has a negligible effect on the power, so it can be ignored.

TYK.3.2 What would a magnification of -0.6 tell us about the nature of the image?
It's negative, so that tells us it's inverted (real), and it's between 0 and -1, so that tells us it's minified.

TYK.3.3 How would you calculate equivalent power of two thin lenses in contact with one another?
Add the two powers together ($F_e = F_1 + F_2$).

TYK.3.4 What is a principal plane?
A principal plane is the location where an equivalently powered lens would need to be placed within a multiple lens system in order to coincide with the secondary (or primary) focal point of the system.

TYK.3.5 What is the difference between back vertex focal length and secondary equivalent focal length?
The back vertex focal length (f_e') is the distance between the back lens and the secondary focal point (F'), whereas the secondary equivalent focal length is the distance between the secondary principal plane (H'P') and the secondary focal point (F').

TYK.3.6 What determines whether we use step-along vergence or Newton's formulae to find image distance with a multiple lens system?

The variable we've been given for object distance determines which formulae to use. If we've been given the object distance relative to the first lens (l) then we use step along, but if we've been given the object distance relative to the primary focal point (x) then we use Newton's formulae.

Chapter 4

TYK.4.1 What is the definition of a thick lens (relative to a thin lens)?

A thick lens takes the refractive index of the lens into account when solving the equations, whereas a thin lens does not.

TYK.4.2 What is the difference between the sag and the edge thickness?

The sag is the height of the segment of the sphere that makes a lens surface, whereas the edge thickness is the literal thickness at the edges of the lens.

TYK.4.3 In an equiconcave lens, does the back surface have a positive or negative radius of curvature?

In an equiconcave lens, the back surface would have a positive radius of curvature.

TYK.4.4 What is a virtual object?

A virtual object is formed when an image acts as a new object for another surface or lens.

TYK.4.5 What causes the resolution of a Fresnel lens to be reduced relative to a 'regular' lens?

Image quality will be slightly reduced due to diffraction occurring at the ridges between each curved ring that makes up the Fresnel lens.

Chapter 5

TYK.5.1 What is the presumed power of the reduced eye?
+60.00D

TYK.5.2 What is the difference between spherical and cylindrical refractive error?

Spherical refractive errors are the same in all orientations, whereas cylindrical refractive errors have a different error along a specific axis.

TYK.5.3 If the far-point of a patient's eye is −25.00 cm, what is their refractive error?

Their refractive error is −4.00DS (L = 1 / −0.25m).

TYK.5.4 Which meridian in a cylindrical lens is written as the 'axis'?

The axis meridian (the axis with no power).

Chapter 6

TYK.6.1 What are the two laws of reflection?
(1) The incident light ray and the reflected light ray lie in one plane.
(2) The angle of incidence (i) is equal to the angle of reflection (i').

TYK.6.2 If an object is 50 cm in front of a plane mirror, where will the image form?

50 cm within the mirror (image distance is equal to object distance in a plane mirror).

TYK.6.3 Describe the nature of an image formed in a plane mirror.

The image is the same size as the object, virtual (upright), reversed and laterally inversed.

TYK.6.4 Explain why the formula for calculating the power (F) of a spherical mirror has a 'minus sign' in it.

Unlike with lenses, mirrors reflect light back in the direction it came, meaning that after reflection, without including the minus sign, all variables would be assigned the opposite (incorrect) sign.

TYK.6.5 If a spherical mirror has a radius of curvature of +20 cm, what is the focal length (f)?
+10 cm (f = r/2)

Chapter 7

TYK.7.1 Using your knowledge of optical systems, can you explain why a P-ray will pass through F'?

Because the incident light is parallel to the optical axis (and therefore suggesting it has zero vergence), and light with zero vergence focuses at the secondary focal point (F').

TYK.7.2 Explain how you could use a ray diagram to decide whether an image distance would be positive or negative.

If the ray diagram shows that the image forms on the right of the lens or mirror, then the distance will be positive, whereas if the ray diagram shows that the image forms on the left of the lens or mirror, then the distance will be negative.

TYK.7.3 In the diagram below, which image is drawn correctly? Explain your answer.

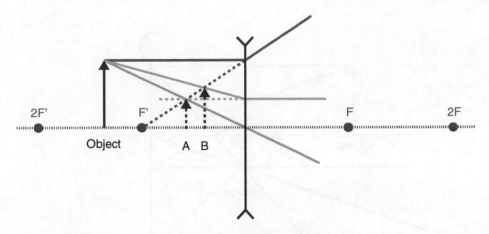

'A' is drawn correctly because it's formed at the intersection of the backwards-projected, refracted rays. The 'B' intersection is incorrect because it is intersecting a refracted ray with an incident ray.

TYK.7.4 Draw a ray diagram to show where an image would form if an object was placed at 2F in front of a positively powered lens.

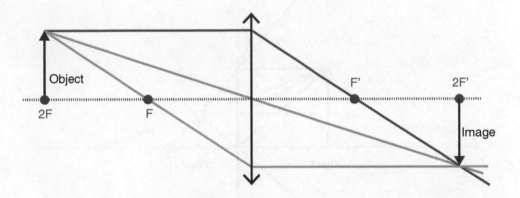

TYK.7.5 Draw a ray diagram to show where an image would form if an object was placed between F' and the lens in front of a negatively powered lens.

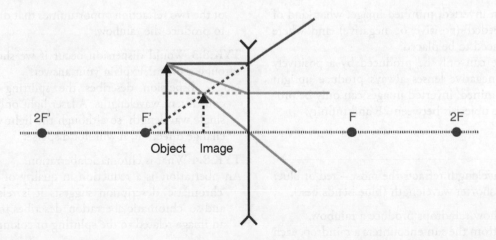

TYK.7.6 Draw a ray diagram to show where an image would form if an object was placed left of C in front of a positively powered mirror.

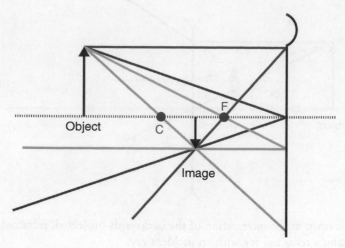

TYK.7.7 Draw a ray diagram to show where an image would form if an object was placed at any location in front of a negatively powered mirror.

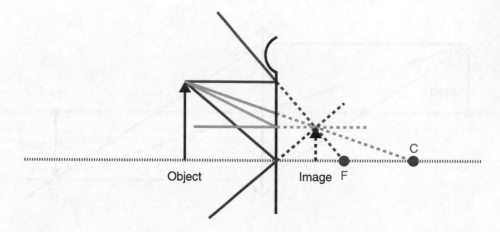

TYK.7.8 To get an inverted, minified image, what kind of lens would be needed (positive or negative) and where would the object need to be placed?

An inverted image can only be produced by a positively powered lens (negative lenses always produce upright images), and minified, inverted images can only be produced when the object is between 2F and infinity.

Chapter 8

TYK.8.1 What wavelength refracts the most – red or blue? Blue because it's a shorter wavelength (blue bends best).

TYK.8.2 Explain how raindrops produce a rainbow.

When white light from the sun encounters a raindrop, each constituent wavelength is refracted slightly different amounts. The light begins to disperse, but when it reaches the other side of the raindrop, some of the light is reflected back again, and so it is then refracted a second time as it leaves the raindrop. It is the combination of the two refraction opportunities that disperse the light to produce the rainbow.

TYK.8.3 Would dispersion occur if we shone a red laser through a prism? Explain your answer.

No – dispersion describes the splitting of light into constituent wavelengths. A laser light only possesses one single wavelength, so although the light will refract and change direction, it will not disperse.

TYK.8.4 What is chromatic aberration?

An 'aberration' is a reduction in quality of an image. The 'chromatic' description suggests it is related to colour, and so 'chromatic aberration' describes imperfections in an image related to the splitting of colours.

TYK8.5 If a person is slightly under-minussed in their glasses prescription, will green or red wavelengths be more likely to focus on the retina?

If a person is under-minussed, their eye is focusing light with too much power. This means that it is likely that all the incoming wavelengths of light will be focused earlier in the eye than expected, and therefore the red wavelengths (which usually focus behind the eye) will be more likely to focus on the retina in this case.

Chapter 9

TYK.9.1 Will light deviate towards the base or the apex of the prism?
Light deviates towards the base (the image deviates towards the apex).

TYK.9.2 What is the 'critical angle'?
A 'critical angle' of incidence describes conditions in which light will leave the surface along the surface itself (indicating an angle of refraction of 90°). It can only occur when moving from a material with a high refractive index to a material with a lower refractive index.

TYK.9.3 If a prism was submerged in water, would it deviate light differently than if it was in air? Explain your answer.
Yes – when light leaves the prism, the amount it is refracted is partly dictated by the refractive index difference between the prism and the surrounding medium. If we alter the refractive index of the surrounding medium, it will change how the light leaves the prism.

TYK.9.4 Would increasing the apical angle increase the power of the prism or decrease it?
Increase.

Chapter 10

TYK.10.1 What is the 'phase' of a wave?
The phase of a wave is defined as the location of a point on the wave within a cycle (measured in degrees).

TYK.10.2 If two identical waves are 180° 'out of phase', what will happen?
Destructive interference will occur, with a net amplitude of zero. This results in no light being produced.

TYK.10.3 What does Huygen's principle predict about light when it gets blocked by an obstacle?
Huygen's principle predicts that the wavelets on the primary wavefronts will permit the light to 'bend' slightly around the obstacle to produce light in the geometric shadow of the obstacle – this is diffraction.

TYK.10.4 If we increased the number of slits in a diffraction experiment from one slit to five slits, what do you think would happen to the diffraction pattern?
The diffraction pattern would have more interference patterns present (as it would be like having five light sources) and so the bright spots within the maxima would get smaller.

TYK.10.5 Why do soap bubbles look multicoloured sometimes?
Soap bubbles are made of a thin film, which means that as incident white light reaches the 'film' of the bubble,

some of the light reflects at the front surface of the film, but some passes through to the back surface. Then at the back surface, some light transmits through, but some is reflected, which means that even though we started with one light source, there will be (in this case), two waves that reflect towards us (the observer). This means that we'll have two waves reaching us, one of which has now travelled a slightly greater distance than the first. These light rays will produce constructive interference if in phase, and destructive interference if out of phase for each of the wavelengths that make up the white light.

Chapter 11

TYK.11.1 What does a focimeter do?
A focimeter determines the spherical power, cylindrical power (and corresponding axis), prismatic power and the optical centre of a lens.

TYK.11.2 What is the graticule?
A graticule is the network of lines in the eyepiece of the focimeter (shown in black in the diagrams) that act as a measuring scale. In this case, the lines represent meridians and degree of prismatic effects.

TYK.11.3 Why is it important to focus the eyepiece before attempting to use a focimeter?
Each observer may have a small amount of uncorrected refractive error, which might make the target appear blurry, even though it is actually in focus. This could lead to errors.

TYK.11.4 If the target falls below the centre of the graticule, would this indicate base-down or base-up prism?
This would indicate base-down prism.

Chapter 12

TYK.12.1 What does 'photometry' mean?
Measurement of light.

TYK.12.2 Describe a 'solid angle'.
A solid angle is a 3-dimensional angle which describes the field of view from a particular point or apex (likened to the angle at the top of a circular cone).

TYK.12.3 What does 'luminous flux' mean and what is it measured in?
Luminous flux defines the measure of power (or perceived power) emitted by a light source and is measured in lumens (lm).

TYK.12.4 Which of the following statements uses photometry terms correctly, and why:
'*The cup is poorly illuminated*' or '*The cup is poorly luminated*'?

'The cup is poorly illuminated' – because illumination describes light falling onto the cup, whereas luminance is the perceived brightness of light coming off the cup.

TYK.12.5 What does a high number of Kelvins (6000 K) suggest about a light source?

It will appear to look 'cold' (towards the blue end of the colour spectrum).

Chapter 13

TYK.13.1 What is an 'optical instrument'?

An optical instrument is any device or equipment, which can alter an image for enhancement or viewing purposes.

TYK.13.2 Could the human eye be classed as an optical instrument? Explain your answer.

Yes – because it refracts light to focus it in a specific place (the back of the eye) and can adjust the power (accommodation of the lens) in circumstances where needed.

TYK.13.3 If we wanted to focus our camera on something very far away, would we choose a 24 mm or 300 mm lens? Explain your answer.

We would choose the 300 mm (longer focal length) lens because it will produce a higher magnification and allow us to see distant objects more clearly.

TYK.13.4 Would you expect a Galilean telescope to have a positive or negative magnification? Explain your answer.

Positive magnification. Galilean telescopes produce an upright image, so the magnification should always be positive (*see chapter 3 for revision on this*).

Chapter 14

TYK.14.1 Define 'unpolarised light'.

Unpolarised light is light that is oscillating/vibrating in all orientations (or a large range of orientations), which means the electric field changes randomly over time.

TYK.14.2 Explain the difference between circular and elliptical polarisation.

Both types of polarisation require two perpendicular linearly polarised waves, but for circular, they need to have the same amplitude and be 90° out of phase, whereas elliptical polarisation can be produced with different amplitudes or different degrees-of-phase difference.

TYK.14.3 What type of light would be emitted through two identically oriented polarising filters?

Polarised light which is polarised according to the orientation of the filters. If both filters are at the same angle, then they will let through the same light.

TYK.14.4 Is light reflected off a lake more likely to be polarised in the horizontal or vertical plane?

Horizontal – when light is polarised by reflection, it is polarised parallel to the surface from which it is reflected. Lakes are usually horizontal!

TYK.14.5 Explain why the sun appears red at sunset.

As the unpolarised sunlight passes through the molecules in the atmosphere, the wavelengths are scattered. This scattering affects shorter wavelengths first, so when the sunlight travels a large distance through the atmosphere (as it does at sunrise/sunset) then more of the wavelengths will be scattered out of the light and sent into the atmosphere. This means that only the longer wavelength light is left, which will make the sun appear red.

Chapter 15

TYK.15.1 Why is it not possible to see the back of a patient's eye without the help of a special device?

The inside of the eye is very dark (meaning you'd need a light to illuminate the inside of the eye to see it), and the pupil is very small, which restricts the field of view.

TYK.15.2 Is a slit-lamp biomicroscope a form of direct or indirect ophthalmoscopy?

Indirect.

TYK.15.3 Why is it advantageous to the clinician to ask the patient to move their gaze when performing ophthalmoscopy?

The field of view when performing ophthalmoscopy is relatively small (even with indirect), so clinicians can ask the patient to change the position of their eyes to allow them to see different parts of the back of the eye.

TYK.15.4 Explain why the anterior angle of the eye is not visible without the help of a special lens.

Because of the refractive index difference between the front surface of the cornea and the air, light from the anterior angle exceeds the critical angle, meaning that it experiences total internal reflection (all the light reflects back into the eye, making it invisible to the external viewer).

TYK.15.5 On a three-mirror goniolens, which mirror would allow the clinician to view the anterior angle?

The D-shape (59°) lens.

TYK.15.6 Explain what an against movement would look like during retinoscopy.

If an against movement is present, the reflex (light from inside the eye) would move in the opposite direction to that of the streak. For example, if the streak was moving from right to left, the reflex would be seen to be moving from left to right.

TYK.15.7 If a clinician performed retinoscopy on a patient at a working distance of 50 cm, what spherical power would they need to account for in the final refractive error?

They would need to account for -2.00DS when determining their final refractive error (L = n/l = 1/0.5 = 2).

TYK.15.8 What equation does applanation tonometry rely on for calculating intraocular pressure (IOP)?

Pressure = force / area

Chapter 16

TYK.16.1 What is an aberration?

An imperfection in the quality of an image – could be from distortion, blurring or both.

TYK.16.2 Which part of a lens induces the greatest amount of aberration?

The periphery (edges) – as distance increases away from the optical centre, aberrations become larger.

TYK.16.3 In terms of Zernike polynomials, what 'order' of aberration is **defocus**?

2 (because it's Z_2^0).

TYK.16.4 Explain how a Scheiner disc can identify the presence of a refractive error.

The Scheiner disc is an occluder with two small, adjacent pinholes. The occluder is placed in front of the patient's eye and a distant (parallel vergence) light is shone at the occlude. The pinholes should then only let through two small spots of light, which, if no refractive error is present, should focus on the back of the eye to form an image of a single spot. However, if the patient's eye is inducing aberrations, then the light will focus incorrectly and will appear as two separate spots of light.

TYK.16.5 Explain how adaptive optics systems can take high-resolution images.

Adaptive optics systems utilise a wavefront sensor and a rapidly deformable mirror to constantly monitor aberrations (sensor) and compensate for them (deformable mirror).

Chapter 17

TYK.17.1 What does OCT stand for?
Optical coherence tomography.

TYK.17.2 Explain how far the mirror in a Michelson interferometer would need to move to produce a path difference of a whole wavelength.

The mirror would need to move a distance equivalent to half a wavelength in order to produce a full wavelength of path difference, because moving the mirror half a wavelength will add (or remove) half from the incident ray and also the reflected ray (totalling a whole wavelength).

TYK.17.3 Explain how a TD-OCT system works.
TD-OCT utilises a low-coherence, near-infrared light source, which is split into two beams (a reference beam and a measurement beam) by a beam splitter. One beam (measurement) will enter the patient's eye, whilst the other beam (reference) will reflect off a moveable mirror. The measurement beam is reflected from the back of the eye with different delay times which are dependent on the optical properties of the tissue and the distance away from the light source. The software within the system can then interpret the interference fringe profiles as they pass through the detector in order to determine the depth of the tissue and produce the nice black-and-white image.

TYK.17.4 Name one difference between a TD-OCT and an FD-OCT system.
Moveable mirror (TD-OCT) versus diffraction grating (FD-OCT).

Low-coherence near-infrared light course (TD-OCT) versus broadband light source (FD-OCT).

TYK.17.5 Name one clinical application of OCT.
Checking the health of the layers of the retina; measuring distances (thickness of cornea, axial length, thickness of retinal nerve fibre layer (RNFL)); measuring the shape of the cornea; checking the fit of a contact lens.

Chapter 18

TYK.18.1 Explain how a pinhole produces an upside-down image.
Light rays have to travel in straight lines, but a pinhole is very small; therefore, light coming off the tip of an object will travel in a straight line through the pinhole and end up near the floor, whilst light rays from the base of the object travel in a straight line through the pinhole and end up near the ceiling.

TYK.18.2 Explain why moving the screen away from the pinhole produces a larger image.
If the object remains still, then the angle of the rays on the other side of the pinhole should remain constant. So, if the screen is closer to the pinhole, it will see more of the scene than if it is farther away.

Chapter 19

TYK.19.1 Explain why the torch looks more yellow as we add more milk.
Adding more milk causes more scattering of the light within the glass. This makes the shorter (blue) wavelengths of light scatter into the milk, causing the torchlight to look more yellow (towards the longer wavelengths) and making the milk look more blue.

TYK.19.2 Explain why using a red light source wouldn't work.
A red light source wouldn't work because it only contains red (long wavelengths). Longer wavelengths are more difficult to scatter (so would require so much milk the light wouldn't be visible through the murkiness) but also lack the full range of wavelengths (as with white light), so there are no blue wavelengths to scatter and make the milk blue.

Chapter 20

TYK.20.1 Explain why the white light produces a rainbow when it passes through the setup described in this chapter.
When white light passes through a prism (a material with two or more refracting surfaces), the individual wavelengths within the white light refract to greater or lesser amounts depending on their wavelength (e.g. red wavelength refracts the least, but blue refracts the most). When the mirror is placed in the tray of water, it turns the tray of water into a prism and splits the wavelengths through dispersion.

TYK.20.2 Explain what you think would happen if you changed the angle of the light approaching our homemade prisms.

As we change the angle of incidence (angle of approaching light), the angle of deviation in the prism changes as well, which means that the dispersed light will move along the paper.

Chapter 21

TYK.21.1 Explain why the distance between the hot spots is equal to half the wavelength of a microwave.

As the amplitude increases upwards or downwards away from the midpoint, the energy also increases, meaning that both the peak and the trough of the microwave profile will produce the highest amount of intensity (heat). Therefore, the microwave will produce two hotspots – one at the peak and one at the trough. The distance between these points is equal to half a wavelength.

TYK.21.2 Explain why we needed to take the turntable out of the microwave for it to work.

The turntable allows the interference produced by the microwave to be evenly spread around the food as it rotates through the hot spots. For this experiment to work we need to make sure the hot spots don't move, so the turntable needed to be removed.

Chapter 22

TYK.22.1 Explain how the human eye can focus distant light onto the back of the eye.

The human eye can focus light because it has a convex front surface (the cornea) with a small radius of curvature, and the cornea has a different refractive index to the air (~1.376).

TYK.22.2 Why did we use water for the refractive index difference?

Water is clear which means the image will still be visible through the 'lenses', and it has a refractive index very similar to that of the human eye (water, 1.333; cornea, 1.376).

TYK.22.3 Explain why the image is sometimes a little distorted near the edges of the 'cornea' in our demonstration (see Fig. 22.7 for an example of this distortion).

These are examples of wavefront aberrations that become increasingly pertinent as light travels through the peripheral edges of a lens. In a way, this makes our homemade 'cornea' even more realistic, as a real cornea also induces more aberrations as light moves away from the optical centre.

TYK.22.4 If we had filled our lenses with glycerine (a viscous, clear liquid of refractive index 1.47), do you think the results would have been the same? Discuss your thoughts.

The experiment would have been a lot stickier (!), but the results would *largely* have been the same, with the flat lens not having any impact on the image, and the 'cornea' producing a magnified image. However, our homemade cornea would have had more power with the glycerine (relative to the water). This is shown in Equation 2.4:

$$F = (n' - n) / r$$

(Let's say our 'cornea' has a radius of curvature of +0.1m; this actual value doesn't matter so much as long as it's constant across both equations.)

With water: $F = (1.333 - 1.00) / +0.10 = +3.33D$

With glycerine: $F = (1.47 - 1.00) / +0.10 = +4.70D$

Chapter 23

TYK.23.1 Explain how constructive interference is produced with two coherent light sources.

Constructive interference is produced when multiple waves arrive in phase (with $n\lambda$ path difference). This results in a larger amplitude of the resultant wave which produces bright light (or visible colour).

TYK23.2 If two coherent waves arrive at a detector 'in phase', what would the path difference be?

To arrive in phase with one another, the waves either need a path difference of 0 (so they've travelled the same distance), or one wave will need to have travelled a multiple of the wavelength ($n\lambda$) to arrive at the same point in the phase.

TYK.23.3 Explain why the interference pattern varies vertically in our experiment.

In this experiment, the film was held vertically in order to ensure that the thickness would vary along the film. This variation occurs because gravity pulls the film downwards, meaning that the film 'pools' towards the bottom of the ring/aperture, thereby making the film thicker towards the bottom. This change in thickness alters the path difference between the ray reflected at the front surface and the ray reflected at the back surface.

TYK.23.4 Why do you think there's no visible interference pattern towards the very top of the film (see Fig. 23.5)?

After a few seconds of being held vertically, the film at the top becomes too thin (~50 nanometres to be precise), so all the wavelengths of light produce destructive interference when reflected back to us at this point (meaning we can just see through the film).

Index